AF577112

Clinical Monitoring Practice

Clinical Monitoring Practice

Second Edition

J. S. Gravenstein, M.D.
Graduate Research Professor
Department of Anesthesiology
College of Medicine
University of Florida
Gainesville, Florida

David A. Paulus, M.S., M.D.
Associate Professor
Department of Anesthesiology
College of Medicine
University of Florida
Gainesville, Florida

With illustrations by

Kelly Crawford, R.R.T.
Department of Anesthesiology
College of Medicine
University of Florida
Gainesville, Florida

Lewis Clark, M.S.M.I.
Learning Resources and Communications
University of Florida
Gainesville, Florida

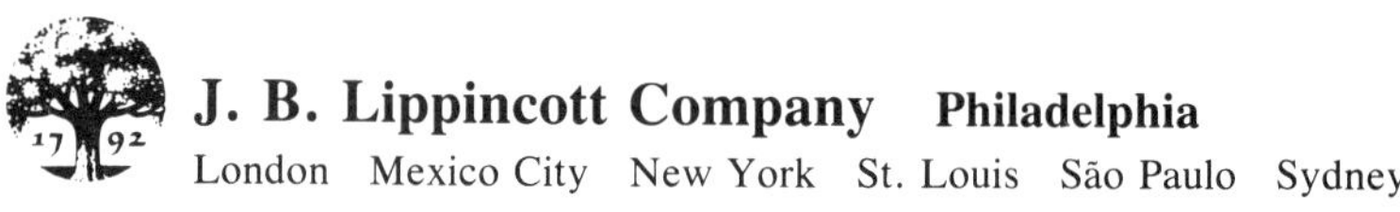
J. B. Lippincott Company **Philadelphia**
London Mexico City New York St. Louis São Paulo Sydney

Acquisitions Editor: *David Barnes*
Sponsoring Editor: *Sanford J. Robinson*
Manuscript Editor: *Michael Scott*
Art Director: *Tracy Baldwin*
Design Coordinator: *Don Shenkle*
Cover Designer: *Joe Netherwood*
Production Manager: *J. Corey Gray*
Production Editors: *Janet Greenwood and Rosanne Hallowell*
Production Coordinator: *Barney Fernandes*
Compositor: *Maryland Composition Company, Inc.*
Printer/Binder: *R. R. Donnelley & Sons Company*

Second Edition

6 5 4 3 2 1

Library of Congress Cataloging-in-Publication Data

Gravenstein, J. S.
Clinical monitoring practice.

Rev. ed. of: Monitoring practice in clinical anesthesia. c1982.
Includes bibliographies and index.
1. Anesthesia. 2. Patient monitoring. I. Paulus, David A. II. Gravenstein, J. S. Monitoring practice in clinical anesthesia. III. Title. [DNLM: 1. Anesthesia—methods. 2. Monitoring, Physiologic. WO 200 G775m]
RD82.G7 1987 617'.96'0287 86-15389
ISBN 0-397-50737-2

The authors and publisher have exerted every effort to ensure that drug selection and dosage and guidelines regarding the use of instruments set forth in this text are in accord with current recommendations and practice at the time of publication. However, in view of ongoing research, changes in government regulations, and the constant flow of information relating to drug therapy, drug reactions, and the use of instruments, the reader is urged to check the manufacturer's directives for each drug or device for any change in indications and dosage and for added warnings and precautions. This is particularly important when the recommended agent or device is new or infrequently employed.

Preface

Physicians, nurses, and technicians responsible for monitoring patients in operating rooms, intensive care units, and recovery rooms are asking with great urgency for clinical information on old and new monitoring techniques and instruments. We have attempted to supply this information in a compact form in *Clinical Monitoring Practice*. In order to respond to the principal concerns of our clinical readers we have stressed practical points and have limited the discussion of theory—both physiologic and engineering—to essentials.

Several new techniques have been established in the last few years. Foremost among them are pulse oximetry and gas monitoring—both capnography and mass spectrometry. The study of evoked potentials has experienced remarkable growth. Alarms have become ubiquitous on electronic monitors, and computers are invading the monitoring field in growing numbers. New methods to measure blood pressure and cardiac output continuously and noninvasively are appearing. The first automated anesthesia record keepers have been produced. Concerns about electrical safety are still with us, understandably enough in light of all the electronic systems that now surround our patients. In addition to discussing all of these developments, we have made many minor improvements on the old chapters. The book still answers many practical questions, among them how to calibrate a transducer, what to do when fetal monitoring is indicated, how to tell the difference between base excess and standard bicarbonate, how to place a catheter into the internal jugular vein, when and how to monitor for air embolism, and how to monitor patients without instruments.

Four years have passed since the first edition of this book was published. During that time several journals and textbooks devoted to monitoring have appeared. Because many experts believe that improved skills and better monitoring equipment will help to prevent mishaps in operating rooms and intensive care units, there is now serious talk about formulating recommendations, guidelines, and standards* that define minimal monitoring conventions. What could speak more clearly to these efforts than the phenomenon of monitoring, which, for the first time in the history of medicine, has been recognized as a field that deserves special attentions. Small wonder, therefore, that clinicians want to stay abreast of the field and that a revised edition of our text has become necessary.

We are very grateful to the many anesthesiologists, surgeons, internists, nurse anesthetists, intensivists, respiratory therapists, engineers, and instrument designers who offered valuable critiques and many excellent suggestions for the revision of the book. Despite their efforts and our best intentions, we assume that we will not have succeeded in eliminating all mistakes.

We owe special thanks to our secretaries and to our editorial assistant, Ms. Christine R. Finnegan, without whose tireless efforts we would not have been able to complete the task.

J. S. Gravenstein, M.D.
David A. Paulus, M.S., M.D.

* Anesthesia Patient Safety Foundation: Newsletter, Spring 1986

Preface to the First Edition

How should I calibrate a pressure transducer? When should I monitor fetal heart tones? Why should I take an x-ray after placing an umbilical catheter in a newborn? What is the difference between base excess and standard base excess? Where can I find the internal jugular vein for insertion of a pulmonary artery catheter? We hear these and many other basic clinical questions when we talk to seasoned clinicians, residents, and young and old nurse anesthetists. Even engineers and technicians are asking about straightforward clinical descriptions of the "how's" and "what's" of monitoring patients in the operating room.

In *Monitoring Practice in Clinical Anesthesia* we have attempted to answer these questions.

Because we wanted to answer questions about practical matters, we have included descriptions of some common monitoring instruments (ECG, blood pressure, Doppler, O_2 and CO_2 analyzers). Because few people have ready access to some important guidelines that affect our practice, we have included statements from the Joint Commission on Hospital Accreditation (on anesthesia and record keeping), the American Society of Anesthesiologists (on trace gases in the operating room), and the National Fire Protection Agency (on electrical safety).

We have kept the book short on theory and long on the "dos" and "don'ts" of practical monitoring. We have also included cross references so that the busy clinician will find it easy to locate material in the text.

All chapters have been reviewed by our friend and critic, Shirley Graves, M.D., of the University of Florida, Department of Anesthesiology, who has made many excellent suggestions and prevented several errors. Many chapters were reviewed by other anesthesiologists, internists, surgeons, engineers, and technicians. Despite these reviews, we fear that a few mistakes will have slipped by. For these we accept responsibility. We hope that the reader will bring them to our attention so that we can eliminate them in a future edition (presumably in exchange for some new errors). Ms. Ann Finnicum and Ms. Sherry Hunt patiently typed and retyped the text; Ms. Lynn Carroll served as our editorial assistant. Without the unselfish help of these many friends, we could not have succeeded.

J. S. Gravenstein, M.D.
David A. Paulus, M.S., M.D.

Contents

Clinical Monitoring Practice

CHAPTER 1

Perspectives on Monitoring

REASONS FOR MONITORING

We anesthetize patients to block their pain and to blot out their memory of the operation. If drugs free of all side-effects were available, during anesthesia we would only need to know the extent to which we have succeeded in blocking pain and in blotting out memory. As every anesthetist knows, the degree of analgesia or amnesia cannot yet be measured. Instead, many variables that have little to do with the state of anesthesia but much to do with the side-effects of anesthetic agents are recorded. Patients do not die from too much analgesia or amnesia; they die from too much anesthetic in the heart, not enough perfusion to the brain, or not enough oxygen in the blood. Therefore, patients are monitored to detect adverse side-effects produced by drugs or clinical actions, common examples of which are hemorrhage, overtransfusion, underventilation, and surgical compression of heart, blood vessels, or lungs.

Monitoring activities could be ranked on a number of scales: for instance, from most to least often used. This scale would start with inspection of the patient, which is done continually and, at least today, would end with recording the evoked potentials. Monitoring could be ranked from least invasive to most invasive, with inspection being the least invasive, and with either catheterization of the pulmonary artery or measurement of intracranial pressure being examples of the most invasive techniques. These activities could also be ranked by cost, historical chronology, or impact on the patient. The importance of each monitored variable could also be a criterion for ranking. This would be of interest because it would be simpler to monitor the essential variables, the ones that make a difference, and forget the others. Certainly, blood pressure is often important as a guide in clinical anesthesia, as are blood gas levels. Some variables rarely affect clinical management but, when they indicate abnormal values, they become most important. An example is the measurement of the concentration of inspired oxygen. An oxygen analyzer should not be necessary to determine whether the oxygen concentration inhaled by the patient is too low, because the oxygen tension can be inferred from the flow meters. However, lagging vigilance is more common than malfunctioning flow meters or gas-delivery systems. The latter can lead to gases other than oxygen flowing out of the oxygen outlet because of some dreadful mistake in the piping from, or the filling of, the cylinders. In this instance, the oxygen analyzer becomes lifesaving. Thus, monitoring is necessary to guard against human errors, which are common, or equipment failure, which occurs infrequently.

INVASIVE VERSUS NONINVASIVE MONITORING

Many anesthesiologists and intensive care specialists shrink from the use of invasive monitoring methods because insertion of a catheter or probe into a vessel represents an operation, inflicts pain, requires anesthesia, carries risks (later discussed in detail with each method), consumes time, depends on skill, and costs more than noninvasive methods. Others say that invasive monitoring methods should be seen in juxtaposition to what the surgical operation will involve: why be squeamish with an arterial or central catheter in a patient who will have to endure a far larger wound and greater trauma at the hands of the surgeon? The decision for one or the other monitoring method is based not on such arguments, but on the question of cost versus benefit.

Recent years have brought a number of new noninvasive monitoring methods that are helping to supplant invasive ones. The pulse oximeter, for instance, reduces the need for arterial blood samples when blood oxygen is to be monitored. Noninvasive methods for estimating the cardiac output may reduce the frequency of placing pulmonary artery catheters.

We grade invasiveness as follows:

1. *Noninvasive:* The monitor is applied to the skin, as exemplified by electrocardiograph electrodes or blood pressure cuffs.
2. *Minimally invasive:* Requires breaking the skin, but only for local application of catheters such as intravenous catheters placed in the back of the hand or the crook of the elbow, or abrasion of the skin, for instance, for placement of cutaneous oxygen electrodes.
3. *Penetrating:* Requires insertion of a probe into a bodily orifice such as the mouth, bladder, or anus, as is done for the placement of esophageal stethoscopes, temperature probes, catheters and the like.
4. *Invasive:* Requires the cannulation of an artery or central vein.
5. *Highly invasive:* Cannulation of a ventricle of the brain or heart, as is done with intracranial pressure monitoring or pulmonary artery catheters.

The ranking of these categories is arbitrary, but in general represents frequency of use (from most to least) as well as risk of complications and cost (from lowest to highest).

ESSENTIAL MONITORING

The question is often asked: what monitors are essential in everyday clinical anesthesia, not for the complicated case, but for a healthy young patient during a routine, minor surgical procedure requiring under 30 minutes of general anesthesia? This can be a more important question than whether or not to insert a pulmonary artery catheter in a patient undergoing cardiopulmonary bypass. For one reason, we see many more minor procedures, and the history of malpractice cases strongly suggests that disasters during simple operations are far more likely to lead to lawsuits than are those occurring during more complex surgical procedures. Secondly, expensive monitoring efforts in common minor procedures will have a greater economic impact than is true for the less common, but highly specialized, procedures.

To answer this question more fully, it is necessary to separate the use of monitoring equipment into two categories:

Monitoring for the Conduct of Anesthesia

In monitoring for the conduct of anesthesia we use monitors for the adjustment of ventilators when the end-expired CO_2 is to be lowered to a desired range in a neurosurgical operation or to bring blood pressure into a desired range for induced hypotension. The thermometer for hypothermia also fits into this category.

Monitoring for the Patient's Safety

The clinician must be concerned with avoiding the development, or correcting already developed, adverse conditions. The list of monitors fitting into the category of routine, uncomplicated cases overlaps with that of the previous category. The adverse conditions we wish to identify and prevent include hypoxemia, arrhythmias, cardiac arrest, hypo- and hypertension, hyper- and hypocarbia, and hypo- and hyperthermia. Although this list could be quickly translated into a series of related monitors, we must take into account the likelihood for each occurrence. For instance, during a minor surgical procedure lasting less than 30 minutes, the chance of undercooling a healthy adult patient can be ignored unless one operates in Siberia under an open January sky. Similarly, in the same time span, hyperthermia, especially a fatal case, will rarely have long enough to manifest itself. Thus, thermometry is a low-priority monitoring variable in brief anesthetics, and many clinicians omit it for such cases. Others include it routinely because thermometry requires little time, effort, or cost. Thus, although the yield is low, the cost per discovered case also remains trivial.

Blood pressure and electrocardiogram (ECG), as well as pressure and oxygen in the breathing circuit, are routinely monitored by the majority of American anesthesiologists and nurse anesthetists. Routine anesthesia for healthy patients could probably proceed without any monitors other than an alert clinician; however, these monitors are invariably called upon in all cases. Even though no one has as yet shown in a statistically sound epidemiologic study that these monitors save lives or reduce anesthetic complications, "community practice" now calls for their inclusion in all patients undergoing general anesthesia. Also strongly recommended is some device that will sound an alarm should the patient become disconnected from breathing circuit and ventilator. For patients under major conduction blocks (subarachnoid, epidural, and major nerve blocks such as axillary or sciatic) the community standard is the same, except that oxygen levels would not be monitored in the patient's respired air. Although we believe that overwhelming agreement exists on the monitors just mentioned, some anesthetists—but not all—would extend the list of essential monitors to include a finger plethysmograph and a precordial or esophageal stethoscope for every patient, and a neuromuscular (twitch) monitor for those receiving intermediate or long-acting muscle relaxants.

Presently, two monitors are gaining fast acceptance in American operating rooms: the pulse oximeter and the capnograph. These two instruments offer rapid information on the adequacy of oxygenation and ventilation (Chap. 6). They are excellent candidates for eventual inclusion in the elite group of "essential" monitors.

A third aid to the anesthesiologist merits watching. It is the automated record (see Chap. 15). The automated record can keep accurate data concerning several variables that allow the anesthesiologist to discern trends and identify typical patterns helpful in the management of difficult patients. The automated record can do this legibly, and it is especially valuable at stressful times, when the anesthesiologist is too busy to keep a record at all. We predict that the automated record will become an essential monitoring agent in anesthetic management.

COST AND EFFECT OF MONITORING

Monitoring systems should provide a certain ratio of expense to benefit, but how expensive or inexpensive, and how effective? We would clearly insist that a monitor should be applied if it costs only 10¢ per application and yet would prevent severe damage to 10% of all anesthetized patients. We would also agree that a cost of $100 per patient to relieve only one out of 1000 anesthetized patients suffering only mild discomfort is unjustified. Between these extremes lies a broad, grey band where the value of monitoring changes from being cost-effective to non-cost-effective. This area shifts relative to time and geography. What might be affordable, and thus cost-effective, in San Francisco, might not be considered so in other parts of the United States or in other areas of the world.

The legal profession presents a different focus in answering the question, "What is affordable?" Its members designate as "negligent" those who omit a monitor, the use of which was well established in the community and would have prevented damage to a patient. Judge Learned Hand has provided an interesting definition of negligence.[2] This well-known jurist said that we are negligent when we fail to accept the cost (C) of preventing damage if this preventive cost would have been less than the cost of the damage (D) multiplied by the probability (P) of the occurrence of damage. This definition designates us as being negligent if we fail to apply a monitor costing no more than $1 per patient if, in one out of 10,000 cases, the monitor could have prevented damage estimated at $2500. (This guideline might be helpful in arguing with hospital administrators and insurance companies when deciding who must pay for the cost of additional monitoring.) In actuality, current expenditures for monitoring are probably lower than those calculated by application of Judge Learned Hand's formula.

How would we calculate the cost of a given monitoring effort, for example, monitoring with a physiologic multichannel monitor? The unit costs $8000, must be replaced in 6 years, and is used for three patients per working day. Assuming 250 working days per year, the unit in its lifetime will be used on 4500 patients, each of whom would have to be charged only $1.80 to amortize the machine. However, disposable electrodes, cables, maintenance, electricity, and administrative costs will increase this sum considerably. These additional, recurring costs are difficult to calculate because individual circumstances have great impact. Often a flat fee that is 10% of the purchase price is applied to cover the recurring cost of the machine. More often than not, the true cost of monitoring efforts is difficult to determine, and rarely, if ever, known.

Not only is it difficult to calculate the actual cost of monitoring, but it may be even more difficult to estimate the potential loss from an accident, as well as to compute the probability of such an occurrence. It is often impossible to establish with rigorous scientific discipline whether or not a given monitor would have prevented an adverse outcome.

Slogoff and Keats studied patients with heart disease who underwent coronary bypass operations.[3] Those who developed evidence of ischemia in the ECG during anesthesia suffered a significantly higher incidence of myocardial infarction after the operation than those patients who remained free of ST segment depression. This important study strongly supports the current standard of care which calls for routine monitoring of the ECG, although, as yet, we have no corollary study of healthy patients undergoing routine, elective operations. It also raises the question as to what we should observe in the ECG. Historically, the ECG was an all-or-none monitor, used to check for myocardial contraction or ventricular fibrillation in cases where the blood pressure had become unobtainable. Later, it became an arrhythmia monitor too, and today it has assumed an additional role as a monitor of myocardial ischemia, as reflected in changes in the ST segment depression (see Chap. 3).

WHAT TO DO WHEN ESSENTIAL MONITORS CANNOT BE APPLIED

An essential monitor can be defined in terms of community standards or by using medical arguments to justify its application.[4] Either method raises important questions when a monitor used routinely in a given case—thus representing the standard of care—cannot be applied for a specific reason.

If the monitoring device is so essential that an elective operation has to be canceled because the device is not available, the patient is inconvenienced, a bed is occupied longer than necessary, and the operating-room schedule is disrupted. A cancellation has an economic and emotional impact, disrupting professional relationships within the institution and undermining the patient's confidence in the institution. It is, therefore, useful to delineate, in advance, what monitoring level is essential and what level is unacceptable.

If a required monitoring device cannot be applied because of clinical circumstances, monitoring will be less than optimal. Can the additional risks imputed be justified? A clearly defined alternative is needed when essential monitoring techniques cannot be used. An example is the use of either the precordial or esophageal stethoscope, which some consider an essential component of routine monitoring. Neither instrument can be used in a patient undergoing a transthoracic esophageal resection, therefore other devices must supplant the functions of the chest stethoscope. The electrocardiogram and invasive blood pressure monitoring can provide continuous information on the patient's circulation. To guard against a ventilator-disconnect accident, a pressure-monitoring device in the breathing circuit of the anesthesia machine or continuous gas analysis of respired gases can be employed. It is prudent to formulate and document in the patient's record, in advance, any deviation from established routine, and to explain what steps were taken to compensate for problems such as the one described above.

Such makeshift compensations for missing essential monitors are more difficult to justify when equipment failure, rather than the patient's condition, is responsible for the lack of proper monitoring. For instance, when an institution uses a mass spectrometer every day to cover a number of operating rooms, what is the proper procedure if the central mass spectrometer fails and all the operating rooms suddenly lack repeated and automatic gas analysis? Here it is helpful to re-examine the basic requirements of essential monitoring. In the mid-1980s these include analysis of oxygen in the respired air, but, as yet, neither capnography nor analysis of other gases. If this situation occurred today, we believe that the operations could proceed as long as there were oxygen analyzers available for every patient, which would be rather easy to accomplish as these analyzers are relatively inexpensive. If an instrument fails that is considered essential for monitoring, such as an electrocardiograph, there is no alternative other than to postpone the operation until the proper monitor can be located. Although such a drastic step could have some negative effects, nothing less will be acceptable—not only in a court of law, but also in the community. We all expect—and accept—in the case of instrument failure, the cancellation of a scheduled commercial airline flight that involves (and inconveniences) hundreds of passengers. By the same token, we must cancel an operation when an essential monitor cannot be located. To do less means exposing the patient to preventable risks. Some hospitals and communities have begun to define in writing their minimal monitoring standards. This is laudable and will make it much easier for an individual clinician to resist pressures to proceed with anesthesia for an elective operation should the minimal essential monitoring equipment be unavailable.

ASSESSMENT OF MONITORING

Measurements made during monitoring should be assessed in terms of their quality and clinical utility. To determine the quality of measurements, their accuracy and precision must be examined (Fig. 1-1).

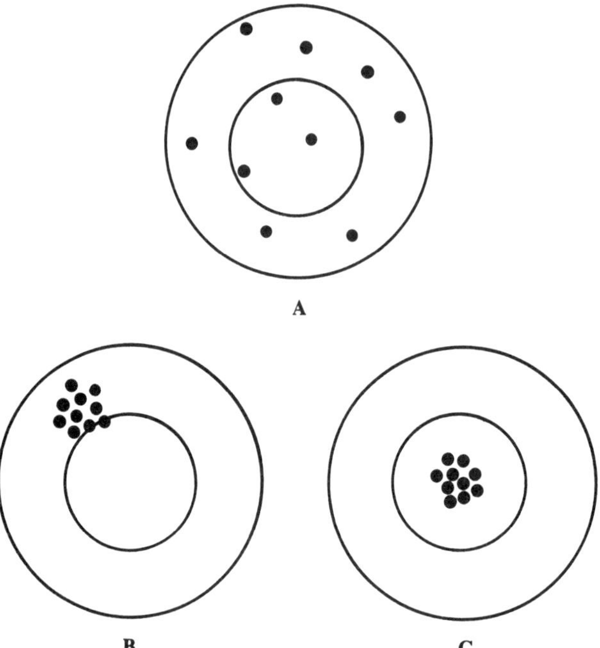

Figure 1-1. Accuracy and precision in target practice: (*A*) inaccurate and imprecise; (*B*) precise but inaccurate; (*C*) accurate and precise.

Accuracy means that the measurement reflects the genuine value. Few measurements made in the operating room are 100% accurate. However, some inaccuracy is acceptable because most values fluctuate, and monitoring, therefore, usually provides only a "snapshot" of changing parameters. It is, for example, not that important to know whether blood pressure was truly 120 torr systolic if, in the next moment and within a few heartbeats, the pressure fluctuates between 115 torr and 125 torr. Under these circumstances, an inaccuracy of the reading by 5% is not clinically significant. Indeed, for most measurements that are monitored repeatedly, trends are more important than accurate measurement of a variable at one given moment.

Trends will become apparent more readily if the measurements are precise. *Precision* means that a given measurement will repeatedly yield the same value. This value may not be accurate, but whatever the inherent error, each repeated reading will contain that same error. Therefore, a slightly inaccurate measurement that can be obtained precisely is of great value to the clinician looking for trends. Some trends become readily apparent from reviewing continuous records of, for instance, heart rate, blood pressure, or temperature. Others are not as easily detected because

Table 1-1. ECG MONITORING OF 100 HYPOTHETICAL PATIENTS WITH A HISTORY OF HEART DISEASE*

		Intraoperative ST Segment Depression During Hypotension		
		Yes	No	Total
Coronary-artery stenosis by postoperative angiogram	Yes	50 true positive	15 false negative	65
	No	10 false positive	25 true negative	35
	Total	60	40	100

* All patients had coronary angiography postoperatively.

great variability of the measurement obscures a trend. Statistical techniques, such as the calculation of cumulative sums (*cusums*), can help.[5] These are not yet directly accessible to the clinician, but modern microprocessors may soon make them more readily available.

Clinical utility encompasses sensitivity, specificity, and predictability. To illustrate these terms, let us assume that we have studied 100 patients who have histories of heart disease and for whom we have recorded the V_5 lead of the ECG during episodes of hypotension during anesthesia. In 60 patients, the ST segment was depressed 1 mm or more. From the coronary angiography of the 100 patients, we know that among the 60 who had ST segment depression, 50 have marked coronary artery stenosis. Among the remaining 40 patients who had no ST segment depression with hypotension, we found 15 with significant coronary stenosis and 25 with normal coronary vessels (Table 1-1).

The *sensitivity* of the test was 77%, which is calculated as follows:

$$100 \times \frac{\text{50 true positives}}{(\text{50 true positives} + \text{15 false negatives})} = 77\%$$

Sensitivity thus looks at *patients with the disease* and reports how many were correctly indentified.

The *specificity* of the test was 71%, which is calculated as follows:

$$100 \times \frac{\text{25 true negatives}}{(\text{25 true negatives} + \text{10 false positives})} = 71\%$$

Specificity thus looks at *patients without the disease* and reports how many were correctly identified.

The *predictability* of the test was 83%, which is calculated thus:

$$100 \times \frac{50 \text{ true positives}}{(50 \text{ true positives} + 10 \text{ false positives})} = 83\%$$

Predictability thus looks at the *patients who had a positive test* and reports how many actually had the disease.

Many activities in anesthesia are carried out without the benefit of knowing either the accuracy and precision or the sensitivity, specificity, and predictability of the measurements. Also, limits have yet to be determined. For instance, it is agreed that an arterial pressure of 40/20 torr must be called *hypotensive*, but there is no consensus exactly where normotension ends and hypotension begins. If the patient's resting pressure is 120/80 torr, is any systolic pressure under 100 or 80 or 70 or 60 torr hypotensive? Where we draw that line will influence the interpretation of our data.[6] Many studies are needed in this area.

REFERENCES

1. Amaranath L, Burke P, Kruel J et al: Why monitor? In Gravenstein JS, Newbower RS, Ream AK et al (eds): Monitoring Surgical Patients in the Operating Room, pp. 19–30. Springfield, IL, Charles C Thomas, 1978
2. Schwartz WB, Komesar NK: Doctors, damages and deterrence. N Engl J Med 298:1282, 1978
3. Slogoff S, Keats AS: Does perioperative myocardial ischemia lead to postoperative myocardial infarction? Anesthesiology 62:107–114, 1985
4. Gravenstein JS: Essential monitoring seen through different lenses. J Clin Monit 2:22–29, 1986
5. Chaput de Saintonge DM, Vere DW: Why don't doctors use cusums? Lancet i:120, 1974
6. McNeil BJ, Keeler E, Adelstein SJ: Primer on certain elements of medical decision making. N Engl J Med 293:211, 1975

CHAPTER 2

Monitoring Without Mechanical or Electronic Instrumentation

Of all monitoring modalities, monitoring without instruments is the most important, since all other methods of monitoring are simply add-ons to this basic form of monitoring. When electronic or mechanical equipment malfunctions, when electrical power fails, when machines become disconnected, there must be a skillful clinician to continue, without instruments, the care of the patient. Just as no airline passenger wishes to entrust his life to a pilot who has not been trained to fly the airplane after the instruments have failed, no patient should be anesthetized by anyone unskilled to monitor without recourse to instruments. Obviously, in the absence of instruments, many measurements can no longer be made, and the assessment of the patient must be based upon estimates and impressions. These skills must be practiced and honed to be done skillfully and competently.

The well-known cartoon ridiculing electronic monitoring in the operating room shows an engrossed anesthesiologist absorbed in the study of an imposing machine with many dials. Behind him is an empty operating room; the patient, surgeons, and nurses have left. In the background one orderly whispers to the other, "Psst, don't tell him that the patient has already left, he's enjoying his work so much." This amusing perspective on computerized monitoring illustrates the concern that the clinician may be distracted from the patient by the proliferation of too many instruments. It admonishes us to look at the patient rather than the computer. On the contrary, instruments, regardless of their sophistication, were designed to allow the clinician to spend more time, rather than less, observing the patient. Good instruments should collect data with a minimal effort on our part, should present these data in a convenient form, and should stimulate us to integrate these data into a picture based upon clinical assessment that relies on traditional diagnosis obtained without the help of instruments.

In summary, the foundation of all monitoring is monitoring without instruments. All data collected with the help of instruments must be viewed as a supplement to the clinical impression gained by observing and examining the patient. Data collected with instruments are extraordinarily valuable, but when the data appear to be incompatible with clinical observation, when doubt about the reliability of the instrument arises, then we have to return to competent monitoring without instrumented assistance.

Monitoring without instruments includes inspection, palpation, auscultation, and percussion. All have a place in anesthesia monitoring and should be practiced.

INSPECTION

In preparation for anesthesia, gas supply, suction, the anesthesia machine, intubation equipment, drugs, monitors, and intravenous (IV) fluids are inspected and checked. The patient deserves no less. His medical record, operation(s) to be performed, laboratory data, drugs ordered and given, nurses' notes, vital signs, and informed consent are checked. Then we inspect the patient himself. In this routine examination we consciously look for important signs that would dictate taking a particular action. This inspection is repeated many times during anesthesia. Intraoperatively, we suggest the following:

Overall Assessment

Scanning of the patient will provide an overall impression of whether or not anything is grossly amiss. Do skin color and chest motion suggest that the lungs are adequately ventilated? Are the ventilator and valves working or is the rebreathing bag on the machine moving? Are the gas settings on the anesthesia machine appropriate? Are IV fluids running? Is the patient in a position that is presumably comfortable and will not lead to nerve damage?

Should you find anything wrong, take immediate action to correct it. If nothing is grossly amiss, proceed to a more detailed examination of special areas.

Assessment of Special Areas

Forehead and Scalp

In lightly anesthetized patients who exhibit some response to painful stimuli but who are curarized, some motion of the forehead sometimes persists to give indication that the patient is responding to the painful stimuli. Has sweat formed on the forehead? It indicates an active autonomic nervous system which, in turn, signifies light anesthesia, the absence of cholinergic blockade, and possibly a rising temperature. During long operations, pressure necroses may form on the forehead (face down position) or the occiput (supine position), particularly in hypotensive patients. Padding with soft material and slightly shifting the head every 20 minutes or 30 minutes help to make this complication less likely.

Eyes

If tears are forming, the patient is lightly anesthetized. Are the eyes moving? This can sometimes be seen even through closed lids. It indicates lack of muscle relaxation and light anesthesia.

If the eyes are not moving, are they centered, that is, does the patient appear to look at an object in the distance? In the absence of muscle relaxants, this indicates the presence of anesthesia but not necessarily a level deep enough to prevent reaction to the surgical incision.

Size of the pupils is important even though it is modified by many drugs; for example, atropine dilates and opiates constrict. It is important to determine whether or not the pupils are dilated and unresponsive to light or whether one pupil is dilated and unresponsive to light. Either indicates an emergency involving the central nervous system.

Check for undue pressure exerted on the eyeball by a face mask, straps, tape, or when the patient lies face down or on his side.

The sclerae should be inspected. Look for injection of the conjunctiva overlying the sclerae. The dilation of small blood vessels will give a reddish appearance to the ordinarily white sclerae. This is common with light anesthesia. The conjunctiva of the lower lid is inspection for its color: pale with hypovolemia or low perfusion; engorged with high venous pressure as in congestive failure; and bluish with poor venous drainage or significant hypoxemia.

These observations are not as easily made after the liberal application of ophthalmic ointment or artificial eye drops used by some anesthesiologists who worry about drying of the open eye during anesthesia. We are concerned about this usually benign routine because, as with any routine, it may occasionally lead to damage. By mistake someone might apply, with dire consequences, an ointment not intended for the eye. Inspection of the eyes is also made more difficult by the application of tape on the upper eyelid. This, again, is intended to keep the eyes closed and to protect the eyes during anesthesia. The application of ointment and tape is useful when the eyes cannot be inspected readily, as in the face down position or when the surgeon works on the face and the eyes are draped. The majority of patients are in the supine position, however, allowing ready inspection of the eyes, and for this reason we prefer to refrain from applying anything to the eyes. Although the application of tape to the upper eyelid is usually benign, on occasion a patient is allergic to the tape or a bit of the very fine skin of the upper eyelid is removed with removal of the tape, causing unnecessary discomfort in the postoperative period.

Edema of the eyelid or conjunctiva (*chemosis*) is common after the patient has remained face down for several hours and also when large volumes of electrolyte solution have been administered.

Nose

The nose is inspected for motion of the alae. Patients in respiratory distress tend to widen their nostrils with inspiration. In adults this is a relatively late sign of respiratory inadequacy that deserves attention; in young children it is an early sign. Inspection of the nose in patients with nasotracheal, nasogastric, or nasopharyngeal tubes is also indicated regularly to make sure that no undue pressure is exerted on the structures composing the nostril. Pressure necrosis or swelling and discomfort may result when these tissues are not monitored during anesthesia.

Mouth

Motion of the lips indicates light anesthesia. If it is associated with inspiration it provides strong evidence of respiratory inadequacy. The lips are examined for color. Cyanosis indicates inadequate perfusion or ventilation. Pallor occurs with vasoconstriction or hypovolemia, and dryness with dehydration, cholinergic blockade, deep anesthesia, and exposure to dry, ambient air. The lips are inspected for trauma that might have occurred with intubation. Make certain that the lip is not caught between the teeth and the oropharyngeal or orotracheal airway. Tape sometimes covers a lip trapped between teeth and an airway, resulting in laceration and hematoma. Tape itself may cause skin trauma. A swollen lip, ulcer, laceration, or perforation may occur, all making for very unhappy patients. The endotracheal tube should be positioned with minimal mouth distortion. Teeth should be inspected for evidence of trauma. Do not let the teeth dry out during long anesthetics. The enamel suffers when allowed to remain dry for hours on end.

The floor of the mouth should be examined to make sure that it is quiescent during ventilation. In a spontaneously breathing patient or in a patient who is making respiratory efforts while his lungs are being mechanically ventilated, contractions of the floor of the mouth with each inspiratory effort demand attention because they give strong evidence of inadequate ventilation.

Ears

The ears are inspected for their position. A kinked pinna under a strap holding a mask in place or in a patient lying on his side will cause considerable discomfort to the patient postoperatively. We have seen an eardrum perforated by a needle. The patient was on his side; the needle had been left on the pillow. Dressings applied carelessly to the head may result in pinna trauma.

Neck

The neck is inspected for its position. Excessive extension may cause occipital headaches and neck pain postoperatively. Venous distention is common under anesthesia even in patients without heart disease. Changes in distention, therefore, need to be noticed and monitored.

Laryngeal motion is an indication of either light anesthesia when it is associated with swallowing or retching, or inadequate ventilation if the larynx moves downward with each inspiration.

Chest

The jugulum is watched for motion. Retraction of the jugulum or the supraclavicular fossae during inspiration of the spontaneously breathing patient occurs with upper airway obstruction.

The thorax is observed for motion with ventilation. The left and right thorax should move in unison with ventilation. If they do not, one of the main bronchi may be obstructed (check bronchial intubation) or a lung may be consolidated or collapsed secondary to fluid or air in the pleural space. Retraction of the intercostal spaces suggests airway obstruction if it is seen during inspiration in the spontaneously breathing patient.

When thorax and abdomen are viewed together in a spontaneously breathing patient, the observable motion should be subtle. There should be no "rocking of the boat" where the abdomen falls when the thorax rises and vice versa, as happens with strained ventilation in the presence of obstruction. Similarly, on expiration in the spontaneously breathing and well-anesthetized patient, the abdominal muscles should remain flaccid. A telltale sign of light anesthesia is the contraction of the abdominal muscles during expiration. This occurs in most patients during light anesthesia or, in the absence of anesthesia, in patients with obstructive lung disease that forces them to use active expiration.

Extremities

The extremities are inspected for position, pressure points, and edema. If infusions or transfusions infiltrate, swelling and discolorations are seen. Venous irritation following the injection of irritating substances shows up as a red streak over the course of a vein. The same reaction is seen after the injection of a substance to which the patient is allergic. For example, erythema of face and blush area is common after atropine injection, and generalized hives indicate a systemic reaction to an antigen.

Wound

Inspection of the surgical wound is part of the monitoring routine. As often as possible, the wound is inspected for color of the blood, pulsation of the content, evidence of muscle tone in the operative field wherever applicable, and content of the operative field. Look for bowel distention or brain swelling, examine the position of the mediastinum in thoracic procedures, and, always, search for ongoing bleeding.

Experienced clinicians can expand this brief survey of inspection. A thorough inspection by the experienced clinician takes less time than it took the reader to skim this discussion.

PALPATION

Just as a thorough inspection is second nature to the clinician, so is palpation, which usually begins with feeling the pulse. This should be done with the index finger lightly applied so that blood flow can continue through the artery. When the pulse is very feeble, use the finger of your free hand to palpate your own pulse to be sure that the pulse felt by the probing finger is not your own. No examiner is beyond making the occasional error of detecting his own pulse instead of the patient's in the tip of the probing index finger.

Palpation of an artery will give an indication of absence or presence of a pulse. With great experience, it might be possible to distinguish between a high blood pressure and a low blood pressure, but to make intermediate determinations is next to impossible. The clinicians of old described different pulse qualities, but how accurate and precise they were is questionable.

Palpation for intraocular pressure, the tenseness of the fontanella in babies, and the tightness of distended jugular veins is sometimes practiced and provides indications for further studies if the palpating finger senses undue pressure.

Palpation of the laryngeal motion is very useful in patients with thick necks in whom slight downward motions with inspiration cannot be seen but can be felt readily. This slight tracheal tug is an indication of some respiratory deficiency that may exist before anesthesia in patients with lung disease or muscle weakness, and is common under anesthesia in patients breathing spontaneously while being weakened by muscle relaxants or anesthesia and suffering some respiratory insufficiency.

The chest motion should be checked in patients breathing spontaneously to make sure that the upper chest rises with inspiration and that both halves of the thorax rise in harmony. After intubation, it is useful to push smartly on the left and then right upper chest while holding a cupped hand over the open endotracheal tube. This quick maneuver reaffirms the position of the endotracheal tube in the trachea and helps to detect an endotracheal tube that is inserted too far. In that case, a puff of air comes out of the endotracheal tube only upon pressing on one side but not on the other. (This test is preliminary and does not replace the careful auscultation of the lungs once the patient is connected to the anesthesia circuit.) It is also useful to palpate the trachea between the cricoid cartilage and the sternum, and then to deflate, and again inflate, the cuff of the endotracheal tube. If the swelling of the cuff cannot be felt, the tube may be down too far; if it can be felt, the tip of the endotracheal tube is likely to be safely above the carina.

Palpation of the upper abdomen for an inflated stomach containing air or liquid is important before induction of anesthesia and after intubation or prolonged artificial ventilation with a mask to discover instances of gastric distention. Palpate the epigastrium again before extubation. Pass a soft catheter into the stomach and aspirate to relieve pressure before extubation. This quick maneuver helps to prevent aspiration. If no gastric tube is needed postoperatively, remove the catheter before extubation.

Palpation of the abdomen can help to detect muscular contraction during expiration, a sure sign of light anesthesia in patients breathing spontaneously.

If, during surgery, you are displaced from your usual position at the head of the table because the surgeon operates on the head or face, position yourself at the side of the patient, where you can feel the patient's abdomen, chest, and neck. If the patient is breathing spontaneously, the coordinated chest and abdominal motion during inspiration and the absence of muscular contraction of the abdominal muscles during expiration will help in gauging the level of anesthesia. Active expiration shows anesthesia levels that are light, and are potentially too light for eye operations or procedures in which a sudden motion of the patient may be dangerous. A quickly contracting diaphragm during inspiration in a spontaneously breathing patient indicates deep anesthesia or respiratory insufficiency with a high CO_2 level. Thus, even without the help of eye signs, palpation of abdomen and thorax can be very helpful in the management of anesthesia.

A distended bladder can also be detected by palpation.

In patients who are at risk of sustaining brachial plexus injuries, for instance, when the head is turned to one side and the opposite arm is extended, palpate between the neck and the clavicle of the extended arm. The smaller this space, the greater our concern should be that the brachial plexus may become squeezed between the clavicle and the first rib.

AUSCULTATION

Auscultation is a relatively recent addition to the anesthesia armamentarium but it is now a firmly established practice. After tracheal intubation and, again, after placing the patient in a new position, both upper lung fields must be listened to in order to assure ventilation of the lungs and to guard against intubation of one bronchus. For intraoperative monitoring, a precordial or esophageal stethoscope is used by many clinicians. The precordial stethoscope most widely used is a heavy metal bell that comes in both a pediatric and an adult size (Fig. 2-1). Its weight is intended to press the bell against the skin. Small disposable circular patches of adhesive are available to glue the stethoscope head to the skin of the chest. Placing a small sandbag or plastic bag with IV solution over the stethoscope can also help to keep the device in place (Fig. 2-2). These convenient devices make auscultatory monitoring easy.

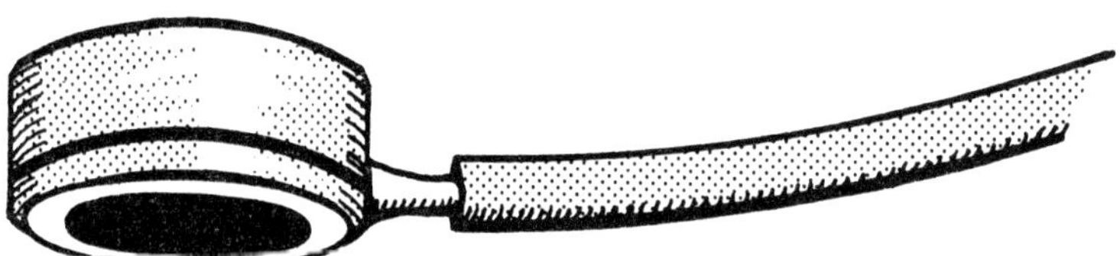

Figure 2-1. Precordial stethoscope. A heavy metal bell can be placed over the precordium for cardiac monitoring or into the jugular fossa for respiratory monitoring.

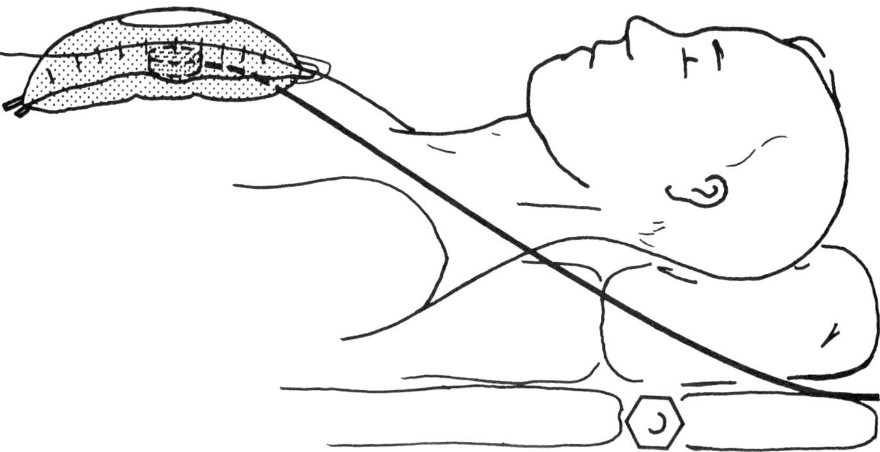

Figure 2-2. Precordial stethoscope. A precordial stethoscope can be kept in place by a 250-ml plastic bag of IV solution.

For all operations in which an endotracheal tube is used, an esophageal stethoscope can be placed. These are simple catheters with a soft balloon; they are advanced into the esophagus until heart and breath sounds are well heard (Fig. 2-3). Some incorporate temperature probes or electrocardiograph electrodes.

The precordial stethoscope is frequently placed over the precordium to monitor heart sounds. Listen for rate and rhythm, and for the muffling of sounds which are easily noticed with significant hypotension and myocardial depression. Monitoring of the precordium may not yield adequate information in severely emphysematous or grossly obese patients, where the heart and breath sounds may be so muted as to be barely perceptible. An esophageal stethoscope helps in these situations. The precordial or esophageal stethoscope is a sensitive, reliable, and inexpensive device, and an excellent adjunct to sophisticated monitoring systems that can be relied upon when other systems fail. In simple, brief anesthetic procedures, the stethoscope may be the single most important device because it allows us to monitor circulation and ventilation continuously without electronics, without lifting our eyes, and without hands!

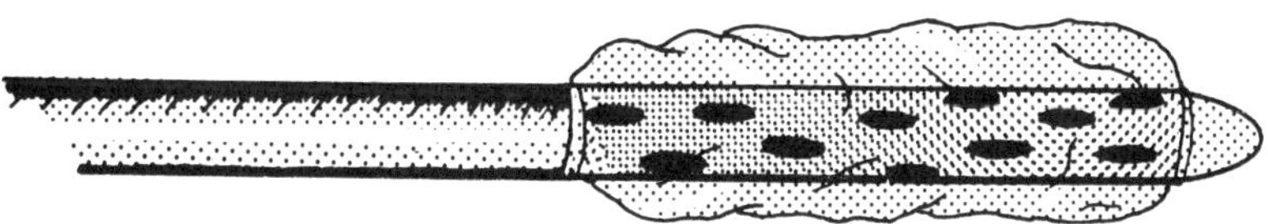

Figure 2-3. Tip of an esophageal stethoscope.

PERCUSSION

During anesthesia, the only areas that warrant percussion are the chest, when hemo-, hydro-, or pneumothorax is suspected, and the abdomen, when air in the stomach is suspected and the air bubbles can be percussed in the epigastrium.

MONITORING DURING TRANSPORT

When the wound is closed, the dressing applied, and anesthesia discontinued, formal monitoring of the patient also stops and is not resumed until the patient is admitted either to the recovery room or to the intensive care unit. Yet, the time of transport is probably more dangerous to the patient than the end of operation or the stay in the recovery room. It is more dangerous than the end of operation, because lifting the patient from the operating-room table to the stretcher may involve drastic changes in position at a time when the patient's homeostatic reflexes are still obtunded and when pooling of blood in dependent vascular beds may lead to sudden hypotension. Transport time is more dangerous than time in the recovery room simply because it is closer to general anesthesia, and recovery from the effect of depressant drugs has not yet had a chance to proceed very far. Hence the paradox: monitoring in the operating room is considered to be essential, as is monitoring in the recovery room, yet monitoring during the phase separating the patient's stay in the operating room from that in the recovery room is often ignored.

To guard the patient against adversity during this transport, a few precautionary steps are in order:

1. Position the patient so that the airway is least likely to become obstructed, either from the tongue falling back or from aspiration of regurgitated material. We recommend for this transport the po-

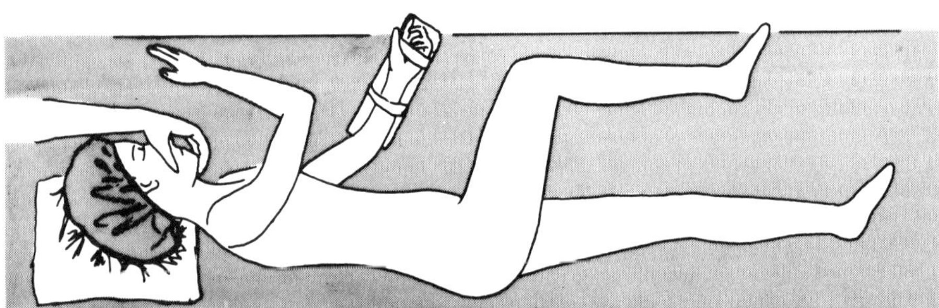

Figure 2-4. Position for transport of unconscious patient. The hand supporting the patient's chin feels every exhalation.

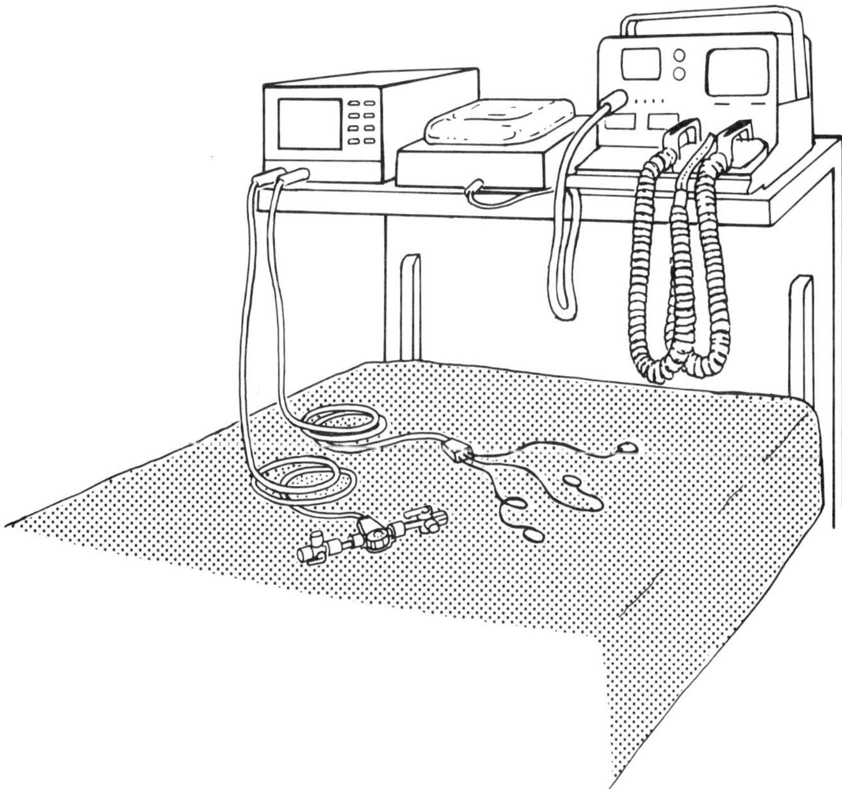

Figure 2-5. A shelf on the foot end of the transport bed supports battery-powered electronic monitoring equipment.

sition shown in Figure 2-4. The patient is placed on his side with the lower leg extended and the upper leg angled 90° at hip and knee. The arms are in front of the patient. The position of legs and arms prevents the patient from rolling on either his back or his face. The position is also comfortable. The occiput is propped up slightly so that the face is dependent. This allows the soft tissues of mouth and pharynx to fall forward. Should mucus or vomitus reach the pharynx, it can flow with gravity out of the corner of the mouth. This lateral position is also more comfortable for the many patients who will have to spend hours lying still on their backs during their operations. Patients who have been operated on in the lateral position should be transported with the operated side down.

2. Stay with the patient while the patient is lifted from operating table to stretcher and during the transport. In addition to continuous

inspection of the patient, place a hand under the patient's chin in such a way that the patient's exhaled breath warms the palm of your hand. In this way you can feel every breath the patient takes, even when inspection of respiratory motion and auscultation of breath sounds are hampered by transport through busy and often noisy corridors. This supporting hand, with the fingers under the patient's chin, serves equally well whether the patient is on his side or on his back. Throughout transport the patient should be rolled feet first, making observation by the clinician possible.

3. Special transport beds are available with a shelf over the foot end that supports battery-powered monitoring equipment (Fig. 2-5). This allows critically ill patients to be monitored electronically during transport.
4. Patients recovering from depressant anesthetics and just recently extubated often hypoventilate, resulting in a hemoglobin desaturation by the time they arrive in the recovery room. When this is a concern, monitor oxygen saturation (see Chap. 6) and administer oxygen by mask or nasal prongs.

CHAPTER 3

The Electrocardiogram

Einthoven, in 1903, invented the string electrocardiograph, a device capable of recording current generated by the heart. It took approximately 15 years for this invention to find its way into the operating room, and even longer before it was generally accepted for routine monitoring.

DESCRIPTION AND APPLICATION

Lead Systems

Einthoven's anatomic electrical triangle, superimposed upon the human torso, provides the basis for placing the electrodes (Fig. 3-1). Electrical activity is represented in the figure as a vector quantity, meaning that electrical activity possesses both a direction and a force that continually change during cardiac activity. Each lead is the vector sum of the leads of the other two sides of the triangle. Consider this mechanical analogy:

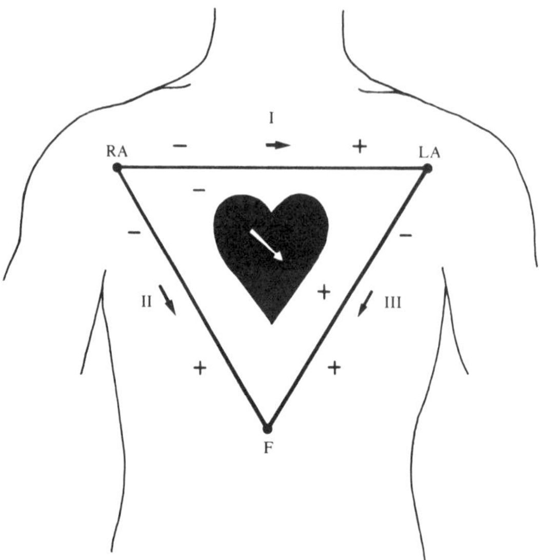

Figure 3-1. Einthoven's triangle. Observe that the right arm (*RA*) is never positive and the leg (*F*) never negative. (The exploring electrode is positive.) Lead I is right arm–left arm, lead II is right arm–left leg, and lead III is left arm–left leg.

Two tugs are pushing a giant ship. Each tug pushes in a certain direction with a certain force. They may be exactly replaced by one tug (perhaps larger) pushing in a certain direction with a certain force. In this way, two forces acting in two directions are replaced with one force in an intermediate direction. The triangle gives rise to the three standard limb leads, which have been used successfully for many years and with which approximately 80% to 90% accuracy in electrocardiographic diagnosis may be achieved. The leads make electrical connections between the following points: lead I connects the left shoulder and the right shoulder; lead II, the right shoulder and the left leg; and lead III, the left shoulder and the left leg. These leads have their own polarities, as shown in Figure 3-1. Observe that the left leg (leads II and III) is always positive and that the right arm (leads I and II) is always negative. It follows, then, that the left arm is positive in lead I and negative in lead III. This is of interest when the electrode is applied over the heart, rather than on a limb. Each lead, when connected to a monitor, measures the electrical potential (voltage) between two points. Whether the leads are connected at wrists and ankles or at shoulders and hips makes no difference. At the center of the triangle thus formed lies the heart.

In 1932, one lead was first placed over the apex of the heart, and from this experiment evolved a system of precordial or chest leads. The

Table 3-1. THREE-LEAD ECG LEAD PLACEMENT

	Standard Leads			Modified Leads						
	I	II	III	IEV	IIEV	IIIEV	I SCAP.V	I CLAV.V	I MAN.V	III CLAV.V
Lead										
RA	RA^-	RA^-	RA	RA^-	RA^-	RA	$Scap^-$	$Clav^-$	Man^-	RA
LA	LA^+	LA	LA^-	V_1^+ or V_5^+	LA	LA^-	V_5^+	V_5^+	V_5^+	CLA^-
F	F	F^+	F^+	F	V_1^+ or V_5^+	V^+ or V_5^+	F	F	F	V_5^+
Selector Switch	I	II	III	I	II	III	I	I	I	III

Note: The nomenclature of modified three-lead ECG electrode placement has been confusing. This table shows the leads occasionally used. In the Modified systems we name the lead selection first, the negative electrode E (for Einthoven) if it is in its standard place, or we list it if modified. We always name the positive electrode last; it is the exploring electrode. Scap = electrode over right scapula; Clav = electrode under right or left clavicle; Man = electrode over manubrium.

In the past, the following terms have been used: CF for IEV_1, CL for $IIEV_1$, CR for $IIIEV_1$, CB_5 for I $SCAP.V_1$, MCR_5 or CS_5 for I $CLAV.V_5$, CM_5 for I $MAN.V_5$, and MCL for III $CLAV.V_1$.

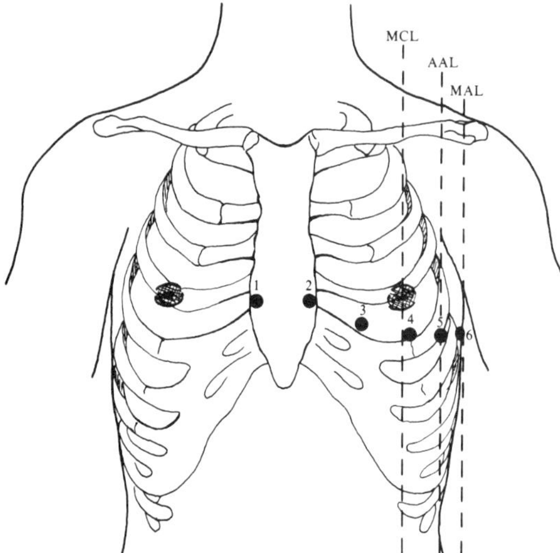

Figure 3-2. The precordial chest leads V_1 through V_6. *MCL* = midclavicular line; *AAL* = anterior axillary line; *MAL* = midaxillary line.

positions over the chest are now named V_1 through V_6, as shown in Figure 3-2. Points 1 and 2 are at the fourth intercostal space just to the right and left of the sternum, point 4 lies in the midclavicular line in the fifth interspace, and point 3 halfway between points 2 and 4. Points 5 and 6 are directly lateral to point 4, but in the anterior and mid-axillary line.

We sometimes have monitors with only three leads, yet we wish to record from a precordial electrode (Table 3-1). This can be done by placing one electrode (the exploring electrode), always the positive one, over the heart, usually at position V_1 or V_5. Since the electrode for the right arm is never positive, it is never used to measure electrical activity over the heart. If we use the left arm electrode over the heart, we need to switch to lead I (*i.e.*, we are measuring between heart and right arm, with the leg serving as ground). If we put the leg electrode over the heart, we have the choice of using either lead II or lead III, thus having either the right arm or the left arm as the negative electrode location while the other serves as ground. We call these leads IEV, IIEV, and IIIEV, depending upon the lead and the choice of electrode over the heart. Our convention is designed to make lead selection and placement simple. In IEV the first number (I) stands for lead I. This alerts the user familiar with the Einthoven triangle (Fig. 3-1) that the left and right arms carry the active leads. The next term (E) indicates that the negative electrode is placed as usual (E for Einthoven). The last term (the left arm lead which is positive in lead I) has been moved to the V position. A subscript to the V (*e.g.*, V_1 or V_5) can indicate which V position was selected.

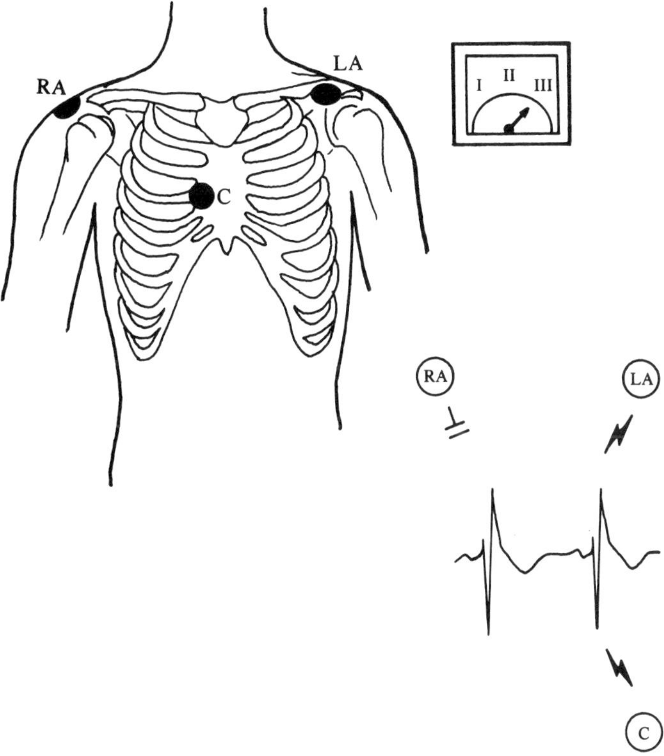

Figure 3-3. Modified chest lead (IIIEV) with right arm serving as ground, the foot electrode placed over the precordium (V_1 position), and the left arm electrode under the left clavicle. Lead selector switch to lead III. Useful for observing conduction defects, such as right bundle branch block.

Kaplan[1a] has recommended a modified chest lead (III CLAV.V_1) with the right arm serving as ground, the leg electrode being placed over the precordium at the V_1 position (to the right of the sternum in the fourth interspace), and the left arm electrode serving as reference (Fig. 3-3).[1b] Instead of putting the electrode on the left arm or shoulder, he suggests placing it under the left clavicle. The selector switch is turned to position III. The chest electrode is positive and serves as the exploring electrode. This particular setting facilitates the observation of conduction defects, bundle branch blocks, and P-wave abnormalities. The leads are summarized in Table 3-1.

Bipolar and Unipolar Leads

The terms *bipolar* and *unipolar* relate to how voltage is measured to generate a signal. The standard limb leads and the three electrode chest leads are bipolar because they measure voltage between two distinct poles.

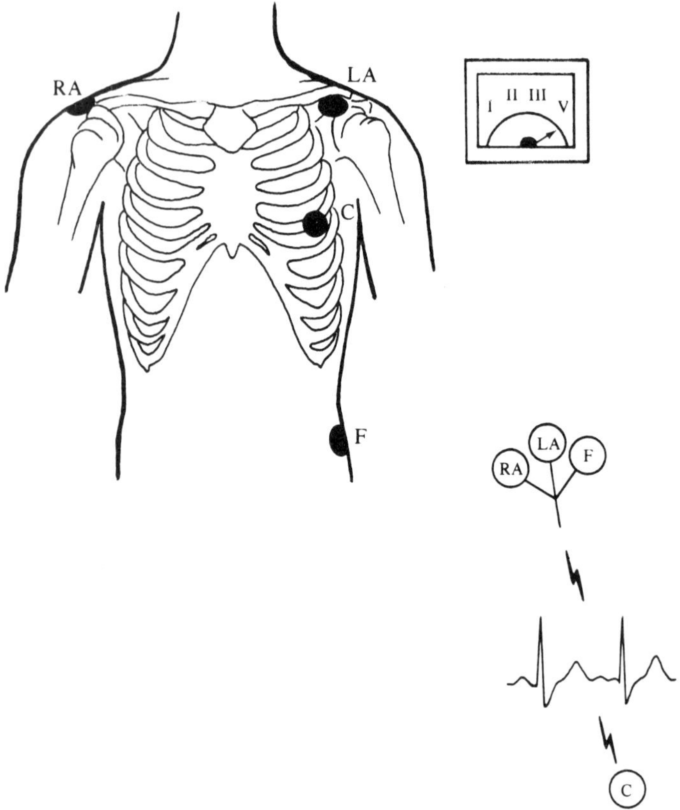

Figure 3-4. The four-lead system is displayed as used in anesthesia. Right arm, left arm, and leg electrodes are combined to form the indifferent electrode; the precordial or chest electrode is placed in position V_5; the lead selector switch is in the V position.

When all limb electrodes are connected through a high electrical resistance (500 ohms), a truly indifferent electrode results (Fig. 3-4). The exploring electrode has maximal influence on the ECG pattern, because the limb leads are combined to provide a general indifferent reference. In this way, the precordial lead system (V-leads) is described as unipolar. The central terminal (indifferent) potential does not change throughout the cardiac cycle, so the potential measured between the central terminal and the precordial exploring electrode is overwhelmingly influenced by the exploring electrode.

It is also possible to have unipolar limb leads. The exploring, positive, active electrode is placed on a limb, and the remaining electrodes are combined to form a central, indifferent terminal. These unipolar, augmented limb leads still have a strong mathematical relationship to the

Table 3-2. AUGMENTED LIMB LEADS*

	Positive	Negative
aVR	Right arm	The remaining leads form a common, indifferent electrode.
aVL	Left arm	
aVF	Left leg	

* The relationship of the bipolar limb leads to the augmented limb leads: lead I = aVL − aVR; lead II = aVF − aVR; lead III = aVF − aVL.

bipolar limb leads; thus, the unipolar, augmented leads can be algebraically summed to derive standard limb leads. The leads and their relationship are shown in Table 3-2.

Most ECG monitors are equipped for electrical standardization, which should be completed before recording ECGs. A signal of 1 millivolt (mV) is thrown into the circuit and causes a deflection that should be 10 mm high (Fig. 3-5). It is sometimes necessary to adjust the monitor in order to obtain a properly standardized signal. This is important when ST segments are monitored, since a 1-mm depression of the ST segment can be diagnostically important. If the machine is not properly calibrated or the correct monitoring mode is not selected, an ST segment depression or elevation may be misinterpreted.

Lead Selection

Table 3-3 summarizes these indications. If the surgical field permits, and if only three electrodes can be used, we use modified chest leads; for instance, to monitor P-waves and the quality of the QRS complex, I SCAP.V_1 or III CLAV.V_1.

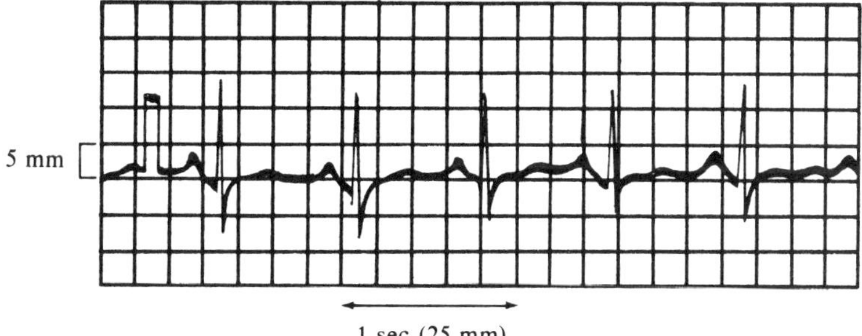

Figure 3-5. The amplitude of the ECG signal is calibrated against a 1-mV test signal which should cause a 10-mm deflection.

Table 3-3. LEAD SELECTION*

Clinical Problem	Preferred Lead Selection
Arrhythmias	
Three-lead system	
With access to chest	III CLAV.V_1
No access to chest	II
Four- or Five-lead system	V_1 or V_5
Ischemia	
Three-lead system	Lead I SCAP.V_1 (see Table 3-1)
Four-lead system	Left arm electrode over V_5, aVL
Five-lead system	
One ECG channel available	V_5
Two ECG channels available	V_5, II
Ischemia†	
T-wave inversion	I, II V_2–V_6
ST depression	All
Injury†	
ST elevation	All
Infarction†	
Q-waves	All except aVR

* Lead selection is determined by the nature of the problem and the surgical requirements.
† Table shows criteria for diagnosis.

CLINICAL INDICATIONS FOR ELECTROCARDIOGRAPHY

The average frequency of abnormal electrocardiographic findings is difficult to estimate. In healthy patients undergoing routine anesthesia, disturbances of heart rate will be common, whereas patients with heart disease will suffer frequent arrhythmias and abnormalities of the ST segment. For routine monitoring in unselected groups of patients the following ranking reflects our clinical experience from most to least common:

1. Changes in RR intervals
2. Tachycardia
3. Bradycardia
4. Shortening of PR intervals to complete nodal rhythm
5. Unifocal ventricular extrasystoles, particularly bigemini
6. ST segment depression
7. Multifocal ventricular extrasystoles

8. Peaked T-waves
9. QT interval lengthening
10. ST segment elevation
11. Widening QRS complexes
12. Ventricular tachycardia
13. Ventricular fibrillation

All of these are of interest to the clinician.

Beat-to-beat changes in RR intervals give excellent information on the vagal tone. Changes in rate displayed as trends are informative as they often reflect changes in cardiac output and signal changes in autonomic activity and myocardial oxygen demand. Shortening of PR intervals is very common; perhaps as many as 20% of patients develop this at some time during the course of anesthesia. Nodal rhythm is usually benign but does go along with changes in ventricular filling and, hence, output and blood pressure. It also signals some ill-understood problems of myocardial conduction (A-V) or irritability (node over sinus).

Occasional, unifocal, premature ventricular contractions (PVCs) are usually benign and common even in asymptomatic patients who are not anesthetized. When PVCs become frequent and particularly multifocal they are viewed with a jaundiced eye as they betray an irritable ventricle. The fear is that they may get worse and lead to ventricular fibrillation. They are usually treated with antiarrhythmic drugs and, where appropriate, by switching the anesthetic agent.

ST segment depression is generally taken as evidence of myocardial ischemia and is therefore considered with great concern. Major problems with current monitoring technology make it difficult to decide whether filtering has either obscured or falsely revealed ST segment depression. There is evidence for both false negatives and false positives with the ECG monitor in the monitoring mode.

QT lengthening occurs in some patients as an inborn or acquired (*e.g.*, drug induced) abnormality. It is dangerous because it can lead to fatal arrhythmias. A rare form of acquired, prolonged QT interval is seen in patients poisoned with fluoride; this is associated with low serum calcium.

ST segment elevation is the hallmark of myocardial infarction. It is fortunately very rare during anesthesia.

Widening of the QRS complexes is typical for bundle branch blocks (BBBs), which sometimes develop during anesthesia, particularly in association with changes in heart rate.

Ventricular tachycardia (VTach) is often the forerunner to ventricular fibrillation.

Thus, ECG monitoring can fulfill many functions. A few of these are discussed in greater detail.

Cardiac Activity

The electrocardiograph serves as an important diagnostic device in situations when no cardiac activity can be detected by auscultation (precordial or esophageal stethoscope), no pulse or blood pressure can be obtained, and the differential diagnosis is as follows:

- Feeble cardiac contractions with insufficient output and unobtainable blood pressure (QRS complexes will be present)
- Cardiac standstill (asystole—no QRS complexes)
- Ventricular fibrillation (irregular ECG—the forerunner of this is often an extreme ventricular tachycardia)

Feeble cardiac activity is sometimes the result of anesthetic overdose. Merely ventilating the lungs with oxygen may suffice to allow redistribution of the anesthetic agent and spontaneous recovery of cardiac activity. Sometimes drug therapy and cardiac massage are also necessary.

When no output exists, it is important to distinguish between asystole and ventricular fibrillation. Although both call for ventilation of the lungs with oxygen and cardiac massage, only ventricular fibrillation will respond to electrical defibrillation.

Arrhythmias

Perhaps more than 50% of all patients develop some rhythm disturbance during anesthesia. Most common are tachycardias during intubation and bradycardias with vagal stimulation. These are usually readily detected with the precordial or esophageal stethoscope, or by a finger on the pulse. The electrocardiographic monitors in the operating room facilitate identification of arrhythmias in three ways:

- An audible "beep" is generated with every heartbeat.
- A digital readout of rate is provided by most modern machines.
- Many machines have alarms that can be set so that a signal will be given when heart rates go above or below a predetermined level. It is important to select alarm levels that are unlikely to be exceeded during ordinary anesthetic procedures, including the episodes of tachycardia that occur with intubation. If the alarm limits are set too close to the ideal average, the alarm will sound when there is no danger. Subsequently the clinician, annoyed by the sound of the alarm, will disable the alarm and, thus, defeat its purpose.

Heart rate is determined by the monitors either from the R-wave of the ECG or from the blood pressure monitor, which is capable of counting beats while the blood pressure is determined automatically. If rate is detected by counting R-waves, the waves must be of sufficient amplitude.

In some machines, it is possible that both R-waves and unusually large T-waves be counted and, thus, an erroneous heart rate may be computed. Other units have an algorithm to suppress recognition of the T-wave. There are also analog methods of determining pulse rate by holding the display of the QRS complex at a certain point on the screen and aligning the R-wave with a scale on the screen. This permits the observer to read the heart rate.

Peripheral pulse sensors based upon a plethysmographic system (see Chap. 4) can also be used to generate a signal for the count of the heart rate.

Dysrhythmias occur with a host of clinical conditions. Under anesthesia dysrhythmias are frequently drug related. For example, atropine, glycopyrrolate, and related drugs can cause bradycardia, tachycardia, and nodal, atrial, or ventricular premature beats. Narcotics, such as fentanyl and morphine, can produce bradycardia. Diazepam sometimes produces bradycardia. Ketamine is often associated with tachycardia. The halogenated anesthetic may produce nodal rhythms, bigemini, and ventricular premature beats. Pancuronium and gallamine produce tachycardia. *d*-Tubocurarine and succinylcholine sometimes produce bradycardia. Vagal stimulation may result in bradycardia. Carotid sinus stimulation, ocular pressure, and mesenteric traction all trigger this response. Sympathetic stimulation and tachycardia are particularly common with tracheal intubation. Heart disease, of course, is associated with a wide variety of rhythm disturbances that may be exacerbated by, but are not typical with, anesthesia.

Ischemia

Generalized hypoxia often causes a marked bradycardia accompanied by hypotension resulting in cardiac arrest. This ominous pattern of bradycardia and hypotension must be recognized as early as possible. The differential diagnosis includes vagal stimulation, which is easily treated by eliminating the vagal stimulus or by giving a vagal blocking drug, such as atropine. Bradycardia and hypotension from hypoxia will not respond well to atropine, if at all, but need to be treated with vigorous ventilation with oxygen.

Ischemia limited to the myocardium, secondary to coronary arterial disease, requires analysis of the ECG waveforms. Not all leads of the electrocardiograph show the typical ST segment changes. Blackburn and his colleagues found lead V_5 to be especially useful in unveiling 89% of ischemic changes.[2] When myocardial ischemia threatens during anesthesia, for instance, in a patient with known coronary atherosclerosis, the five-lead system with the V-electrode over position 5 is recommended.

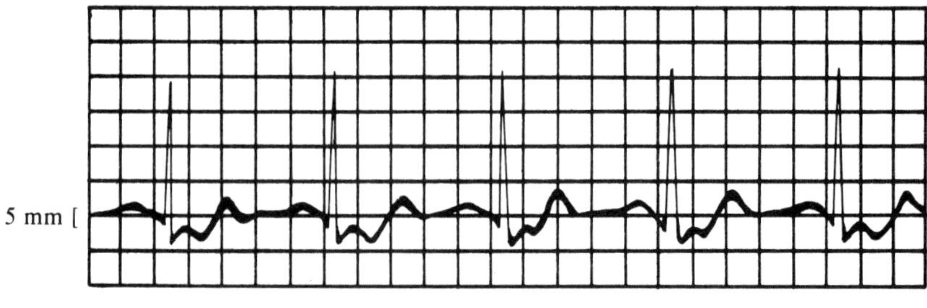

Figure 3-6. Ischemia is suspected with ST segment depression. Depressions of 1 mm or more are often indicative of myocardial ischemia. The ECG signal must be properly calibrated (1 mV = 10 mm deflection) to allow diagnosis of 1-mm ST segment depression.

Sometimes it is necessary to protect the precordial lead with a Steri-drape*, or something equivalent, to divert the flow of prep solution.

If it is possible to record two ECGs simultaneously, we follow Kaplan's suggestion of using standard leads V_5 and II.[1b] This combination allows us to monitor the anterior surface of the heart (lead V_5) and the inferior portion (lead II) simultaneously. Where dual channels are not available for monitoring or recording these leads, it is easy to switch from lead II to V_5 occasionally to keep track of developments.

Not all monitors possess five leads. If only three electrodes are available, a modified chest lead I or III is used (see Table 3-1). Lead I is used for monitoring the anterior wall of the heart and lead II is selected for the inferior wall. Regardless of the lead monitored, standard criteria for ST segment depression are used. The electrocardiographic signal is properly amplified so that a 1-mV signal gives a 10-mm deflection. If, in an ECG standardized in this way, the ST segment drops below the isoelectric line (Fig. 3-6) by 1 mm or more, the concern for possible ischemia must be strong. ST elevation of more than 1 mm may also signify myocardial injury or pericarditis even though some normal patients, particularly black patients, may have ST segment elevations in the chest leads without evidence of ischemia.

The T-wave is examined for its direction, height, and shape. Normally, it is upright in leads I, II, and V_2 through V_6, and inverted in aVR. A reversal in direction of this repolarization wave is suggestive of myocardial injury or infarction. A sudden change in T-wave direction is to be considered with alarm. Sharply pointed T-waves are also noted with suspicion. The height of the T-wave in the standard leads is less than 5 mm,

* 3M, Surgical Products Division, St. Paul, Minnesota.

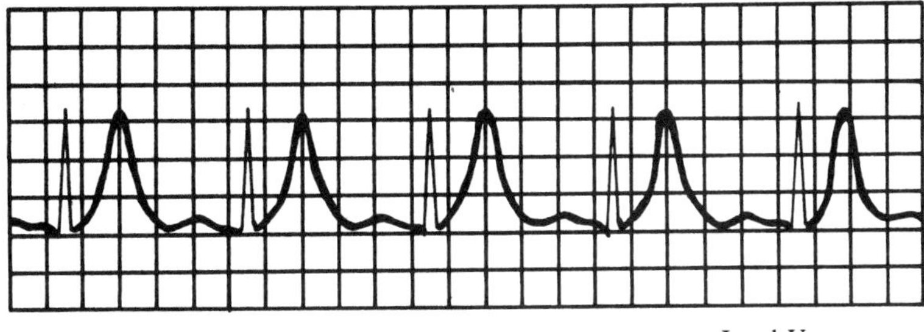

Figure 3-7. Hyperkalemia in adults causes peaked T-waves.

but in the precordium it is not above 10 mm. If these limits are exceeded, myocardial ischemia or infarction is to be considered.

Electrolyte Changes

In adults, high, spiked T-waves occur with elevated serum potassium levels (Fig. 3-7). Children sometimes may have peaked or notched T-waves and, in the precordial leads, even inverted T-waves that are quite normal.

With hypokalemia (Fig. 3-8), one first sees a prolongation of the QT interval, which is measured from the origin of the QRS complex to the end of the T-wave. This convention of measuring the QT interval is important because the interval changes with heart rate. The normal QT interval is less than half the preceding RR interval. With hypokalemia, T-waves may become inverted and the ST segment may sag.

Hypocalcemia also produces a prolonged QT interval (Fig. 3-9), but the T-wave usually remains normal.

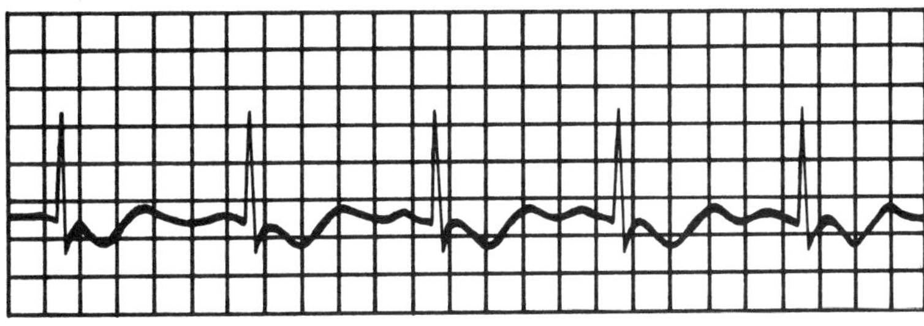

Figure 3-8. Hypokalemia is associated with a prolonged QT interval, inverted T-wave, and sagging ST segment.

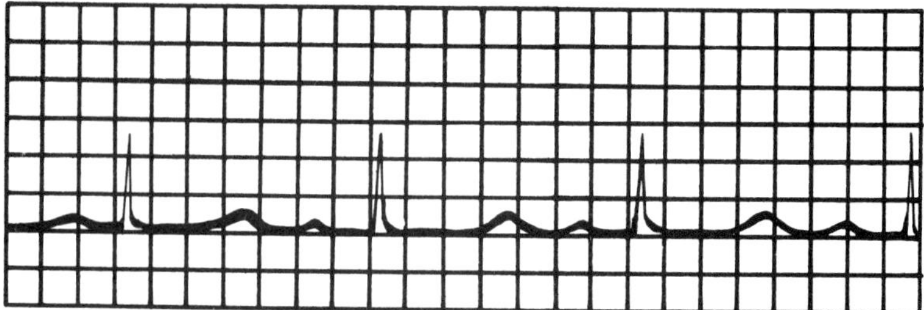

Lead II

Figure 3-9. Hypocalcemia typically causes a prolonged QT interval.

During the administration of potassium, during artificial ventilation of a patient with low potassium levels (which can further lower the serum potassium levels; see Chap. 14), and during the administration of calcium, the ECG should be monitored for these changes. Leads II, V_4, or V_5 are frequently suitable.

Pacemaker Function

The last use of the ECG is to check pacemaker function. There are two types of pacemakers, demand and nondemand, also known as either synchronous or asynchronous.

Asynchronous pacemakers send an electrical signal to the heart with absolute regularity, independent of intrinsic cardiac electrical activity. Even during electrocautery, the unit continues to discharge. Intraoperatively, this is an advantage. A disadvantage is that it may discharge during repolarization, which may lead to ventricular fibrillation, a rare event. Competition between the electronic and biologic pacemakers may occur unless the patient is in complete heart block. Asynchronous pacing is done through either the right atrium or the right ventricle.

Synchronous pacing makes use of the cardiac electrical activity to govern the pacemaker. Two common types are used: ventricular-inhibited and atrial-triggered pacemakers. Ventricular-inhibited pacemakers sense the QRS complex and are interrupted by it. They do not compete with intrinsic electrical activity but stand ready to deliver a pulse should no QRS activity develop within the specified time period.

Atrial pacemakers sense the P-wave, wait a bit, then stimulate the ventricle. Should a P-wave not be sensed, the device returns to the asynchronous mode.

Sometimes sequential pacemakers are used in which both the atrium and ventricle are wired. If the P-wave is not sensed, then the atrium is sent a signal followed shortly by a signal to the ventricle to contract. This well-timed atrial contraction should improve ventricular filling.

Implanted synchronous pacemakers may all be converted to an asynchronous function by placing a magnet adjacent to them.

Just as cardiac function is, in part, monitored by the ECG, so too is pacemaker function observed. In most leads, the pacemaker spike of electrical activity can be observed. If it is regularly followed by consistently appearing cardiac electrical activity, the pacemaker is said to be "capturing." Some transvenous devices allow pacemaker signal current to be adjusted. By varying the current, we can define rather precisely the amount of current to cause capture. Not all electrocardiograph leads will pick up pacer activity, but by checking several leads, including V_5, a satisfactory lead should be discovered.

CLINICAL APPLICATION OF ECGs

Skin Preparation

To establish a good electrical contact, the electrical resistance of the skin must be minimized. Careless preparation for monitoring fails to reduce the high electrical resistance encountered between skin and electrode, and jeopardizes the attainment of a useful ECG. Removing excessive body hair may help. Be careful not to abrade the skin, since "roughing" the skin is painful and unnecessary. Thoroughly cleanse the site with saline, soap and water, alcohol, or, ideally, a degreasing agent. Whichever method is chosen, be certain that the patient is not allergic to any agent used and that the skin is allowed to dry thoroughly.

Electrode Selection

Now that satisfactory adhesive electrodes are available, needle electrodes should be avoided. Use silver/silver chloride electrodes to be certain of adequate electrical conduction. All electrodes applied to a patient should be of a uniform make to avoid generating a batterylike effect. Check the expiration date on the package. Just before applying the electrode, be certain there is a gel-filled sponge on it, and that it is moist. It may take up to 15 minutes for a good contact to be established as the gel soaks into the skin. ECG paste eliminates the wait. Dry electrodes may be used if ECG paste is applied to the electrode. Apply the center first so that the adhesive holds the gelled area tightly against the skin.

An ECG backpad is currently available. It has four electrodes that are affixed to a plastic adhesive pad. Unfortunately, this provides a nonstandard lead. Neither is the placement of the pad standardized. These units offer no flexibility in lead selection and cost approximately twice as much as four separate electrodes.

Cables

Only use cables either supplied by the manufacturer or approved by the manufacturer of the monitor. An improper cable will cause trouble during electrocautery or defibrillation; approved cables frequently have series resistors in them to prevent surges of current from damaging the monitor. Before each use, the cable should be inspected for breaks in the insulation, as well as for sharp bends that may result in breaks. Be certain the contacts at the end of the cables to which the electrodes attach are clean and appropriate for the electrodes used.

Lead-Fault Indicator

A lead-fault indicator signal, available on some devices, alerts the clinician to an open circuit in the cable or the attachment wires, insufficient paste or gel on the electrodes, one or more disconnected electrodes or electrode attachment wires, no selection of an ECG (by using one of the ECG selector switches or by activating two or more selector switches simultaneously), or excessive direct current in one or more of the electrodes.

Mechanical Faults

Once the monitor is connected and the cables properly placed, a satisfactory waveform should be obtained. A quick check includes the items below.

Trace

Is the unit turned on and connected to a power source? Most battery-powered units will operate on line power while recharging the battery. If a mode selector switch is present, check to be certain an ECG selection has been made. Also, the electrical outlet must be supplied with electricity, a point not that easily checked in an operating room with safety plugs.

TRACE INTENSITY

The intensity of the cathode ray tube display of any monitor can vary. The intensity may be so diminished as to make the trace invisible. To be certain that this is not the problem on monitors so equipped, turn the intensity knob until satisfactory image brightness is obtained.

TRACE POSITION

An adjustment knob for trace position is available on some units. By slowly changing the setting from one extreme to another, a waveform may appear anywhere between the top and the bottom of the screen. Most units handle this task automatically.

TRACE FREEZE

If the button that freezes the trace is activated, the waveform will not disappear from the screen and will not move. To see an active waveform, merely unfreeze the trace.

FLAT TRACE

If the ECG signal from the patient is not amplified sufficiently, a "straight line" may result. First check the patient, then the machine, for instance, by increasing the QRS amplitude.

Module

Make certain the switches activating the ECG display are in the proper position. One part of a monitor may be turned on, but another part may be turned off. In some units, the monitor is constructed of parts or modules. If modules are not adequately plugged into the monitor, function will occasionally be lost. If this is a possibility, turn off the power, pull out the module, and then reinsert it.

Artifacts and Interference

Electrocardiographic monitoring in the operating room is complicated by many factors, including artifacts that may simulate arrhythmic and nonarrhythmic abnormalities. These may get displayed on the oscilloscope and distort the true electrocardiogram. At times, artifactual arrhythmias have even led to institution of inappropriate therapy. Most artifacts and interferences can be easily resolved by analyzing the path the signal must traverse from patient to monitor.

Artifacts

Among the most easily diagnosed but sometimes the most difficult artifacts to resolve are those caused by loose electrodes or broken leads. These artifacts may actually simulate Q-waves and sometimes inverted T-waves. Although a lost electrode is easy to demonstrate, a broken lead is much more difficult to identify. Some ECG monitors have built-in cable testers. The distal end of the cable is connected to the monitor and, if the lead is broken, its very high resistance will cause a large voltage drop.

Another place where high resistance may occur is at the connection between either the lead and the monitor, or the lead and the electrode. A dried or missing electrode pad can be particularly frustrating if suspicion arises after the lead is hidden under sterile drapes and access is lost. Also, moisture, grease, or dirt may interfere with the electrical equipment.

The oxygenator used during cardiopulmonary bypass may simulate ventricular tachycardia or other arrhythmias. Even if the pump is not operating, but the oxygenator is, electricity may be transmitted by the electrochemical potentials from the oxygenator.

An automatic infusion pump in the operating room also can cause artifacts. One infusion system has been shown to generate a waveform resembling that of paroxysmal ventricular contractions with variable coupling. Grounding of this system may help to eliminate the artifact.

A respiratory variation may occur, particularly on the frontal plane of the electrocardiogram, and may show up in leads III and aVF. This respiratory pattern or variation may be present during either assisted or spontaneous breathing. A pneumothorax may further change the respiratory variation in the electrocardiogram by shifting the frontal QRS complex to the right.

Occasionally, an aide restraining the patient may cause an artifact. This occurs when the electrical signals from the patient and the person restraining the patient combine, resulting in rather bizarre artifactual arrhythmias.

Responses within the patient may cause artifacts; for instance, involuntary contraction of muscles during electrocautery may simulate atrial flutters. The shivering or restless patient may also alter ECG patterns. A combative youngster makes ECG recording difficult and frustrating.

Interference

ELECTROCAUTERY

Electrocautery, which actually preceded the electrocardiograph into the operating room, may generate considerable electrical noise, which Doss and his colleagues have analyzed extensively.[3] They found that the radio-frequency component of the noise ranged between 800 kHz and 2000 kHz. This range comprised the largest portion of interference to the electrocardiograph preamplifier. A second source was the frequency of the alternating current line which, in the United States, is 60 Hz. Equipment supplied with alternating current is always a potential source of 60-Hz interference, also known as 60-cycle interference. A third component of noise was in the low-frequency range between 0.1 Hz and 10 Hz. This comes from electrosurgical units making or breaking contact intermittently with the patient's tissue. If currents from the electrosurgical unit directly activate striated muscle fibers, they too will cause noise that the ECG monitor will pick up. Some manufacturers have confronted this problem and are making units available that automatically suppress this source of exasperation.

MOVEMENT

Because it is loose or not placed over bone, an electrode moving on the skin may result in interference. If interference appears, press each electrode against the skin and observe the quality of the signal. Alternatively, try other leads. Discovering that one good lead exists frequently indicates electrode malfunction or insufficient skin contact in the others. Reprepare the skin, replace the electrode, or do both.

GROUNDING

Be certain that beds and other equipment near the monitor and the patient are properly grounded; otherwise, the signal will show 60-cycle interference.

OTHER CAUSES

A power cable crossing or running in close proximity to the electrocardiograph cable, loose electrodes, and electrocautery may all contribute to 60-cycle interference. Equipment that causes high interference, even a transmitter for a communication system, may be near the patient. Inadequate preparation of the skin before the application of the electrode may cause the baseline to wander. Another cause may be inadequate penetration of the gel into the skin; a good conducting pathway depends on this penetration, which may take 15 minutes to complete. Dry electrodes and poor skin preparation are the most prevalent causes of 60-cycle interference. The baseline may wander if the patient is moving about considerably, or with poor electrode placement, or with respiratory motion. There are other sources of interference from equipment in the operating room, including x-ray machines, air conditioning, vacuum and pressure pumps, fluorescent lights, and electric blankets.

Filters

An electronic filter reduces the amplitude of a signal over a certain frequency range.[4] Filters are available to eliminate the noise and are included in many monitors. Additionally, many monitors give a choice between a *diagnostic* or a *monitor* frequency mode. In the diagnostic frequency mode, a filter screens out only frequencies under 0.14 Hz. In the monitor mode, the filter eliminates frequencies under 4 Hz. The diagnostic mode gives better traces but is more susceptible to baseline wander. The baseline can be established with additional filtering, but a certain price is paid.

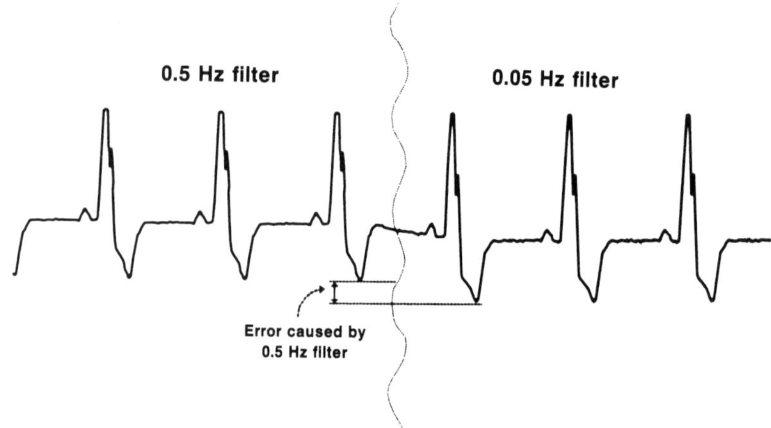

Figure 3-10. The effect of filtering a simulated ECG is shown. The first complexes on the left were recorded with an 0.5-Hz filter, the last three with an 0.05-Hz filter. Observe that the ST segment depression becomes visible only after replacing the 0.5-Hz filter with an 0.05-Hz filter. (Courtesy of P. T. Weinfurt, PhD)

In the monitor mode, P-waves and T-waves may decrease in amplitude and ST changes may be obscured or falsely suggested. Switching back to the diagnostic mode will unmask this artifact, if it is present. Figure 3-10 shows a possible effect of switching from diagnostic to monitoring mode.

REFERENCES

1. Kaplan JA: Cardiac Anesthesia, a, pp 129–130; b, pp 149–150. New York, Grune & Stratton, 1979
2. Blackburn H, Taylor HL, Okamoto N et al: Standardization of the exercise electrocardiogram—A systematic comparison of chest lead configurations employed for monitoring during exercise. In Karvonen MJ, Barry AJ (ed): Physical Activity and the Heart, pp 101–133. Springfield, IL, Charles C Thomas, 1967
3. Doss JD, McCabe CW, Weiss GK: Noise free electrocardiographic data during electrosurgical procedures. Anesth Analg 52:156, 1973
4. Tayler DI, Vincent R: Artefactual ST segment abnormalities due to electrocardiograph design. Br Heart J 54:121–128, 1985

CHAPTER 4

Arterial Pressure

The repeated or continuous measurement of arterial pressure during anesthesia has become an essential monitoring practice in the United States. Although it is difficult to say how the monitoring of arterial pressure improves the anesthetic care of our patients,[1] a number of observations have linked arterial pressure to organ function and mortality. Organs such as the brain, the heart, and the kidney require minimal pressure for perfusion, and organ failure must be feared if the patient suffers prolonged hypotension with pressures below this critical level. Unfortunately, many factors influence the critical level and no universally applicable limits can be stated. In hypertensive patients, Goldman correlated a blood pressure reduced by 33% for 10 minutes or longer with an increased risk of postoperative cardiac complications.[2]

In studies of the autoregulation of cerebral blood flow, the lower limit of mean arterial pressure assuring adequate brain blood flow is usually set at around 60 torr. In the young this level will be lower, whereas in those with established hypertension and atherosclerosis it will be higher.

Another approach looks at the lowest pressures that can be recorded during a normal day. These pressures usually occur during physiologic sleep in the small hours of the night and may be 15% lower than the pressures measured in a resting, supine, and awake person, for instance, the morning before the operation. Thus, the assumption that arterial pressure may be safely allowed to fall 15% below preanesthetic values intraoperatively can be defended.[3]

Of course, extensive clinical experience with induced hypotension has taught us that pressures well below this level can be tolerated, provided they do not sink and stay below the levels required for organ perfusion. This can be monitored by watching the electrocardiogram for evidence of ischemia of the heart (see Chap. 3), the production of urine for evidence of renal dysfunction (see Chap. 14), and the size of the pupil or the electroencephalogram (EEG) or evoked potentials (see Chap. 10) for evidence of an adequately perfused central nervous system.

Just as it is difficult to define the limit between normal blood pressure and hypotension, so is it difficult to delineate hypertension. Based on epidemiologic studies, internists arbitrarily define hypertension as those arterial pressures at rest that are associated with an increased mortality of 50% or more. These values are as follows: for men under 45 years, 130/90 torr; for older men, 140/95 torr; and for women, 160/95 torr. In the course of a normal day, the blood pressure of a healthy person will exceed these values, for instance, with exercise, excitement, or in the operating room during intubation under light anesthesia. Hypertensive patients will show greater elevation in response to such challenges and higher resting values than are the case for normotensive patients.[3]

UNITS OF PRESSURE

Poiseuille introduced the convenience of the mercury manometer. To this day, blood pressure is still measured in millimeters of mercury (mm Hg). Recently, the international system of units (SI units) has been adopted by a number of countries and millimeters of mercury are being replaced by pascals or millibars. With the advent of space travel, a pressure recording system that is independent of gravity was necessary; for this, the torr was introduced.

Definitions needed to convert pressure measurements follow:

$$1 \text{ atmosphere} = 1{,}013{,}250 \text{ dynes/cm}^2$$

$$1 \text{ torr} = 1/760 \text{ of } 1 \text{ atmosphere}$$

$$1 \text{ torr} = 1333.2 \text{ dynes/cm}^2$$

$$1 \text{ torr} = 1 \text{ mm Hg}$$

$$1 \text{ mm } H_2O \text{ (at 4°C)} = 98.06 \text{ dynes/cm}^2$$

$$1 \text{ mm } H_2O = 0.0735 \text{ torr}$$

$$1 \text{ millibar (mb)} = 100 \text{ newton/meter}^2 \text{ (N/m}^2\text{)}$$

$$1 \text{ mb} = 0.75 \text{ mm Hg}$$

$$1 \text{ mm Hg} = 1.33 \text{ mb}$$

$$1 \text{ pascal (Pa)} = 1 \text{ N/m}^2$$

One hectopascal (hPa) and 1 kilopascal (kPa) are 100 Pa and 1000 Pa, respectively. A blood pressure of 120/80 mm Hg or 120/80 torr can also be expressed as 15.9/10.6 kPa. Tables 4-1 and 4-2 provide help for the conversion of torr into kilopascals and of millimeters of water into torr.

SYSTOLIC, MEAN, AND DIASTOLIC PRESSURES

Systolic pressure is the peak pressure and *diastolic* is the lowest pressure of one cardiac cycle in the arterial vascular system. Systolic pressure is generally lower in the aorta than in distal large arteries such as the femoral or brachial artery because reflected waves and the complex, physical properties of the elastic, branching vascular system distort the pressure wave as it travels from the root of the aorta into the periphery. Although the differences between systolic pressure in the root of the aorta and in a large peripheral artery in young people may amount to more than 10 torr (the periphery being higher), the differences in diastolic pressures are not as pronounced.

The *mean arterial pressure* is *not* the sum of the systolic plus the diastolic pressure divided by two. It is a measurement that integrates the area under the pressure curve to obtain a true mean. This is usually done electronically or can be estimated with one of two formulas:

$$\text{mean arterial pressure} = \text{diastolic pressure} + \tfrac{1}{3} \text{ pulse pressure*}$$

$$\text{mean arterial pressure} = \frac{\text{systolic pressure} + (2 \times \text{diastolic pressure})}{3}$$

The result is the same. This estimate suffices in clinical practice, but in investigations a more accurate mean arterial pressure is needed. The relationship between systolic, mean, and diastolic arterial pressures is shown in Figure 4-1.

* *Pulse pressure* = systolic pressure − diastolic pressure.

(Text continues on p. 50)

Table 4-1. CONVERSION OF TORR INTO kPa*

	0	1	2	3	4	5	6	7	8	9
0	0.00	.13	.27	.40	.53	.67	.80	.93	1.06	1.20
10	1.33	1.46	1.60	1.73	1.86	2.00	2.13	2.26	2.39	2.53
20	2.66	2.79	2.93	3.06	3.19	3.33	3.46	3.59	3.72	3.86
30	3.99	4.12	4.26	4.39	4.52	4.66	4.79	4.92	5.05	5.19
40	5.32	5.45	5.59	5.72	5.85	5.99	6.12	6.25	6.38	6.52
50	6.65	6.78	6.92	7.05	7.18	7.32	7.45	7.58	7.71	7.85
60	7.98	8.11	8.25	8.38	8.51	8.65	8.78	8.91	9.04	9.18
70	9.31	9.44	9.58	9.71	9.84	9.98	10.11	10.24	10.37	10.51
80	10.64	10.77	10.91	11.04	11.17	11.31	11.44	11.57	11.70	11.84
90	11.97	12.10	12.24	12.37	12.50	12.64	12.77	12.90	13.03	13.17
100	13.30	13.43	13.57	13.70	13.83	13.97	14.10	14.23	14.36	14.50
110	14.63	14.76	14.90	15.03	15.16	15.30	15.43	15.56	15.69	15.83
120	15.96	16.09	16.23	16.36	16.49	16.63	16.76	16.89	17.02	17.16
130	17.29	17.42	17.56	17.69	17.82	17.96	18.09	18.22	18.35	18.49
140	18.62	18.75	18.89	19.02	19.15	19.29	19.42	19.55	19.68	19.82

150	19.95	20.08	20.22	20.35	20.48	20.62	20.75	20.88	21.01	21.15
160	21.28	21.41	21.55	21.68	21.81	21.95	22.08	22.21	22.34	22.48
170	22.61	22.74	22.88	23.01	23.14	23.28	23.41	23.54	23.67	23.81
180	23.94	24.07	24.21	24.34	24.47	24.61	24.74	24.87	25.00	25.14
190	25.27	25.40	25.54	25.67	25.80	25.94	26.07	26.20	26.33	26.47
200	26.60	26.73	26.87	27.00	27.13	27.27	27.40	27.53	27.66	27.80
210	27.93	28.06	28.20	28.33	28.46	28.60	28.73	28.86	28.99	29.13
220	29.26	29.39	29.53	29.66	29.79	29.93	30.06	30.19	30.32	30.46
230	30.59	30.72	30.86	30.99	31.12	31.26	31.39	31.52	31.65	31.79
240	31.92	32.05	32.19	32.32	32.45	32.59	32.72	32.85	32.98	33.12
250	33.25	33.38	33.52	33.65	33.78	33.92	34.05	34.18	34.31	34.45
260	34.58	34.71	34.85	34.98	35.11	35.25	35.38	35.51	35.64	35.78
270	35.91	36.04	36.18	36.31	36.44	36.58	36.71	36.84	36.97	37.11
280	37.24	37.37	37.51	37.64	37.77	37.91	38.04	38.17	38.30	38.44
290	38.57	38.70	38.84	38.97	39.10	39.24	39.37	39.50	39.63	39.77
300	39.90	40.03	40.17	40.30	40.43	40.57	40.70	40.83	40.96	41.10

* To convert torr (mmHg) into kPa, find torr value on left margin and top line. A blood pressure of 128, 101, 95 torr (systolic, mean, and diastolic) is 17, 13.4, 12.6 kPa.

Table 4-2. CONVERSION OF mmH_2O INTO TORR*

	0	1	2	3	4	5	6	7	8	9
0	0.00	.07	.15	.22	.29	.37	.44	.51	.59	.66
10	.74	.81	.88	.96	1.03	1.10	1.18	1.25	1.32	1.40
20	1.47	1.54	1.62	1.69	1.76	1.84	1.91	1.98	2.06	2.13
30	2.21	2.28	2.35	2.43	2.50	2.57	2.65	2.72	2.79	2.87
40	2.94	3.01	3.09	3.16	3.23	3.31	3.38	3.45	3.53	3.60
50	3.68	3.75	3.82	3.90	3.97	4.04	4.12	4.19	4.26	4.34
60	4.41	4.48	4.56	4.63	4.70	4.78	4.85	4.92	5.00	5.07
70	5.15	5.22	5.29	5.37	5.44	5.51	5.59	5.66	5.73	5.81
80	5.88	5.95	6.03	6.10	6.17	6.25	6.32	6.39	6.47	6.54
90	6.62	6.69	6.76	6.84	6.91	6.98	7.06	7.13	7.20	7.28
100	7.35	7.42	7.50	7.57	7.64	7.72	7.79	7.86	7.94	8.01
110	8.09	8.16	8.23	8.31	8.38	8.45	8.53	8.60	8.67	8.75
120	8.82	8.89	8.97	9.04	9.11	9.19	9.26	9.33	9.41	9.48
130	9.56	9.63	9.70	9.78	9.85	9.92	10.00	10.07	10.14	10.22
140	10.29	10.36	10.44	10.51	10.58	10.66	10.73	10.80	10.88	10.95

150	11.03	11.10	11.17	11.25	11.32	11.39	11.47	11.54	11.61	11.69
160	11.76	11.83	11.91	11.98	12.05	12.13	12.20	12.27	12.35	12.42
170	12.50	12.57	12.64	12.72	12.79	12.86	12.94	13.01	13.08	13.16
180	13.23	13.30	13.38	13.45	13.52	13.60	13.67	13.74	13.82	13.89
190	13.97	14.04	14.11	14.19	14.26	14.33	14.41	14.48	14.55	14.63
200	14.70	14.77	14.85	14.92	14.99	15.07	15.14	15.21	15.29	15.36
210	15.44	15.51	15.58	15.66	15.73	15.80	15.88	15.95	16.02	16.10
220	16.17	16.24	16.32	16.39	16.46	16.54	16.61	16.68	16.76	16.83
230	16.91	16.98	17.05	17.13	17.20	17.27	17.35	17.42	17.49	17.57
240	17.64	17.71	17.79	17.86	17.93	18.01	18.08	18.15	18.23	18.30
250	18.38	18.45	18.52	18.60	18.67	18.74	18.82	18.89	18.96	19.04
260	19.11	19.18	19.26	19.33	19.40	19.48	19.55	19.62	19.70	19.77
270	19.85	19.92	19.99	20.07	20.14	20.21	20.29	20.36	20.43	20.51
280	20.58	20.65	20.73	20.80	20.87	20.95	21.02	21.09	21.17	21.24
290	21.32	21.39	21.46	21.54	21.61	21.68	21.76	21.83	21.90	21.98
300	22.05	22.12	22.20	22.27	22.34	22.42	22.49	22.56	22.64	22.71

* **To convert mm H_2O pressure into torr,** find mm H_2O on left margin and top line. A central venous pressure of 8 cm H_2O (80 mm) is 5.9 torr.

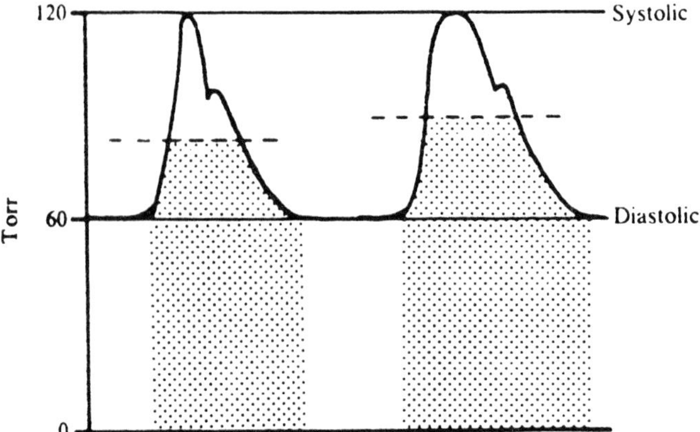

Figure 4-1. Systolic and diastolic arterial pressures may be the same but mean pressures may differ depending upon the area under the curve described by the blood pressure. Mean pressure is indicated by the broken line.

WHICH PRESSURE SHOULD BE RECORDED?

Systolic arterial pressure is considered by some to be the most important pressure variable. During anesthesia, more often than not, mean and diastolic pressures parallel systolic pressure when rising and falling. Systolic pressure reflects hypertension and hypotension. It also reflects the oxygen requirement of the heart because a high pressure generated by the heart is associated with a high consumption of oxygen. The "rate–pressure product" is obtained by multiplying systolic pressure by heart rate. A high heart rate and a high systolic pressure mean the heart requires significantly more oxygen than either a low heart rate and a high pressure, or a low heart rate and a low pressure. High rate–pressure products (above 15,000) are undesirable in patients with coronary artery disease. Remember, however, that the same rate–pressure product may reflect widely different conditions. A product of 15,000 can be produced by 100 (heart rate) × 150 torr systolic pressure, which may tax the myocardium far less than 150 (heart rate) × 100 torr systolic pressure.

Mean arterial pressure reflects the driving pressure pushing blood into an organ. Mean pressure is also used in the calculation of total peripheral resistance (see Chap. 5). Unlike systolic pressure in the recumbent patient, mean pressure is always lower in the peripheral arteries than in the root of the aorta. Invasively measured, mean pressure is less sensitive to the artifacts of the measuring system than systolic pressure.

Diastolic arterial pressure is often emphasized in studies of hypertension. The sustained diastolic pressure is thought to be an important variable in the diagnosis of hypertension. Myocardial perfusion depends on diastolic pressure because most perfusion occurs during diastole, when the cardiac muscle is relaxed. During systole, the contracting myocardium occludes many of its own blood vessels. Thus, a high diastolic arterial blood pressure provides a better myocardial perfusion than a low diastolic arterial pressure.

Diastolic arterial pressure does not always parallel systolic pressure. For example, during hypercarbia, systolic pressure rises more than diastolic.[4] With increased intracranial pressure, the pulse pressure (the difference between systolic and diastolic) also widens. In shock, pulse pressure diminishes; measurements of only systolic or mean arterial pressure cannot show changes in pulse pressure and, therefore, cannot convey the typical picture of vasoconstriction and hypovolemia. Hence, diastolic arterial pressure is of interest during anesthesia.

Ream gives an excellent discussion of these features,[5] and we agree with his conclusion that, in clinical anesthesia, all three arterial pressures—systolic, mean, and diastolic—should be monitored.

FACTORS AFFECTING BLOOD PRESSURE

Many factors play on the arterial blood pressure. The autonomic nervous system and drugs affect the function of the heart and the peripheral vascular resistance. Hemorrhage and infusion therapy alter blood volume and, depending on the fluids given, change the viscosity of the blood. The following are also factors that can affect arterial blood pressure.

Ventilation

Ventilation influences blood pressure. During spontaneous breathing, vagal activity changes rhythmically with every breath, causing a slowing of heart rate with expiration. This physiologic phenomenon will allow more runoff after systole and, therefore, a lower diastolic arterial pressure.

Systolic pressure is also influenced by breathing, being normally a little (a few torr) lower during inspiration. In patients with obstructive lung disease, asthma, cardiac tamponade, or shock, this phenomenon is exaggerated and systolic pressure may decrease by 10 torr or more during spontaneous inspiration. This is called the *paradoxical pulse*.

During positive pressure ventilation, blood pressure may rise a little during early inspiration but then falls markedly, particularly in patients with low blood volume and low central venous pressures (Fig. 4-2).

Position

Arterial pressure varies with the position of the patient. Imagine a supine, lifeless statue with a vascular system of rigid pipes pressurized to 100 torr

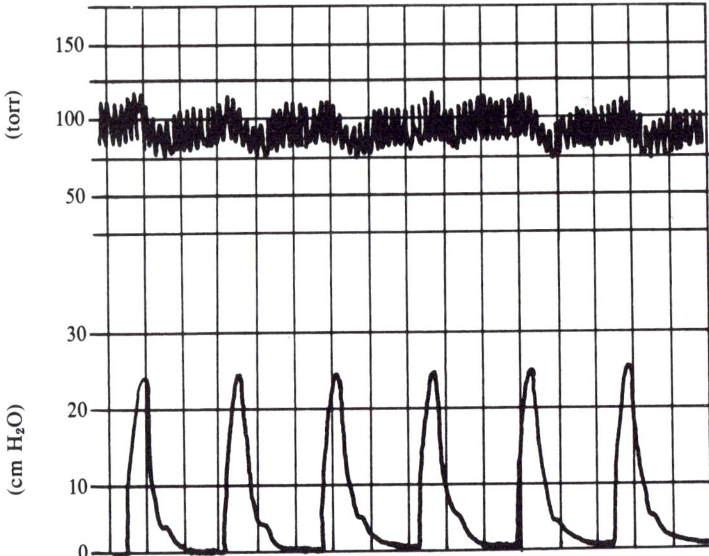

Figure 4-2. During positive pressure ventilation, blood pressure varies. It usually rises a little during early inspiration but then falls markedly, particularly in patients with low blood volume and low central venous pressure. This tracing comes from a patient undergoing a hysterectomy under enflurane anesthesia. Top trace is arterial pressure recorded in the brachial artery, bottom trace is airway pressure.

and with all vessels and the heart equally horizontal. Under these circumstances, the pressure, whether measured in the toe, in the head, or in the chest, would be 100 torr. Righting the statue would cause the pressure in the feet to be higher by the weight of the water column resting on the feet. The pressure in the head would still be 100 torr.

Now imagine a system with elastic pipes and a pump that drives fluid into the head and feet, as in the human vascular system. The heart lifts the column of blood from the heart to the head; in addition, the pump must overcome the vascular resistance of the head. The blood pressure in the root of the aorta of a standing man may show a mean of 90 torr, while that of the head will then be 90 torr minus the weight of the fluid column extending from aorta to head. Figure 4-3 shows typical pressure relationships for a person who is lying down and a person who is standing with one arm at his side and the other held high above his head.

When mean pressure falls, a point will be reached when that pressure no longer suffices to push blood past the vascular resistance offered by tissue. This is important in an anesthetized patient in the sitting position. In healthy patients, the cerebral perfusion pressure requires approxi-

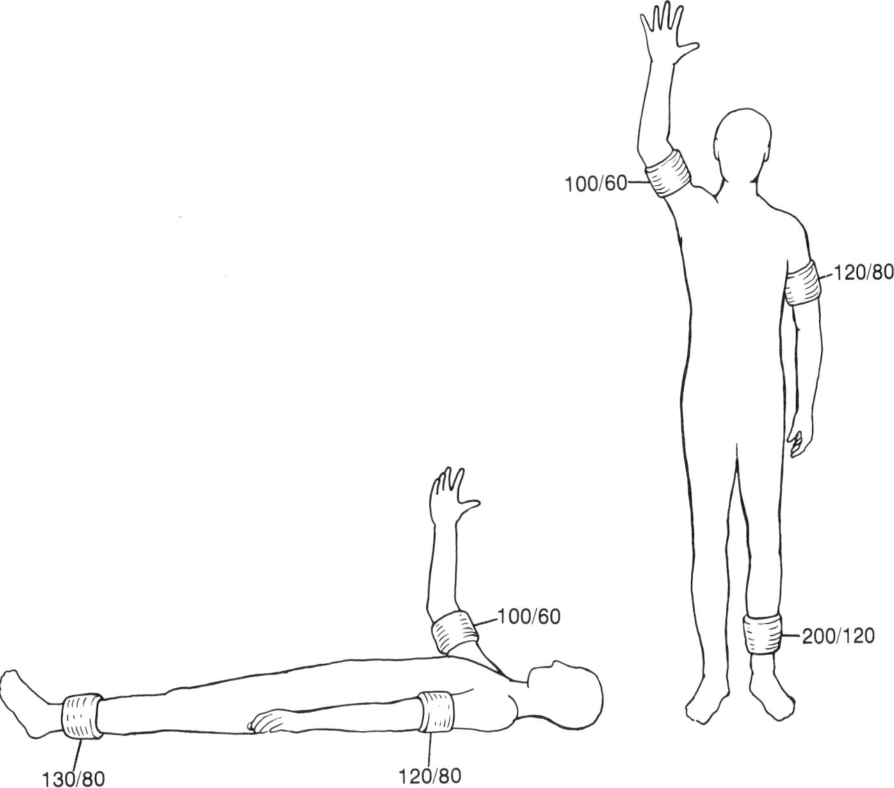

Figure 4-3. Position influences blood pressure. Values are in torr for systolic and diastolic arterial pressure.

mately 60 torr mean pressure. If we record blood pressure at heart level, in other words, roughly 20 cm or 30 cm below the brain of a sitting patient (Fig. 4-4), these 20 cm or 30 cm must be taken into account when the cerebral arterial pressure is computed. Assume we measure 90/60 torr at heart level and a mean pressure of 70 torr. In the brain, the arterial pressure would be about 20 torr lower (assuming a vertical difference of 28 cm between heart and brain). The mean arterial pressure in the head, then, would be approximately 50 torr, lower than acceptable for many patients. Use Table 4-2 to convert millimeters of water (mm H_2O) into torr to estimate this difference. Ignoring the difference between the relative densities of water and blood, 28 cm of H_2O (or blood) equals 21 torr. To measure blood pressures invasively under these circumstances, the pressure transducer is prudently kept at the level of the brain so that no calculations are needed to arrive at a reasonable estimate of blood pressure in the brain.

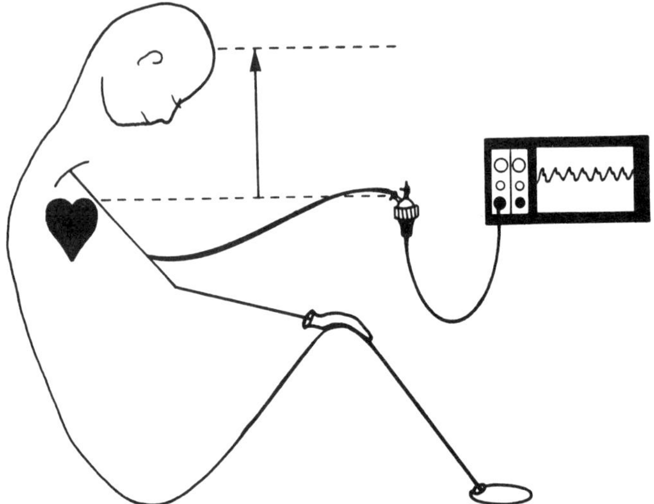

Figure 4-4. The relationship of the transducer to the pressure that is to be measured. When measuring pressure at the level of the heart, the transducer is placed at the level of the heart. In patients in the sitting position, monitoring of the mean arterial pressure in the head is frequently necessary. It is lower than the mean arterial pressure near the heart. Placing the transducer at the level of the head and adjusting its zero level in that position allows monitoring of arterial pressure in the head. It makes little difference which artery is cannulated for arterial pressure monitoring.

Age

Newborn babies may have systolic pressures of 60 torr, premature newborns even lower. Systolic pressures in children are often around 90 torr, but many adults live normal lives with resting pressures in that range. With advancing arteriosclerosis, often parallel to age, systolic pressures rise. Elderly patients with normal vessels may have systolic blood pressures around 120 torr.

NONINVASIVE VERSUS INVASIVE MONITORING OF BLOOD PRESSURE

Arterial blood pressure can be measured noninvasively or invasively. Invasive monitoring methods are significantly more expensive than noninvasive ones. Table 4-3 gives a breakdown of the factors that determine this cost. Some factors may differ from one hospital to another, but invasive monitoring will cost about ten times as much as noninvasive monitoring, whenever the two are compared.

Although the expenses for blood pressure monitoring may pale when

Table 4-3. COST ESTIMATES OF INVASIVE VERSUS NONINVASIVE ARTERIAL PRESSURE MONITORING

	Invasive	Noninvasive
Cost of pressure module (invasive) or oscillometric blood pressure monitor	$4000.00	$2000.00
Maintenance (10% of cost)	$400.00	$200.00
Life expectancy	7 years	7 years
Number of times used per day	1	3
Number of days used per year	200	200
Cost per case	$3.14	$0.52
Cost of cuffs or transducers, catheters, tubing, fluid, tape per case	$26.00	$0.50
Time to apply	10 min	1 min
Cost of personnel per case	$10.00	$1.00
Cost for operating room time	$10.00	$1.00
Total cost per case	$49.14	$3.02

seen in the context of the entire cost of an operation, they are not trivial. Several functions of invasive arterial monitoring can be assumed to a certain degree by noninvasive methods, which Table 4-4 summarizes. In the following discussion of blood pressure measurements, we will first examine noninvasive methods—both old and new—and then invasive ones.

Noninvasive Monitoring

Discontinuous Methods

All methods that call for the inflation and deflation of a cuff and the detection of the systolic pressure several beats before the diastolic pressure can be sensed suffer from an inherent weakness because the natural variability of blood pressure will affect precision. On the one hand, we may—by chance—catch a fleetingly high systolic reading, a reading that happens to stand out and does not represent the average systolic blood pressure of the patient. On the other hand, we may get a distorted pulse pressure, the difference between systolic and diastolic blood pressure, if we take readings as the blood pressure is changing. The distortion occurs when systolic and diastolic pressures cannot be determined for the same heartbeat. If the blood pressure varies, as it often does spontaneously or with artificial ventilation, we may catch a low (or high) systolic pressure and, by the time the diastolic pressure is determined a few beats later, both systolic and diastolic pressure may have risen (or fallen) by 10 torr or 20 torr (Fig. 4-5).

Table 4-4. ARTERIAL BLOOD PRESSURE AND GAS MONITORING

	Method		
Indication for Monitoring	**Arterial Catheter**	**Alternative**	**Remarks**
Rapid changes in blood pressure	Beat–beat intra-arterial pressure tracing	Penaz method (see below)	Penaz method may fail in patients with poor peripheral circulation and in infants and children
*p*H shift	Arterial blood gas analysis	Venous blood gas analysis (Chap. 6)	Venous blood gas can give data on metabolic acid–base derangements
P_{CO_2} shift	Arterial blood gas analysis	End-expired CO_2 (see Chap. 6) or cutaneous CO_2 (see Chap. 6)	Respiratory CO_2 monitoring gives breath-to-breath data, but will not show an alveolar–arterial gradient
P_{O_2} shift	Arterial blood gas analysis	Pulse oximetry (see Chap. 6) or cutaneous P_{O_2} (see Chap. 6)	Pulse oximetry gives beat-to-beat data on O_2 saturation; fails with poor circulation and gives no information on $P_{aO_2} > 100$ mm Hg. Cutaneous P_{O_2} can give data on high P_{O_2} but not beat-to-beat, and fails with poor circulation

With these methods, continuous readings are not obtainable; instead, measurements spaced two or more minutes apart must be used. When drugs are administered that act rapidly—in less than a minute—discontinuous measurements become inadequate and continuous noninvasive or invasive recordings are necessary. In general, we need to monitor at twice the rate at which the phenomenon requiring observation occurs. If blood pressure changes significantly over 4 minutes, measurements

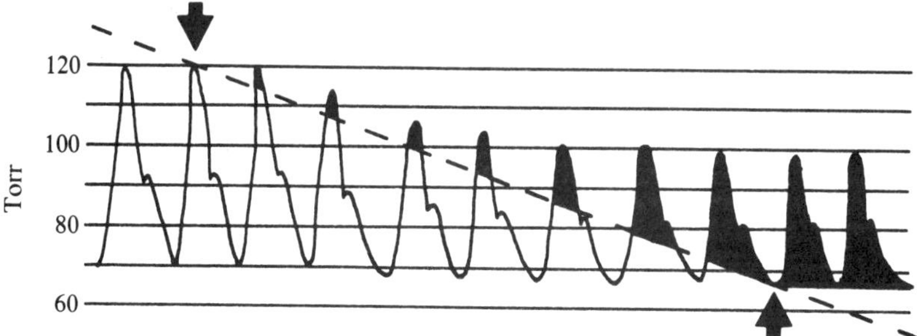

Figure 4-5. With noninvasive methods, systolic arterial pressure is determined for one beat and diastolic arterial pressure for a later beat. The pulse pressure may, therefore, be distorted if the arterial pressure changes as, for instance, with ventilation. A high systolic and low diastolic arterial pressure are shown and consequently an exaggerated pulse pressure. If systolic pressure were measured during the low phase of pressure, then a falsely narrow pulse pressure might be recorded.

should be made every 2 minutes. For most clinical situations, the above standard is a reasonable and readily attainable goal. Of course, with a cardiac arrest or sudden massive hemorrhage, the rate of change is much faster.

The oldest and most frequently used noninvasive method calls for the application of a cuff around the upper arm and a stethoscope above the brachial artery, just under the cuff. The cuff is inflated to above systolic pressure and gradually deflated, while the examiner listens for sounds, called *Korotkoff sounds,* in the artery. Several features of this method and its modifications must be observed.

CUFFS The cuff must be neither too wide nor too narrow for the extremity around which it is wrapped. If it is too wide, the pressures obtained are erroneously low. Conversely, a cuff that is too narrow causes spuriously high readings. Figure 4-6 shows that the inflation of the cuff causes a bell-shaped compression of the underlying tissue. If the cuff is too narrow, the bell is too small to compress the artery unless extra pressure is applied. Because the pressure of the cuff must squeeze the artery shut, extremely sclerotic arteries with calcified walls produce false readings. In patients with these hardened, diseased vessels, blood pressure measured by a cuff is higher than intraluminal blood pressure measured invasively. Often, it may not be obtainable by the cuff method at all.

The cuff should be 20% wider than the diameter of the limb on which it is used. On the average, it should be 12 cm to 14 cm wide for the upper arm of a normal adult. The cuff should be applied firmly, not loosely, to the arm; otherwise, recording tends to be falsely high.

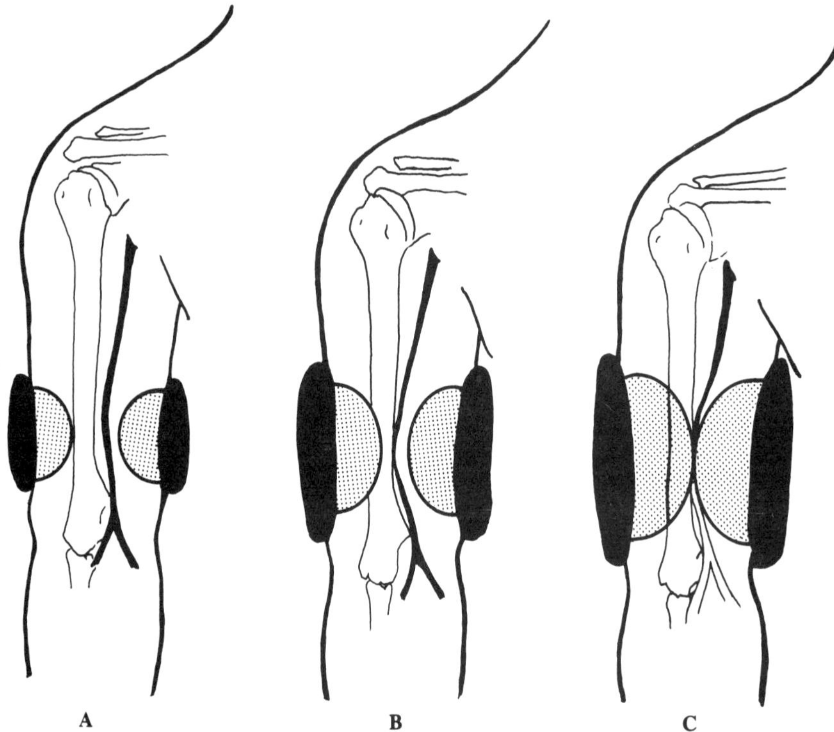

Figure 4-6. The width of the blood pressure cuff encircling the upper arm influences the pressure reading. Three cuffs, all inflated to the same pressure, are shown. The narrowest cuff (*A*) will require more pressure, and the widest cuff (*C*) less pressure to occlude the brachial artery for the determination of systolic pressure. Therefore, a large overestimation of systolic pressure can be the consequence of using a cuff that is too narrow. The wider cuff may give an underestimation of the systolic pressure, but the error with a cuff 20% too wide is not as great as with a cuff 20% too narrow.

If possible, do not apply the cuff to a limb that is used for an intravenous infusion. Measuring blood pressure not only interferes with transfusion therapy, but hematomas and swelling of the arm result in back pressure and may cause erroneous pressure readings.

Have assorted cuffs available, from tiny ones suitable for infants to gargantuan sizes for the obese and for instances when pressures must be measured at the thigh. Cuffs come in different forms and models. They should be easy to wash and have a convenient fastener, such as a self-fastening band.

The cuff houses a matching inflatable rubber bladder. Pediatric-sized bladders in adult-sized blood pressure cuffs will give grossly exaggerated blood pressures when used on an adult. Bladders that encircle the arm are preferred,[6,7] even though many clinicians will find a bladder acceptable if it is the proper width and encircles no less than half the limb.[8] The bladder must lie over the artery.

Cuffs may be applied to the upper arm, the lower arm, the thigh, or the calf. With an automatic oscillometric machine, accurate mean arterial pressures can be obtained with the cuff applied just above the ankle. When an ideally fitting cuff is not available, use the next wider, rather than narrower, cuff.

MANOMETERS The mercury manometer is the standard device. Because its mercury reservoir has a larger diameter than its graduated column, the manufacturer must calibrate the column to account for changing levels in the reservoir, the diameter of which may be ten times or more greater than that of the vertical tube. After pressure is applied and mercury is forced out of the reservoir into the column, the difference between the levels in the reservoir and in the column is determined. Maintenance of the mercury manometer requires that the reservoir is filled so that at zero pressure the mercury column rests at the zero mark. Certain precautions have to be taken. Make sure that the vent on top of the vertical tube is open so the mercury column can rise without compressing an air bubble, which would cause erroneous readings. The mercury manometer must stand vertically or, if it is slanted, the column has to be appropriately calibrated.

The aneroid manometer with a circular pressure gauge serves well in anesthesia. If properly maintained, the units are sufficiently accurate for clinical use. However, they should be checked regularly against a well-maintained mercury manometer. When checking an aneroid manometer, make measurements of the entire range of pressures to be sure the instrument is working linearly. A routine schedule, for instance every 4 months, to calibrate all aneroid manometers in a department of anesthesia is useful.

STETHOSCOPES A number of different types of stethoscopes are in use, most of them flat, so that they fit under the cuff. Usually, the stethoscope is applied distal to the cuff or slightly under the cuff to listen for Korotkoff sounds. A convenient stethoscope widely used in anesthesia has a wide plastic or rubber head that is molded to fit the curvature of the arm and is placed under the blood pressure cuff. Since this cup is so wide (Fig. 4-7), accurate placement of it is not as critical as with narrow-head stethoscopes that must be positioned exactly over the artery. The wide cup is placed entirely under the blood pressure cuff but must be under the distal third rather than under the center or upper half of the cuff, so that the Korotkoff sounds can be determined reliably.

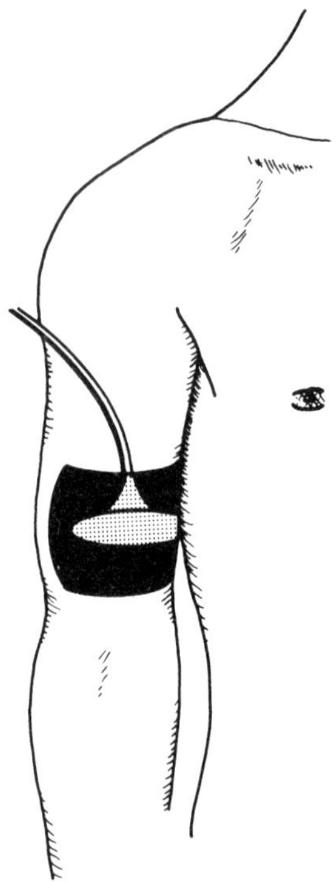

Figure 4-7. The wide, molded stethoscope that fits under the distal third of the blood pressure cuff is comfortable and easy to place.

THE MANUAL METHOD

Measuring blood pressure with a monaural stethoscope (Fig. 4-8) to detect Korotkoff sounds during anesthesia is much more difficult than in the ideal setting of the physician's office. Ordinarily, blood pressure is measured on the upper arm; the lower margin of a properly sized cuff should lie about 2.5 cm (1 inch) above the antecubital space. Do not inflate the cuff more than 20 torr or 30 torr above systolic pressure in conscious patients, and particularly in children. It hurts.

Deflate the cuff at a rate of 2 torr to 3 torr per heartbeat. Do not reinflate the cuff in the middle of a blood pressure recording to double-check a systolic or diastolic reading. This practice leads to systematic errors because, when a cuff is halfway inflated below systolic but well above venous pressures, blood sequesters in the arm, the arm swells, and the next recording will be erroneous.

Classically, five Korotkoff sounds are described in phases:

- Phase one occurs at the first sound, described as a "faint, clear tapping sound which gradually increases in intensity."

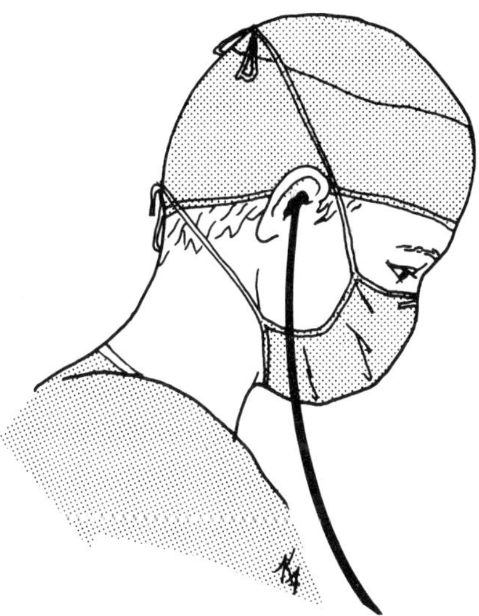

Figure 4-8. The monaural stethoscope is widely used in anesthesia. The earpiece can be fashioned out of dental acrylic material using a cast of the external part of the external ear canal. Even simpler, a piece of soft rubber tubing can serve as an earpiece. Wearing an earpiece regularly may lead to accumulation and inspissation of earwax, with loss of hearing until the wax is removed.

- Phase two is heralded by a swishing murmur.
- Phase three probably coincides with mean arterial pressure; the sounds are crisp and loud.
- Phase four is recognized when the sound is abruptly muffled and has a soft, blowing quality.
- Phase five marks the end of all sound.

An auscultatory gap (a Korotkoff sound *below* systolic pressure cannot be heard) sometimes separates phase one and phase two. This gap occurs particularly in some hypertensive patients and may range up to 40 torr. Missing the gap can lead to a serious underestimation of systolic pressure. Therefore, palpate the radial artery on the arm in which you measure the pressure and feel for a pulse before you hear a "systolic pressure." If you feel a pulse, systolic pressure lies higher and the patient has an auscultatory gap.

The American Heart Association recommends that the systolic (phase one) and *two* diastolic pressures be recorded, the first and second diastolic pressures corresponding to phases four and five. If the two levels are identical (phase four = phase five), we still are encouraged to note both. During anesthesia, this is not done. It is often difficult or impossible to hear anything but the beginning and end of blood pressure sounds (phases one and five), so this is all that is clinically recorded.

ELECTRONIC METHODS

Automated, noninvasive measurement of arterial blood pressure is possible with mechanical devices that inflate the cuff and record the pressure automatically. A number of different types are on the market. Some employ a microphone applied to the artery to detect Korotkoff sounds or subaudible sounds; some use Doppler crystals to detect arterial wall motion or blood flow. Others let the oscillations in the cuff be transmitted through the tubing to the transducers housed in the unit and then calculate systolic and diastolic, as well as mean, blood pressures. All units are sensitive to interference, such as a surgeon leaning on the cuff while blood pressure is being measured. Some have complex algorithms used to determine and reject noise artifacts; this feature is very important to anesthesiologists. Before purchasing a unit, apply the cuff to the arm of a volunteer and test the machine. See what happens to its accuracy when, during recording, the body is moved as it might be during an operation, the arm is bumped, or a bone or the cuff is tapped. The human brain is well equipped to recognize and reject erroneous noises, but, for electronic units, noise presents a major hurdle. The ability to reject noise is particularly important in units that have automatic alarms. If noise is rejected poorly, the units will give an alarm when they should not, and the alarm will then be disconnected by an annoyed clinician, defeating the very purpose of the alarm.

Most devices that measure blood pressure noninvasively and automatically allow a cycle of recording as often as every minute or as infrequently as every 30 minutes. Remember, however, that 2 torr or 3 torr per heartbeat is the recommended rate of cuff deflation; to go from 200 torr to 50 torr, therefore, requires approximately a minute. To measure blood pressure every minute hurts the conscious patient, and in the unconscious patient measuring pressure this often for too long will interfere with blood flow to the arm.

Ulnar nerve and radial palsy after anesthesia have been linked to the use of automatically inflated blood pressure cuffs.[9,10] When placing the cuff proximal on the upper arm, the cuff should be situated so that the tubing supplying the cuff cannot press on a nerve. This can be accomplished by letting the tubing emerge from the proximal end of the cuff, as is customary in anesthesia. Switching the machine on while the patient is still awake allows the patient to report paresthesias should they develop during inflation of the blood pressure cuff and, thus, provides an opportunity to find a comfortable, safe position for it. (Patients with little muscle mass are at greater risk of pressure damage.) This will also generate useful baseline data for blood pressure and heart rate before induction of anesthesia.

A faster rate of deflation decreases the accuracy of the method. Assuming that true systolic pressure is 99 torr and that the cuff is deflated from 100 torr to 90 torr between two beats, the systolic pressure will be read as 90 torr, 10% lower than true. Particularly during anesthesia, when hypotension is feared, there is a tendency to use bleed rates of blood pressure cuffs that are far too fast. Bleed rates can be continuous or stepwise-linked to heart rate. In either case, fast bleed rates (or large steps) cause inaccuracy.

The oscillometric and automatic devices operate on similar principles, which must be understood to recognize the limitations of the units. Improper operation increases errors; therefore, the manufacturer's recommendations should be followed religiously. These vary somewhat from company to company. Guidelines common to all equipment follow:

1. Use a cuff of proper size.
2. Squeeze the air out of the cuff before applying it.
3. Wrap the cuff snugly around the arm. For very obese patients with cone-shaped upper arms, using the forearm or the calf just above the ankle is sometimes preferable.
4. Avoid moving the limb being used. Most units have algorithms designed to reject artifacts produced, for instance, by moving the patient's arm or by tapping the cuff or its tubing. However, these algorithms prolong measurement or, with some instruments, prevent the deflation of the cuff, so it becomes inflated again before the diastolic pressure is reached. This is not desirable.
5. Most units have alarms. They serve an important function. Do not deactivate them; set them at reasonable limits. If something goes wrong and circumstances show that the alarm was disconnected, unpleasant questions are bound to be raised.
6. Even a smart machine needs calibration. Set rigid schedules (by service contract with vendor or by using in-hospital personnel) to have units checked and calibrated, and keep a log of such service.

MICROPHONES Korotkoff sounds can be detected with an electronic stethoscope applied to the artery. The sounds are amplified and can be converted electronically into automatic readings of systolic and diastolic blood pressures. These units function satisfactorily within normal ranges of blood pressure but have the same limitations as the auscultation of Korotkoff sounds. An auscultatory gap may be missed, or the unit may fail to work in severely hypotensive patients or those with significant vasoconstriction. Noise artifacts pose another problem with electronic stethoscopes.

Automated blood pressure devices have provisions for preventing overinflation. When first applied, they generally stop inflation at 160 torr or less. When the device discovers that this pressure falls below the systolic pressure of the patient, the machine automatically reinflates the cuff to a higher value. All devices stop inflation at a maximal level that varies with the brand of the unit, but it always is well above 200 torr. In pediatric units, the level to which the cuff is inflated on first application usually lies lower (often at around 125 torr) than is true for units intended for adults, and the upper limit for inflation is also lower, although it may still be above 200 torr.

The speed of deflation also varies somewhat from manufacturer to manufacturer. Some adjust the rate as a function of pressure and switch to a slower rate of deflation at lower pressures.

When the automated devices give data that are inconsistent with the clinical picture, it is important to remember that machines can fail. The electronics may malfunction, or some foreign material (e.g., rubber from the tubing), may obstruct the conduits.[11]

DOPPLER DEVICES Upon deflation of the cuff, the return of blood flow can be detected with a Doppler device (see Chap. 11). This is an electronic unit that detects either movement of the artery or blood flow through it. If the probe is applied as shown in Fig. 4-9, it will be more responsive to the flow of blood. By turning the probe through 90°, it becomes more sensitive to the motion of the arterial wall. Doppler probes can be applied to any artery and tuned so that every pulse is audible (Fig. 4-9). If a proximal blood pressure cuff is inflated to above systolic pressure, sound disappears. As the cuff is slowly deflated, systolic pressure is identified when sound resumes. Diastolic pressures are not easily identified.

One unit, the Arteriosond,* has an automatic device based on the Doppler principle. It senses wall motion of the artery and gives an audible signal with each heartbeat, starting with systolic pressure and ending with diastolic. A digital read-out is also provided. An array of Doppler crystals has to be placed over the brachial artery. It is necessary with this instrumentation, as with all other Doppler devices, to apply a special contact jelly or a soapy solution to the electrode to eliminate an air interface. Do not use electrolyte paste; it damages the probe. The Arteriosond works well but is sensitive to motion artifact.

PLETHYSMOGRAPHY Other devices use a plethysmograph applied to the finger. The plethysmograph employs a light and a photoelectric cell to detect changes in the volume of the finger (Fig. 4-10). In older models

* Roche Medical Electronics, Inc., Cranbury, New Jersey (a division of Hoffman-LaRoche)

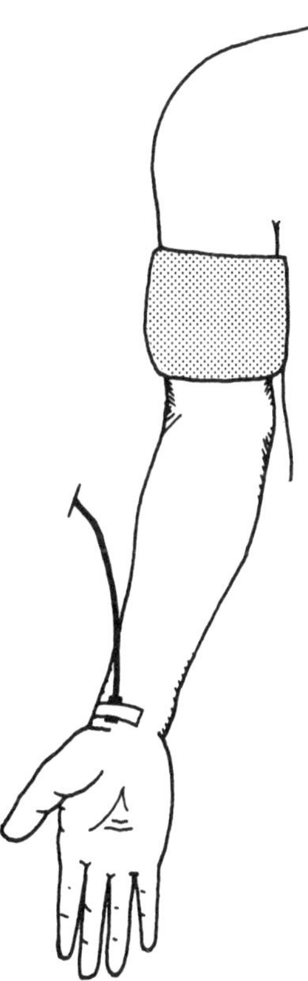

Figure 4-9. A Doppler probe is attached to the radial artery. It gives a signal with every heartbeat until a cuff around the arm exceeds systolic pressure.

(prior to 1976), burns from the heat of the incandescent light have been reported in cases when perfusion of the finger was reduced secondary to shock or hypotension and the light produced relatively excessive heat. In newer units the problems of excessive heat have disappeared. Some models are applied to the finger with a spring-loaded clip. Make certain that they are not too tight, causing ischemia of the finger.

OSCILLOMETRY In busy clinical practice, Korotkoff sounds are sometimes difficult or impossible to hear. Clinicians then look for oscillations of the aneroid manometer. Because the pulse impinges on the inflated cuff proximal to the occluded artery, these oscillations begin as the cuff is deflated well before systolic pressure is reached. A marked increase in the amplitude of the oscillations identifies the point when the blood first begins to flow through the artery under the still-inflated cuff, which is the point of systolic blood pressure. The amplitude of the oscillations

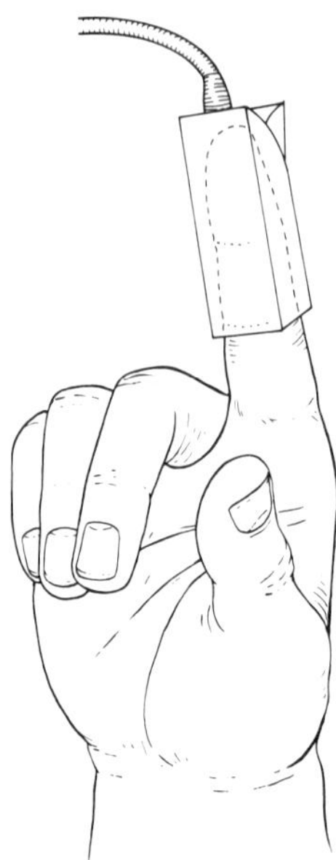

Figure 4-10. A finger plethysmograph gives a signal with every heartbeat. The pulsatile signal stops when the cuff around the arm exceeds systolic pressure.

continues to increase and reaches a peak that coincides with the mean blood pressure. Then the oscillations decrease and finally disappear well below diastolic pressure. Thus, the amplitude of the oscillation changes as the pressure passes from systolic to diastolic values. When a mechanical–electronic device is used to determine blood pressure by oscillometry, the machine must be programmed with an algorithm (a prescription or rule) that allows the unit to recognize these changes in amplitude.

The oscillometric–automatic technique determines systolic and diastolic pressures in a roundabout way, yet the results are satisfactory and the accuracy of the method is probably ±10% or better.

In clinical practice, the oscillometric technique, when performed by hand and eye, is unreliable. Unfortunately, the technique is frequently used for patients with low blood pressure when other noninvasive and nonautomatic methods fail. The clinician bleeds the cuff and watches for the first jiggle of the manometer needle, which he accepts as systolic pressure, though the true systolic pressure tends to be much lower (Fig. 4-11).

SUBAUDIBLE SOUND The arterial wall begins to oscillate briefly with each heartbeat as a blood pressure cuff is deflated below systolic pressure. These oscillations cease with, or a little below, diastolic pressure. The

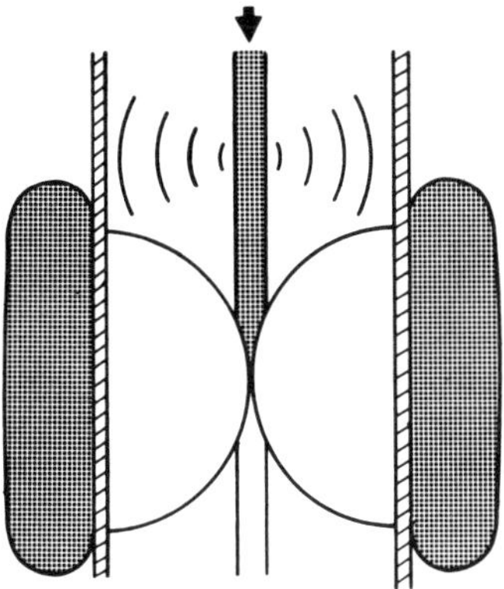

Figure 4-11. A cuff around the arm is inflated above systolic pressure to occlude the artery. The pulsations of the artery proximal to the cuff are transmitted to the cuff and cause an oscillation of the pressure gauge, easily detected on an aneroid manometer. Thus, a pulsating needle on the pressure gauge in the absence of Korotkoff sounds or other evidence of flow distal to the cuff does *not* represent systolic blood pressure.

oscillations can be detected by suitable amplification and rendered audible. Using these subaudible sound waves, the Infrasonde* unit determines systolic and diastolic blood pressures noninvasively. The unit requires manual inflation of the cuff and produces a sound reminiscent of the Korotkoff sound. Pressures are read on an aneroid manometer, just as is done with the cuff and stethoscope method.

Figure 4-12 shows a summary of these noninvasive methods. Channel 1 represents the pressure in the blood pressure cuff which was inflated to over 150 torr and deflated at a rate of about 4 torr per heartbeat. Channel 2 shows the Korotkoff sounds resulting in a blood pressure reading of 117/78. Channel 3 charts the Arteriosonde with Doppler returns. Channel 4 shows the Infrasonde using subaudible sound frequencies and channel 5 details one of the oscillometric machines. Channel 5 clearly shows that oscillations in a properly applied cuff appear well before systolic pressure is reached and persist after diastolic pressure. The algorithm in the machine, however, recognizes the changes in amplitudes that occur when systolic and diastolic pressures exist. Only the oscillometric system can estimate a mean arterial pressure by identifying the peak amplitudes at the lowest cuff pressure. Channel 6 shows that the "return of flow" method, that is, the appearance of a pulse in the finger, can give only systolic pressures, which are often lower than systolic pressures under the cuff.

* Infrasonde, Sphygmetrics, Inc., Woodland Hills, California.

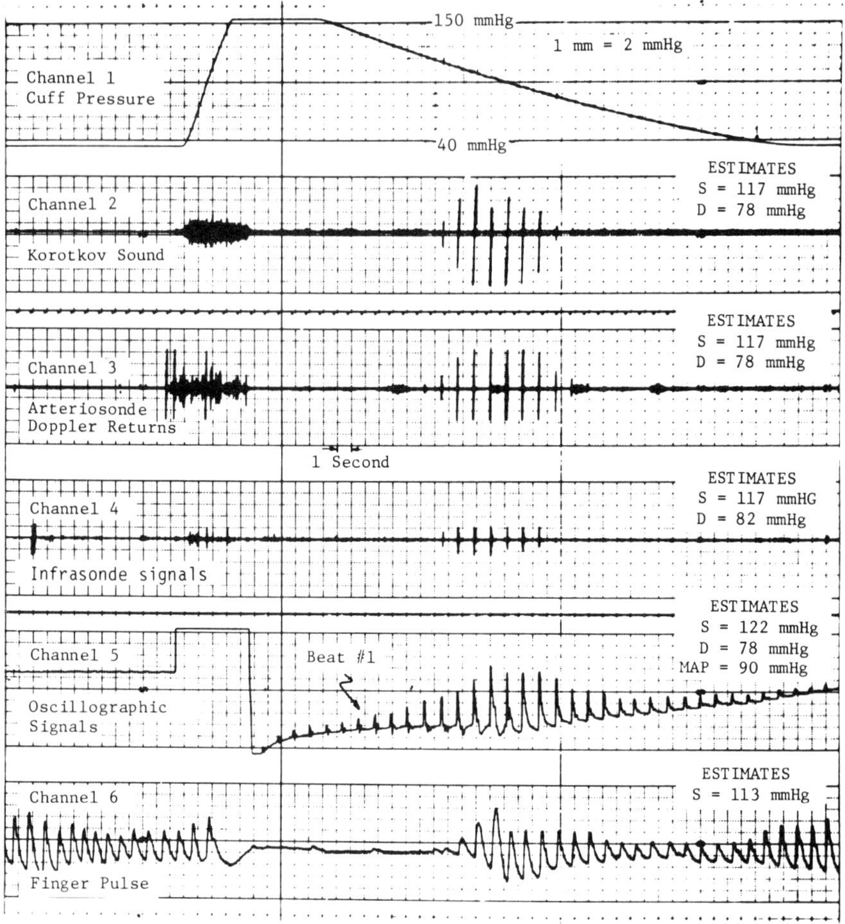

Figure 4-12. Simultaneous recording of blood pressures using different noninvasive methods. *Channel 1* shows initial high pressure in the cuff around the arm and then deflation at a rate of about 4 torr per heartbeat. *Channel 2* traces the appearance of Korotkoff sounds and a blood pressure reading of 117/80 torr. *Channel 3* marks the returns by a Doppler probe from the Arteriosonde. *Channel 4* traces the subaudible sound frequencies detected by the Infrasonde, and *Channel 5* marks the recordings provided by one of the automatic oscillometric machines (in this instance, the Dinamap machine). *Channel 6* shows the signal provided by a finger plethysmograph. (Gravenstein JS, Newbower RS, Ream AK, et al [eds]: Essential Noninvasive Monitoring in Anesthesia. New York, Grune & Stratton, 1980. With permission of Apple Howard, Ph.D.)

FLUSH METHOD

In the past, systolic pressure of infants was often recorded by blanching the arm, then inflating a cuff around the arm, and releasing the pressure slowly until the area distal to the cuff became flushed, indicating return of circulation. This method is neither accurate nor precise.[12] With Doppler probes, oscillometric devices,[13] or infrasound, blood pressures can be determined, even in small infants, much better than with the flush method.

The Penaz (Continuous) Method

The "newest kid on the block" concerning blood pressure monitoring offers what few people thought possible, namely a noninvasive method that reports systolic, mean, and diastolic blood pressures with every heartbeat. The method, first realized by the Czechoslovakian physiologist Penaz,[14] is based on the following, elegant approach.

With every heartbeat the volume of the digital arteries—and with them the volume of the finger—increases a little during systole and falls during diastolic runoff. This well-known phenomenon has been observed by thousands of anesthesiologists who have applied a plethysmograph to a finger of one of their patients. Indeed, the plethysmogram looks like a blood pressure tracing obtained invasively, and it shows systole, the dicrotic notch, and diastole. Penaz wrapped a small blood pressure cuff around the finger and applied just enough external pressure to equal the pressure inside the artery. Thus, cuff pressure equals intra-arterial pressure.

This is the principle. The trick, however, is to find a way to determine at which point internal and external pressures match. This can be done by keeping the pressure at such a level that the vessel wall is unloaded, that is, the vessel's volume will not change during a cardiac cycle because internal and external pressures are kept equal, and thus transmural pressure is kept at zero.

Now for the technical approach. The plethysmogram is monitored with the help of a light source and a photo-cell incorporated in a little blood pressure cuff wrapped around the finger. The point at which the arterial wall is unloaded is estimated by determining several pressure–volume relationships during a cardiac cycle and setting an operating point that may lie close to mean arterial pressure. A small computer now tracks the plethysmographically-determined volume and attempts to keep this volume constant by letting more or less pressure flow into the finger cuff: a brilliant solution to a dream thought impossible for many decades!

The finger, of course, has to be maintained under a pressure equal to mean arterial pressure as long as the device is operated. This is surprisingly well tolerated, even though the fingertip distal to the cuff tends to turn a little dusky as venous return is impeded.[15] The device has been kept on a single finger of patients for up to 7 hours without harm, and has even been used successfully during cardiopulmonary bypass.[16] Of course, it will fail when vasoconstriction in the digital arteries prevents pulsations, at which point it is time to seek blood pressure information by other means. It must be remembered, however, that even radial pressures obtained through an indwelling catheter may give data that do not reflect aortic pressures, for instance, after cardiopulmonary bypass in children.[17]

The mean arterial pressure in a finger must be a little lower than that in the arm, which must be lower than that in the aorta, otherwise blood could not flow from the heart to the periphery. Pressures in the thumb may mirror radial arterial pressure more closely than do pressures in the fingers. When peripheral vessels constrict, for instance, after cardiopulmonary bypass, and particularly in children with active vascular responsiveness, the peripheral readings may show significantly lower values than would be found in the aorta. But these phenomena would also hold true in a comparison of pressures in radial-to-femoral arteries.[17]

The Penaz method is now commercially available.* The cuff, which is the principle of operation, and the monitor are shown in Figures 4-13 and 4-14.

Invasive Monitoring

Invasive arterial monitoring is now well established because it provides not only continuous measurement of blood pressure but also ready access for the analysis of arterial blood gases.

Is It Safe to Cannulate the Artery?

The most commonly cannulated artery is the radial artery, and a commonly performed test to establish the presence of collateral circulation through the ulnar vessel is Allen's test.[18] It requires the active participation of the patient, in which he must clench his fist tightly to blanch the skin of his hand, and during which the wrist must not be flexed or extended, which would stretch the arteries. Both the radial and ulnar arteries are then occluded by the fingers of the clinician. (The radial artery is best occluded not at the radial styloid process, but more proximally, where the tip of the catheter is expected to lie.) The patient opens his hand, then the ulnar, but not the radial, artery is opened by releasing the pressure. If the volar arch in the palm of the hand forms an anastomosis between the radial and ulnar arteries, as is usual, the hand turns pink in

* The Finapress, Ohmeda, Inc., Madison, Wisconsin.

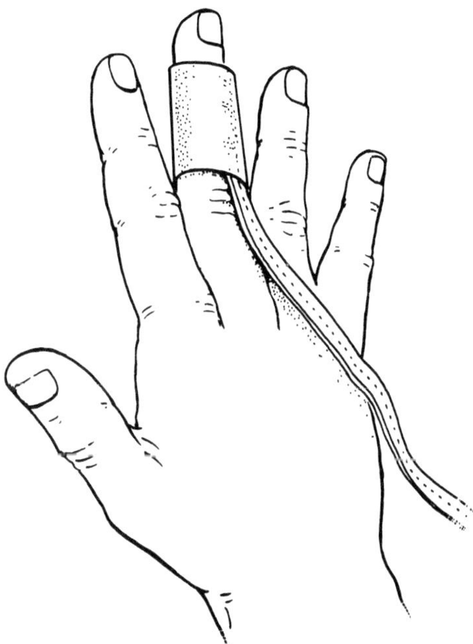

Figure 4-13. The Penaz continuous and noninvasive blood pressure method. A small inflatable cuff is wrapped around the finger. Incorporated in the cuff are a light source and a sensor to monitor the plethysmogram.

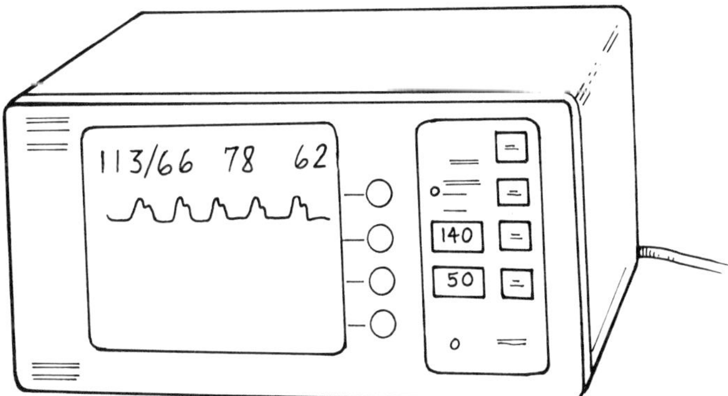

Figure 4-14. The Penaz monitor. Under the tradename Finapress, Ohmeda (Madison, Wisconsin) manufactures a blood pressure monitor based on the Penaz principle. It offers continuous but noninvasively obtained systolic, diastolic, and mean arterial pressure measured in a finger. Heart rate is also reported and alarms can be set.

5 seconds. If an adequate anastomosis doesn't exist, only the area of the hand supplied by the relieved artery turns pink; the other part of the hand remains blanched for 10 seconds or longer.

In the unconscious or uncooperative patient, occlude the artery with two fingers, one proximal and one more distal on the radial artery. Then ease the distal finger, but not the proximal one, and feel for a pulse distal, but close, to the radial occlusion. A pulse indicates a patent volar arch. Alternatively, the Doppler probe, a finger plethysmograph or pulse oximeter transducer can be applied to the index finger to test the adequacy of distal flow during the occlusion of the radial artery. The Doppler probe sometimes helps to locate vessels and monitor flow in obese patients whose vessels may be difficult to palpate.

One may also apply the Doppler probe to the princeps pollicis artery, which arises from the radial artery. Occlusion of the radial artery will lead to a disappearance of the Doppler signal from the artery if collateral circulation from the ulnar artery is absent.[19]

Anesthesiologists assumed, not unreasonably, that a patient with evidence of inadequate collateral circulation (as judged, for instance, by an unfavorable Allen's test) would be at risk of suffering circulatory complications in the fingers and hand should the cannulation of the ulnar or radial artery lead to the prolonged occlusion of the vessel and ischemia to tissue distal to the occlusion. The value of Allen's test was questioned by Slogoff and co-workers, who reported in 1983 on their experience with 1699 patients who required cannulation of the radial artery for monitoring.[20] With a Doppler probe they measured the flow in the vessels the first day, and again 7 days later, after removal of the cannulae. The authors stated:

> Although partial or complete radial artery occlusion after decannulation occurred in more than 25% of the patients, no ischemic damage to the hand or disability occurred in any of the patients. Neither duration of cannulation nor the size or material of the cannulae were determinants of abnormal flow. Abnormal flow was significantly related to female sex, the presence of hematoma, and the use of extracorporeal circulation. The radial arteries of 16 patients whose Allen's test results showed abnormalities were again cannulated and neither abnormal flow nor ischemia followed. In 22 patients, the ulnar artery was cannulated after multiple punctures of the ipsilateral radial artery and ischemia did not follow. We conclude that in the absence of peripheral vascular disease, the Allen's test is not a predictor of ischemia of the hand during or after radial artery cannulation; that when decreased or absent radial artery flow follows cannulation it is of no consequence; and that radial artery cannulation is a low-risk, high-benefit monitoring technique that deserves wide clinical use.[20]

This study by Slogoff and his colleagues, which originated at a highly respected medical center in Texas, challenges a number of clinical caveats. These are:

1. Do not leave the catheter in place for more than 20 hours.[21]
2. Do not use large-bore catheters in slender vessels.[22]
3. Do not use polypropylene catheters.[23]
4. Do not use tapered catheters.[24]
5. Prevent multiple punctures of an artery which would militate against cannulating the ulnar vessel in the hand if cannulation of the radial (or vice versa) artery had failed after multiple attempts.[25]

The study by Slogoff and co-workers[20] reconfirms the frequency of thrombosis (about 25%) after cannulation of a peripheral artery and the fact that most of the thrombi will recanalize spontaneously. Occlusion of the artery with a thrombus may occur during the monitoring session[18] or, and this is perhaps more common, hours after decannulation.

We still apply Allen's test and feel reassured when it indicates a good collateral circulation (even though rare ischemic problems have arisen in patients with a favorable Allen's test, as for instance reported by Ghandi and Reynolds[19]). An unfavorable test will predispose us toward being stricter with our indications for invasive monitoring. We accept the study by Slogoff and co-workers[20] as reassuring to the patient who requires arterial cannulation, but we advise against the abandonment of other clinical practices that are time-honored and reasonable. It is not necessary to puncture the artery of a patient with a large catheter if a smaller one will do; if multiple attempts at cannulating a vessel in one hand have failed, it is better to switch to the other hand than risk damaging the only remaining good vessel in the one hand. The excellent results from the above-mentioned study notwithstanding, serious complications do occur, and patients have suffered the loss of fingers or required operative intervention to re-establish blood flow that was interrupted by thrombosis, intimal damage, or external (by hematoma) compression of a cannulated artery. Fortunately, these complications are rare (perhaps less than 1 in 1500, if we extrapolate from the data from the Texas study).

It must be remembered that other than local conditions can result in ischemia to the hand. Therefore, it is prudent to check the brachial and axillary arteries before attributing ischemia of the hand to cannulation of the radial or ulnar vessels.[26]

Spaccavento and Hawley[27] have reviewed the epidemiology of infections secondary to the prolonged cannulation of arteries. They write that *only* (our italics) 10% of reported nosocomial infections were related to invasive arterial monitoring, and that the mortality of such infections ranges from 20% to 40%. The sources of infection were transducer domes and catheters. This study contrasts to the report by Slogoff and his colleagues,[20] who described their relatively relaxed method of inserting cath-

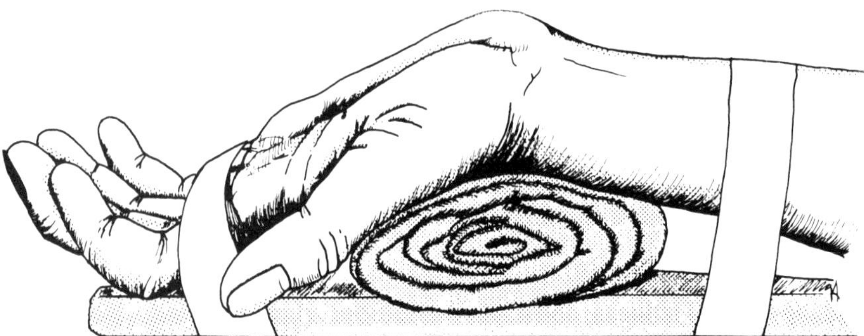

Figure 4-15. For cannulation of the radial artery, a towel is placed under the wrist and the hyperextended hand is fixed to a small arm board. After cannulation of the artery, hyperextension is no longer needed and the hand should be fixed in a more comfortable position. Only with steel needles (*e.g.*, the Cournand needle) is it necessary to maintain the wrist in the hyperextended position.

eters (not employing a rigorous surgical technique) and the subsequent absence of infections (their patients received broad-spectrum antibiotics preoperatively). Finally, we must mention that sometimes the effort to prevent infection can cause harm. Thus, for newborns the Food and Drug Administration has warned against the intravascular use of flush solutions containing preservatives.[28] Several fatalities in premature infants have been attributed to benzyl alcohol (0.9%) in flush solutions.

Selection of Artery for Cannulation

Some anesthesiologists cannulate the brachial (or occasionally the axillary) rather than the radial or ulnar artery, or a femoral artery rather than the dorsalis pedis or anterior peroneal artery. Others insert, into the radial artery (percutaneously), long (100-cm) catheters that are advanced into the subclavian artery.[29]

The brachial artery is easily palpated. For cannulation, hyperextend the arm, palpate the artery proximal to the biceps tendon, and cannulate the vessel about 1 cm proximal to it. Higher up, the vessel lies in soft tissue and is more difficult to catch with a needle.

For cannulation of the radial or ulnar artery (whichever is more prominent), the wrist is hyperextended by putting a support, for example, a rolled towel, under the wrist and then strapping the hand to a small board (Fig. 4-15). Overextending the wrist may compress the arteries, making cannulation more difficult.

Pyles and co-workers[30] describe the cannulation of the dorsal radial artery, which is an extension of the radial artery. After having given off its palmar branch to the volar arch, it emerges in the snuff box on the dorsum of the hand between the bases of the first and second metacarpals. Here the vessel lies quite superficially under the skin and is readily palpated. The fact that the dorsal radial artery is distal to the anastomosis in the palm may be thought to be advantageous, because occlusion of the vessel will not jeopardize the supply of radial blood to the fingers fed by the digital arteries arising from the superficial palmar arch. In the case of thrombosis of the dorsal radial artery, however, the backup of the blood supply through the palmar arch is not available. The vessel is easily palpated, but cannulations fail more often than is true for the radial artery proper, perhaps because the dorsal branch is smaller and its course more tortuous. The arteries of the foot are easily identified by palpation. Plantar flexion of the foot and toes is helpful. Cannulation of the dorsalis pedis artery is performed wherever the artery is most prominent and superficial, usually in the mid-dorsum of the foot. Moorthy[31] has described the cannulation of the anterior peroneal artery, which in adults is a suitable alternative to the dorsalis pedis artery when manual compression of the dorsalis pedis artery indicates poor collateral circulation. In a few patients (perhaps 3%), compression of the anterior peroneal artery will cause the pulse in the dorsalis pedis artery to disappear. In that instance, the dorsalis pedis artery arises from the anterior peroneal artery and no advantage is realized by cannulating the anterior peroneal artery instead of the dorsalis pedis. In the majority of patients, however, occluding the anterior peroneal does not affect pulsation in the dorsalis pedis artery, which then can serve as a suitable alternative if an artery in the foot or leg has to be used for monitoring. The vessel is not always readily palpated and is not easy to cannulate. It lies on the anterior lateral aspect of the lower leg, a little medial to the upper border of the lateral malleolus.

Gordon and colleagues[32] have described their experiences with the cannulation of vessels other than the radial and ulnar arteries. They were successful in cannulating brachial, axillary, femoral, dorsalis pedis, and superficial temporal arteries. For the larger vessels (brachial and femoral) they used a guide wire (see the Seldinger technique, Chap. 5), and, for the others, direct percutaneous cannulation with catheters matched to the size of the vessels was utilized. At this time, we have no evidence that one route exposes the patient to greater danger than another.

Techniques of Cannulation

CLINICAL CONCERNS DURING CANNULATION

Persistent anesthesiologists who have tried repeatedly to accomplish a difficult cannulation of a vein or an artery—or, for that matter, a major nerve block or conduction anesthetic—have reduced many a patient to tears. How often have we heard the physician (or ourselves) say, "Just a little longer (stab, push) . . . we are almost done, just another moment (push, stick, stick)." These needles hurt. Skin and arteries are endowed with sensory nerves, and, to make matters worse, the circumstances under which these procedures are carried out generate anxiety all by themselves, without the additional pain of the cannulation. Therefore, it would be much pleasanter for the patient if all vessels could be cannulated during general anesthesia, but often that is not advisable or feasible because the patient needs to be monitored during induction, or treated in the intensive care unit. Several steps can be taken to diminish the pain and terror the patient experiences when someone tries to invade one of his major vessels with a needle and catheter:

1. Use local anesthesia liberally. We prefer 0.5% or 1% lidocaine without epinephrine.
2. Use a small needle (25-gauge or smaller) for the skin.
3. Do not inject intradermally as that is particularly painful; instead, inject subcutaneously, but close to the skin.
4. Wait long enough to give the anesthetic a chance to take effect. It helps to massage the local anesthetic to distribute the drug. That is also reassuring to the patient and it consumes the time necessary for the drug to work.
5. Premedicate the patient. Waller and co-workers,[33] for instance, studied patients with heart disease and recorded changes in vital signs during the cannulation of arteries and central veins. They found no change in these variables during the cannulation. Their patients, however, were taking propranolol preoperatively and were premedicated with 5 mg to 10 mg diazepam *per os*, and 0.1 mg/kg morphine sulfate and 0.3 mg to 0.4 mg scopolamine intramuscularly. Despite the administration of these drugs, 5 of the 20 patients required additional medication during the cannulation. For this the authors used intravenous morphine and diazepam, in the average a little over 4 mg of each drug. If the clinician must resort to heavy premedication, he must be wary of oversedating the patient. General anesthesia with proper attention to ventilation and circulation should be preferred to a patient overmedicated and unresponsive!

TECHNICAL TIPS

Once a vessel has been chosen for cannulation, the artery is palpated and its course determined by further palpation. If desired, the course of the artery may be marked with a pen on the skin. The area is then prepared with an iodine-containing (or equivalent) solution or with alcohol.

Next, we fill a plastic Teflon catheter that comes mounted over a steel

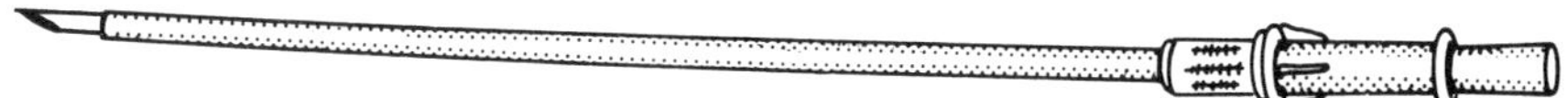

Figure 4-16. Catheters used for intra-arterial monitoring of blood pressure come mounted over steel needles. The needle is withdrawn after the catheter has been placed.

needle (Fig. 4-16) with heparinized saline. Other anesthesiologists prefer to connect the catheter–needle assembly to the pressure-recording device so that they can observe the appearance of a pressure waveform on the oscilloscope, which signals entry into the vessel and facilitates cannulation. Inserting the catheter, particularly a small one, through tough skin without the end of the catheter peeling away from the needle shaft is sometimes difficult (Fig. 4-17). This can be avoided by making a hole into the skin wheal with a large-bore needle (18-gauge to 16-gauge) and then inserting the catheter assembly through the prepared hole.

Morray and co-workers[34] have used a Doppler flow probe in infants to assist in the identification of the artery to be cannulated. With the Doppler flow probe,* they first locate the area of maximal flow slightly proximal to the intended site of cannulation. After inserting the arterial needle–catheter assembly through the skin, the assembly is advanced toward the Doppler probe. As the needle tip comes to lie under the probe and on top of the artery, the Doppler tones become high-pitched, or they disappear; then the needle is pushed into the vessel and the catheter advanced over it. This method can also be used in adults in whom the identification of the artery by palpation leaves uncertainties.

There are three techniques for inserting the catheter into the artery. One method is to spear the artery with the needle at almost a 90° angle. The needle and catheter are then withdrawn slowly until blood comes out of the needle, which indicates that its bevel lies in a vessel. At that point, the hub of the assembly is lowered and the catheter is pushed over the

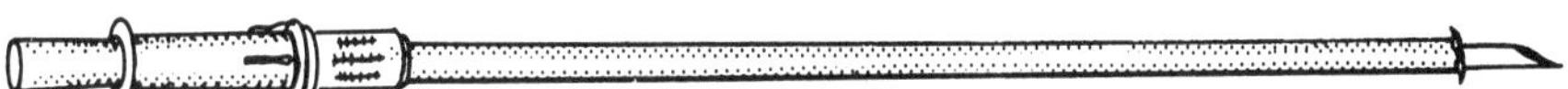

Figure 4-17. The tip of the catheter is tapered to facilitate insertion of needle and catheter through the skin and into a vessel. However, when the skin is tough, the tip of the catheter may peel away from the needle. If such a catheter were to be used for arterial monitoring, the artery would be damaged. To avoid this occurrence, make a hole in the skin with a large needle and then insert the arterial needle–catheter assembly through the prepared hole in the skin.

* Ultrasonic Doppler Flow Detector, Parks Electronics Laboratory, Beaverton, Oregon

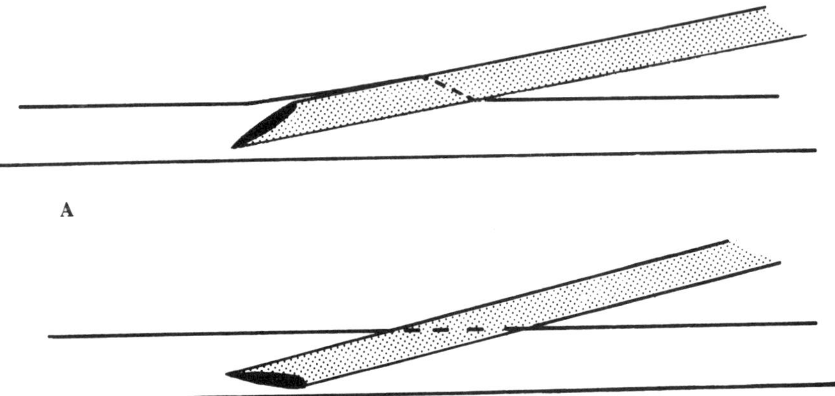

Figure 4-18. The insertion of a needle into an artery or a vein can be accomplished with a bevel-up (*A*) or a bevel-down (*B*) approach. Both have proponents and a little dogma to sustain them.

needle into the artery. This technique has been criticized because it leaves two holes in the artery, one unnecessarily. Also, the technique may lacerate the intima of a small vessel, because during withdrawal the hub of the needle is lowered as soon as blood flows through the needle, then the needle is advanced into the artery. At this moment, the cutting point of the needle may still be embedded in the arterial wall, particularly if the vessel is narrow; lowering the hub and advancing the needle will now cut the posterior wall of the vessel or its intima with or without arterial muscle. Damage of the arterial musculature may set the stage for the formation of an aneurysm.

The second and third methods of inserting the catheter into the artery are related and differ only in how the bevel of the needle is held relative to the artery. The techniques call for palpation of the artery with two fingers to ascertain the direction of the vessels. The catheter is then inserted through the needle hole in the skin until the distal, palpating finger feels, under the skin, the needle tip above the artery. At this point, the hub of the needle is raised slightly and the needle, with a small, sharp, advancing motion, is pushed into the lumen of the artery. The needle is then advanced a little further so that the tip of the catheter lies within the artery. The hub of the needle is then grasped and the catheter is pushed over the needle into the vessel, sometimes with a rotating motion. Using the second method, the bevel faces upward (Fig. 4-18A). The argument is that the artery can be more easily entered and the lumen of the artery can be lifted a bit to advance the needle tip and the catheter into the vessel.

With the third method, the needle is inserted with the bevel down (Fig. 4-18B). The argument is that the needle will be less likely to go right through the vessel and, therefore, cannulation is easier.

All three methods have skillful proponents. The individual clinician has to decide which method works best. We favor either the second or third method, because we believe that one hole in an artery is less likely to produce complications from hematoma or clot formation than two holes.

An alternative method employed by many cardiologists follows the recommendations made by Seldinger. Convenient, disposable sets with guide wires for the percutaneous cannulation of arteries are available from different manufacturers (see also Chap. 5).

HOW TO PREVENT THROMBOSIS

Because of the high incidence of thrombosis, we recommend continuous infusion with heparinized saline through all arterial catheters (Fig. 4-19). Not only does this reduce the chance of thrombosis, but the quality of the recording improves (no damping from partially blocked catheters). It takes only a few milliliters of saline and a vigorous flush to push a thrombus into the aorta; hence, the thrombus can embolize to vital organs.[34] When a thrombus forms, always aspirate and remove the thrombus before flushing the catheter with fresh saline. Systems available to flush the arterial tubing continuously (250 units to 500 units heparin in 250 ml saline; 1 ml to 3 ml per hour) do not significantly affect the accuracy of pressure recordings.[36]

While reducing the likelihood of clot formation, many of the infusion devices introduce new concerns. The unit shown in Figure 4-19 is typical. Its bag filled with heparinized saline is pressurized to 300 torr. A drip chamber in the tubing (often simple intravenous tubing) leading from the bag to the catheter transducer assembly allows the user to monitor the flow rate of heparinized saline. Distal to the valve constricting the flow to a few milliliters per hour, the pressure drops to that of the patient. Consequently, some of the air in the drip chamber under high pressure will go into the solution, only to come out of the solution again when the pressure drops in the tubing leading from the valve to the patient. The formation of tiny bubbles in this tubing after hours of use is a common occurrence. Another danger is related to an inappropriate use of the system, causing air to be infused into the arterial system of the patient. For this reason, many physicians insist on the inclusion of air filters in the tubing distal to the drip chamber; however, this will not prevent the formation of tiny bubbles secondary to the pressure difference in the infusion tubing in front of (300 torr), and behind (arterial), the rate-limiting valve.

Ideally, the heparinized saline can be infused with a motor-driven pump that could be regulated without requiring such high pressures or a

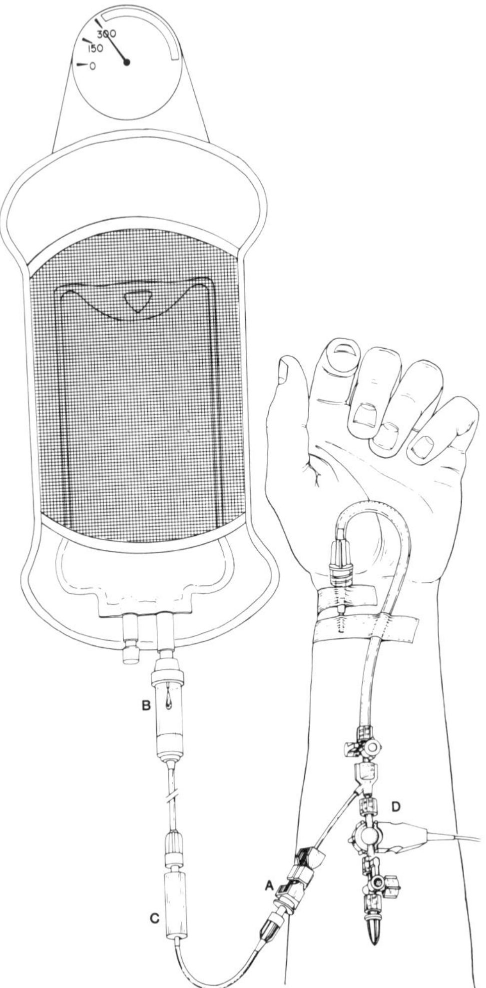

Figure 4-19. Commerically available systems allow the infusion of 1 ml to 3 ml/min of solution into an intra-arterial catheter. The solution, containing heparin (1–3 units/ml), is put under pressure well in excess of systolic blood pressure. The units also permit a rapid flushing (*A*) of the arterial catheter. When the flush option is used often, one does not know how much fluid has been infused into the artery. It is desirable to incorporate a drip chamber (*B*), which permits the detection of a faulty valve leading to excessive flows. Note the air filter (*C*) in the system. Shown here is a disposable pressure transducer (*D*).

drip chamber in which the rate of flow is monitored. In pediatric monitoring such infusion pumps are already in use. For umbilical arterial monitoring the infusion rates are often set at 30 ml/hr, not only keeping the system patent, but at the same time providing for the administration of maintenance, or replacement, fluids.

Small doses of heparin, given to reduce the postoperative incidence of deep vein thrombosis and pulmonary embolism, may also work to the advantage of cannulated arteries. Pretreatment with aspirin[36] has been claimed to reduce the incidence of arterial thrombosis from 39% to 13%. The patients were treated with 600 mg oral aspirin with supper the evening before arterial cannulation. We do not know whether this increases the surgeon's difficulties with hemostasis.

Invasive Monitoring in Infants

When radial catheterization is feasible, the technique and precautions are similar to those described above. Since smaller catheters have to be used, air bubbles are more of a problem. In small infants, a cutdown may be necessary. Smith[38] recommends a nontapered 22-gauge Teflon catheter and the continuous, slow infusion of heparinized Ringer's solution (rather than saline). We use 24-gauge catheters. Since small catheters thrombose more readily than large ones, and since in an infant it takes very little flushing solution to push a clot or an air bubble from the radial artery to the brain, prevention of clot formation and air bubbles is particularly important. Always try to aspirate clots; do not embolize them. When taking blood samples, let the arterial pressure fill the syringe. Vigorous aspiration of a tightly fitting catheter may damage tender intima by pulling it into the catheter hole.

In newborns, the umbilical artery is cannulated. This is a dangerous procedure because thrombosis of celiac, renal, or mesenteric arteries may result. Smith[38] estimates serious complications to occur in up to 2% of neonates so cannulated. Shnider and Levinson[39] recommend that a 3.5- or 5-French catheter be advanced into the umbilical artery so that the tip lies distal to the origin of the celiac, mesenteric, and renal arteries, just above or at the bifurcation of the aorta. This point may be reached by advancing the catheter no more than 2 cm ($\frac{3}{4}$ inch) beyond the point at which blood can first be aspirated.

Others recommend measuring the distance from umbilicus to shoulder and then, after consulting a chart, advancing the catheter more or less depending on the size of the infant.[40] Some advocate a cutdown when cannulation fails or the catheter perforates the vessel.[41]

Cole and Rolbin[42] suggest a technique for catheterization of the umbilical artery that first makes use of a 16-gauge, catheter-over-needle cannula that is introduced into the umbilical artery of the cord (which should be left 10 cm or longer during the delivery). The needle of this assembly should stay in the cord and not be advanced beyond the margin of the skin, to avoid perforating the tender vessels. The needle is then withdrawn; the cannula remains and serves as a conduit for the advancement of a 3.5-French umbilical artery catheter. Once the catheter is properly placed, the cannula is withdrawn. A heavy silk suture is tied around the cord proximal to the point of entry into the vessel to guard against bleeding and dislodging. We recommend cannulation as soon after birth as possible, because arterial spasm makes cannulation very difficult within 10 to 15 minutes of birth. Of course, the procedure requires sterile technique.

Whichever method is used, an x-ray examination is required to assure positioning of the catheter tip at the level of L4 in the aorta as the bifurcation usually lies at that level. To avoid exposure to x-rays and visualize the bifurcation directly, Houston and colleagues placed catheters with the help of ultrasonic imaging.[43]

When heparinized Ringer's solution is infused at 1 ml to 3 ml/hr, the amount of fluids and heparin—although insignificant for an adult—has to be taken into account. If the only solution administered intra-arterially to the infant comes from a continuous flushing solution, the amount of 1 ml to 3 ml/hr is insignificant. However, with intermittent, manual flushing, as is necessary after sampling arterial blood, significant overhydration may result. Keep track of the amount of blood taken and solution flushed into the artery. For adults, we use 500 units of heparin for 250 ml solution (*i.e.*, 2 units/ml). In newborns this can be reduced to 1 unit/ml, which would mean giving a newborn about 3 units of heparin per hour. The usual doses for anticoagulation of a patient's blood are about 300 units/kg body weight. Heparin has a half-life, depending on dosage, of 1 hour to 3 hours. A concentration desired for anticoagulation, such as during cardiopulmonary bypass, is approximately 2 units to 3 units per milliliter of blood. Thus, even in newborns, heparin should not lead to systemic complications. However, in infants of low birth weight, heparin and the preservative benzyl alcohol in heparin in the intravascular flush solution have been suspected of contributing to intraventricular hemorrhage. In patients at risk, the heparin can be omitted from the flush solution.[43a,43b]

Transducers

A wide variety of transducers are available, including small units that attach to the arm, bulky units that are kept in holders next to the patient and disposable assemblies (Fig. 4-20). The fidelity of recordings differs little with one type of transducer or another. Before buying a transducer, determine how well it can record the baseline for hours on end without drift. Some transducers drift badly, particularly when temperature changes.

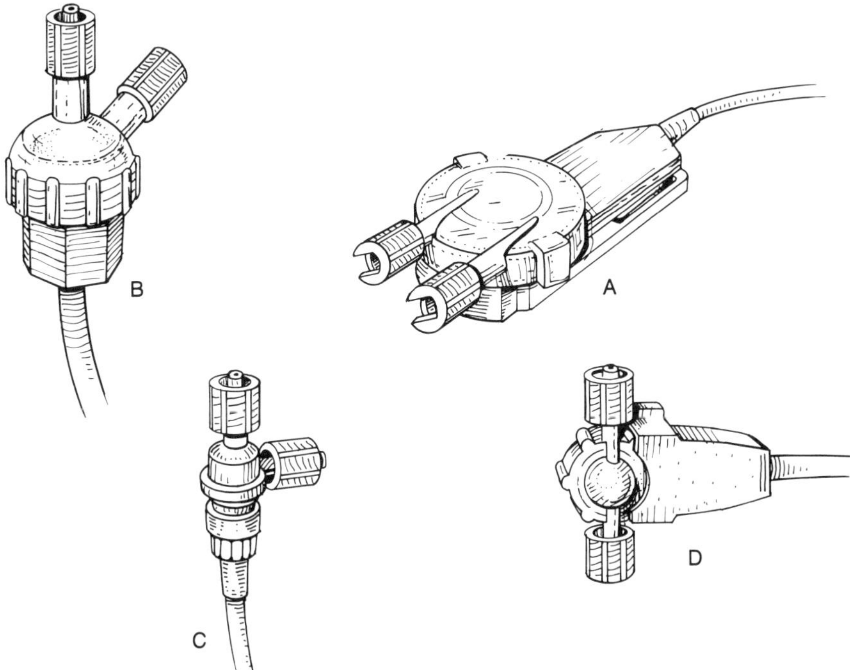

Figure 4-20. Common pressure transducers. *Counterclockwise from top right*: (*A*) flat pressure transducers (Hewlett-Packard, Waltham, Massachusetts) that can be strapped to the arm of the patient; (*B*) typical transducer with plastic, disposable dome; (*C*) small transducer with very small fluid volume above the pressure sensitive diaphragm; (*D*) disposable pressure transducer.

A number of companies have now made available disposable transducers (see Fig. 4-20). This astonishing development, made possible through modern microcircuitry, confronts the clinician with the need of calculating for his particular hospital the cost of acquisition and manpower for the older, reusable transducers, compared to the price of the new, disposable units. The convenience for the user and the reduced liability for contamination that the disposable transducers offer is difficult to express in monetary terms, but obviously many American hospitals have found these advantages great enough to switch to them. The disposable transducers are packaged in sterile form, many already equipped with a pressure drip assembly for the continuous infusion of heparinized saline. Other units occupy a middle position; they are reusable, but their life expectancy is much shorter than that of the traditional transducers.

The ideal assembly, containing at its tip a pressure transducer and chemical sensors for P_{O_2}, P_{CO_2}, and pH so tiny that they can be advanced into an artery, will become available in the future. Size, cost, and problems with clotting need to be improved. At this time, for prolonged monitoring, we use catheters that are connected to transducers removed from the patient.

Physics of Invasive Monitoring

Invasive measurements are not inherently more accurate than noninvasive ones. Indeed, considerable errors can occur with the finest equipment. Many years ago, Fry reviewed the problems besetting invasive recordings; this review is a classic and we recommend it to those seeking details.[44]

STATIC

The system must be able to measure accurately the pressure applied to it. This is typically checked by connecting the system to static pressure for an hour or more. Neither the baseline (atmospheric pressure) nor the static-pressure signal should vary at all. Of course, perfection cannot be expected, but drift, inaccuracy, or imprecision should be slight enough to affect the measurements insignificantly; 1% or 2% inaccuracies are usually acceptable. Changes in temperature can cause the transducer to drift or inaccuracies to exceed tolerable limits. Check how thermal changes (between room and body temperatures) affect the static accuracy of your system. If these changes are significant, either do not use the transducer or maintain it at a constant temperature.

Changes in the pressure of the cardiovascular system occur rhythmically. In studying the shape of the curve as the pressure rises to its peak and then decays, two problems confront us.

KINETIC ENERGIES If the tip of the intra-arterial catheter faces the bloodstream, kinetic energy is detected, which would not happen if only the pressure impinging on the wall of the artery could be measured. Clinically, we can do little about this phenomenon. Arterial catheters with holes in the side, rather than the tip, have been recommended but are not practical. Thus, our recording, particularly of high pressures generated by a vigorous heart, reflects some kinetic energy.

NATURAL FREQUENCY The measuring system has some elasticity and can oscillate. Imagine a diving board: if you jump up and down on it, it oscillates more and more; but to accomplish this, you must jump at the frequency that is inherent in the board (*i.e.*, its natural frequency). If you want to measure how much your weight deflects the diving board, you would not jump on it. The same applies for blood pressure measurements. You do not want to strike the natural frequency of your system lest it

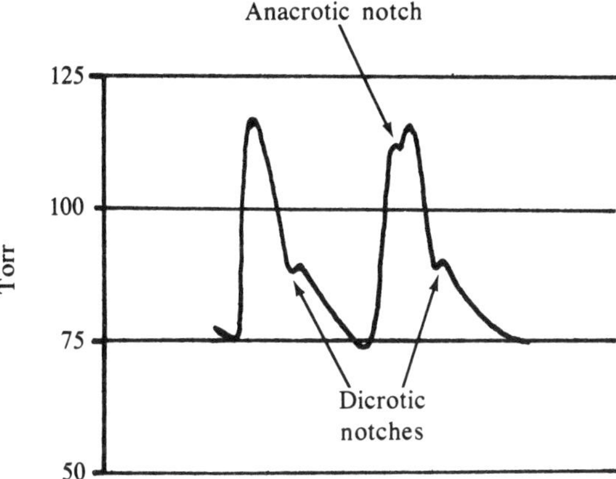

Figure 4-21. The shape of the arterial pressure wave can change rapidly. Note the development of an anacrotic notch.

start "ringing" or oscillating and, thus, distort the measurements. This brings up two additional questions.

What are the frequency components of arterial blood pressure? These are determined by dissecting a blood pressure waveform (using a Fourier analysis) into its harmonics. The idea here is that each point on the pressure curve is the sum of a host of oscillations, some with large and others with small amplitudes, all of them uniquely related to each other. The heart's contraction moves the system. An incredibly complex interplay of factors, then, conspires to shape the pressure curve. The diameter, elasticity, length, and branching of vessels, the composition of blood, pressure wave reflections, and, most importantly, the physics of the measuring system all affect the shape of the pressure curve. Sympathetic discharge, straining, as with the Valsalva maneuver,[45] blood loss, or cardiac depression can dramatically change these forces, causing the shape of the blood pressure curve to have or lose an anacrotic notch (a catch in the upslope), as seen in Figure 4-21. Ordinarily (but not invariably), the natural frequencies in the physiologic system (excluding the blood pressure measuring system) lie predominantly below 24 Hz (24 oscillations/sec). If the artery were connected to a recording system with a natural frequency of 12 Hz, and if the blood pressure contained 12-Hz harmonics of large amplitude, the system would ring.

How can we determine the natural frequency of our recording system? One way is to use a sine-wave generator (commercially available but expensive) to produce different frequencies and amplitudes of waveforms. Thus, the input to your system is known and the output can be recorded. A typical graph, shown in Figure 4-22, reveals a system with faithful

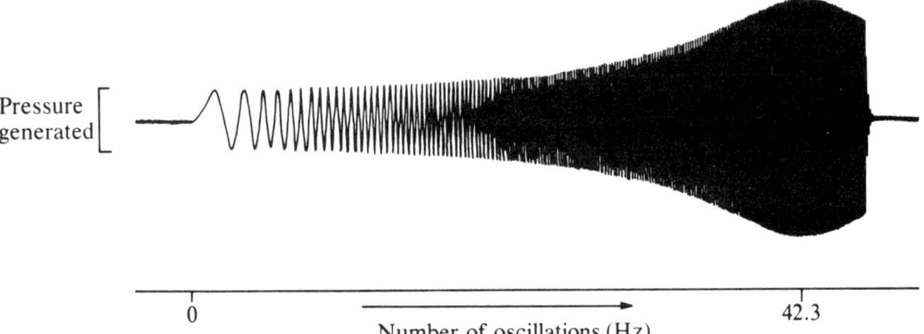

Figure 4-22. The pressure recorded by an arterial pressure-monitoring system including pressure transducer, extension tubing, stopcocks, and flushing assembly is shown. At zero a pressure generator is switched on. The pressures generated are faithfully reflected by the pressure transducer initially but, as the frequency of the pressure pulses increases (without changing the pressures themselves), the clinical system begins to oscillate and significantly exaggerate the signal to it. Maximal oscillations occurred in this instance at 42.3 Hz. This point of maximal oscillation is called the *natural frequency* of the measuring system. A pressure-monitoring system with such a natural frequency would be acceptable for clinical use even though it is capable of "ringing."

output until the frequency rises to 42.3 Hz, at which point the system begins to oscillate, exaggerating the input signal. This system is deemed acceptable for clinical use.

Within reach of everyone who has an electronic monitoring system is a simpler, homemade frequency-testing method (Fig. 4-23). Take a 5- or 6-ml plastic syringe, remove the plunger, drill a hole into the side of the barrel close to the end (5-ml mark), and fit a stopcock to the hole with a little glue to prevent leaking. Fill the syringe with water to, but not above, the drilled hole. Now fit a toy balloon (don't forget to reimburse the child who supplies it) to the end of the syringe. A rubber membrane or glove can also be used. Connect the tip of the syringe with the system to be tested. Be sure to include exactly the same tubing, stopcocks, and flushing devices that are used clinically. Remove all bubbles and connect the tubing to the pressure transducer. Now attach to the stopcock a blood pressure bulb (or another source of compressed gas) and inflate the balloon until it is tight. Record the pressure generated on rapidly running paper (use maximal speed, *e.g.*, 100 mm/sec).

Now, with a knife blade, pop the balloon so that it will quite suddenly deflate. You will get a tracing similar to that shown in Figure 4-24.

For a quick check in the operating room one can also set the system aringing by quickly exposing it to a sudden jolt. Systems incorporating a high pressure infusion drip with heparinized saline usually have some means for flushing the catheter with considerable pressure. Such a sud-

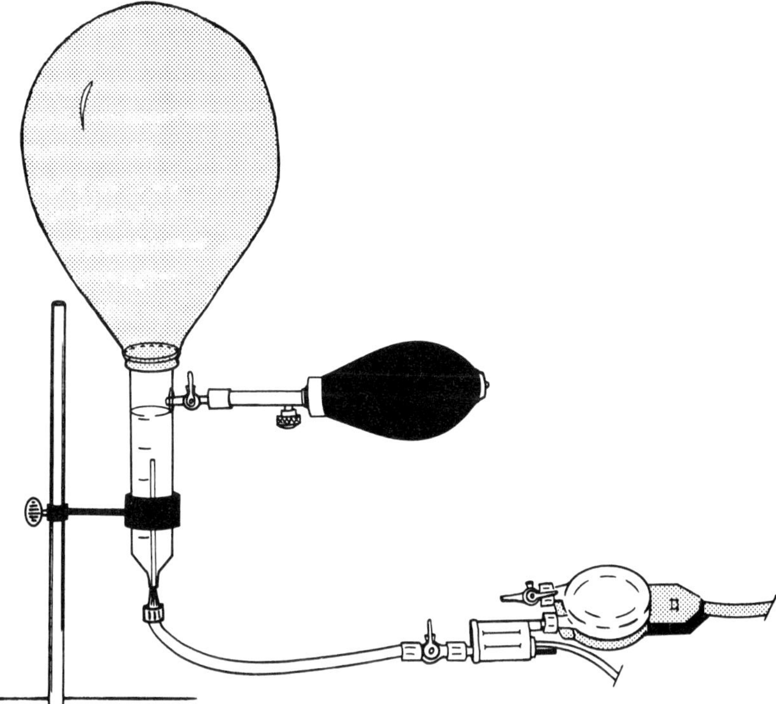

Figure 4-23. A homemade system to determine the natural frequency and damping of a blood pressure recording system. A 5-ml syringe is used. A hole is drilled into the side of the barrel close to the end. This is armed with a stopcock through which pressure can be applied, as demonstrated with the bulb from a blood pressure manometer in this figure. The end of the syringe is covered with a toy balloon, rubber glove, or rubber membrane. The blood pressure recording system, including the extension tubing, stopcocks, and arterial cannula to be used, is attached to the tip of the syringe. The arterial catheter projects into the syringe, which is filled with water to, but not above, the pressure source. Pressure is then applied until the balloon is tight. The pressures used should be within the operating range of the pressure transducer. When the system records a stable pressure of, for instance, 50 torr, the balloon is ruptured suddenly. A small hole with a needle will not suffice; a knife blade will yield the most accurate results. This sudden release of pressure will result in oscillations that are recorded on rapidly running paper.

den, short-lived rise and decline of pressure triggers oscillations in the system as shown in Fig. 4-25. These can be observed on the oscilloscope screen or recorded on a strip-chart recorder. This clinical test serves as a quick visual assessment of ringing and damping.[46]

From the strip-chart recording, determine the natural frequency and

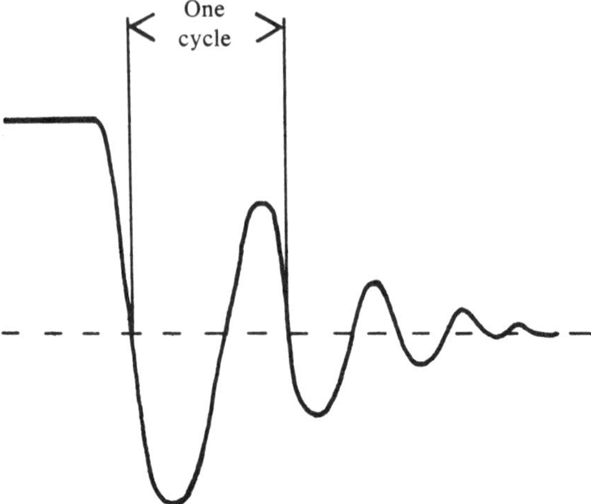

Figure 4-24. Pressure oscillations recorded after popping the balloon (see Fig. 4-23). The natural frequency of this system is determined by the following formula:

$$\text{natural frequency} = \frac{\text{paper speed (mm/sec)}}{\text{length of 1 cycle (mm)}}$$

the damping factor of your system:

$$\text{natural frequency (fn)} = \frac{\text{paper speed (mm/sec)}}{\text{length of 1 cycle (mm)}}$$

This formula assumes that the system is underdamped, as most clinical systems are. With a damping coefficient less than 0.3, the natural frequency will be within 10% of the true value. Larger damping coefficients require a correction factor.[44]

DAMPING

Although we want a brisk response to any change in pressure, we also want the system to come to rest quickly after registering the new pressure. A severely damped system will never overshoot, whereas an underdamped system can. How quickly the over-oscillation dies down is expressed by β (beta), the damping coefficient. A β value of 1 means that the system does not resonate at all, even at its natural frequency; unfortunately, the system also responds sluggishly to change.

An underdamped system (*e.g.*, β = 0.2) permits oscillation at the natural frequency of the system.

An optimally damped system should lie somewhere in between (β value of 0.6 to 0.7). Remember, this is a compromise between two extremes, and, as is true of most compromises, it is not perfect.

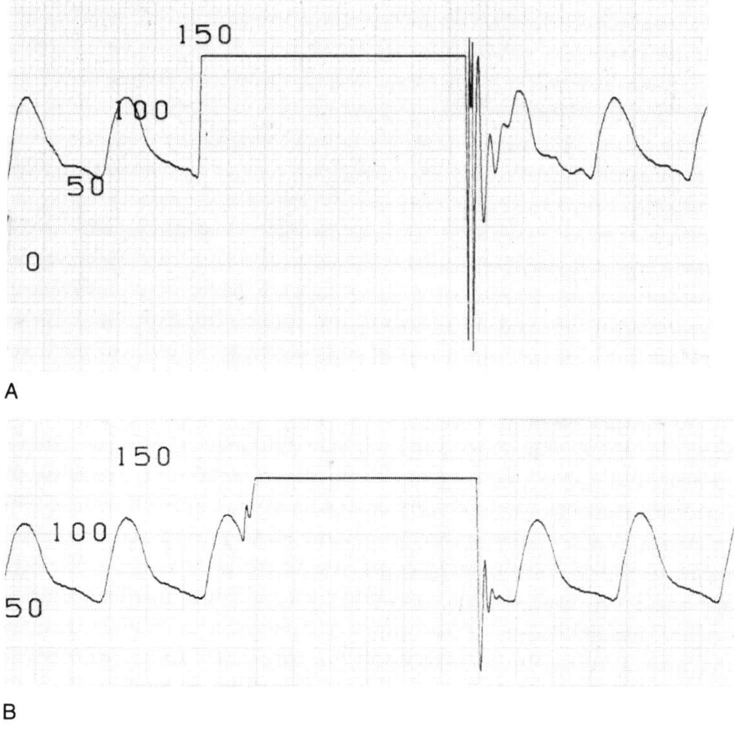

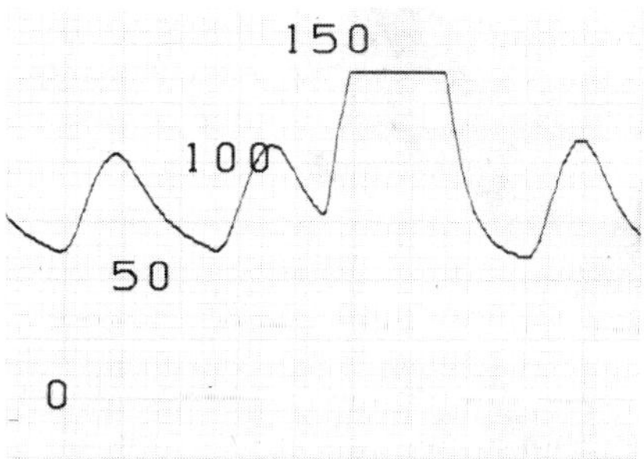

Figure 4-25. Flushing the arterial catheter to assess natural frequency and damping. In the operating room, quickly flushing the arterial catheter with pressurized, heparinized saline generates high pressure in the system. When the flushing finally stops, the system oscillates according to its natural frequency and damping coefficient. In panel *A*, several oscillations were observed on paper moving at 25 mm/sec. These oscillations could also be analyzed by running the paper at 100 mm/sec, as shown in Figure 4-24. Panel *B*, after removal of 1.2 mg tubing, shows evidence of mild damping. Panel *C*, following addition of an air bubble into tubing, shows marked damping.

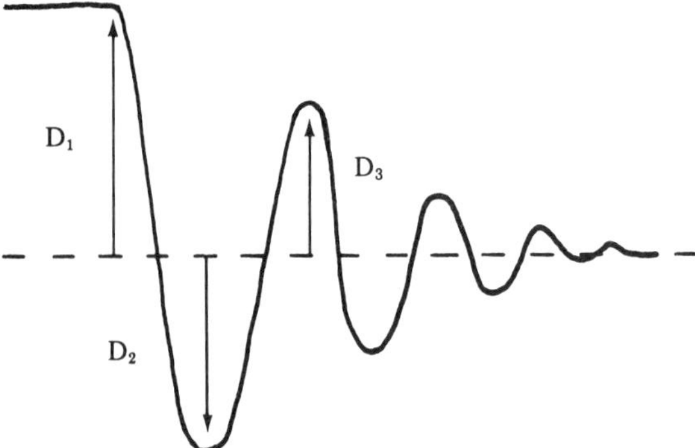

Figure 4-26. To determine the damping ratio, the record obtained from the balloon-popping experiment (Figs. 4-23 and 4-24) is used. The ratio of D_2 to D_1 is expressed as a percentage. See Figure 4-27 to obtain the damping factor.

THE DAMPING COEFFICIENT The record obtained with the balloon experiment provides the necessary data. Be sure that the pressure in your system is such that the recording pen can travel fully through the arc of its swings without clipping at the top or bottom, and that the transducer will record negative and positive pressures equally well. Label the oscillations as shown in Figure 4-26 and use this formula:

$$\beta = \sqrt{\frac{\left(\ln \frac{D_2}{D_1}\right)^2}{\pi^2 + \left(\ln \frac{D_2}{D_1}\right)^2}}$$

A simple method of using this formula is illustrated in Figures 4-26 and 4-27. For example, if D_1 is 6 cm and D_2 is 3 cm, the amplitude ratio D_2/D_1 is 0.5 and the damping coefficient is 0.215.

In summary, you have an excellent system if the natural frequency of your system is very high (over 80 Hz) even though the damping coefficient is low. There is little chance that ringing will occur since it is unlikely that such a high frequency will be encountered in clinical use. The lower the natural frequency of your system (15 Hz), the more important the damping coefficient becomes; a β value of 0.6 or 0.7 is desirable. Many clinical systems have natural frequencies between 10 Hz and 20 Hz and a damping coefficient below 0.3. All of these systems will ring when conditions allow. Ringing is very common, particularly at high heart rates, and usually leads to an overestimation of systolic pressure, sometimes by 20 torr or 30 torr. Figure 4-28 shows commonly used ar-

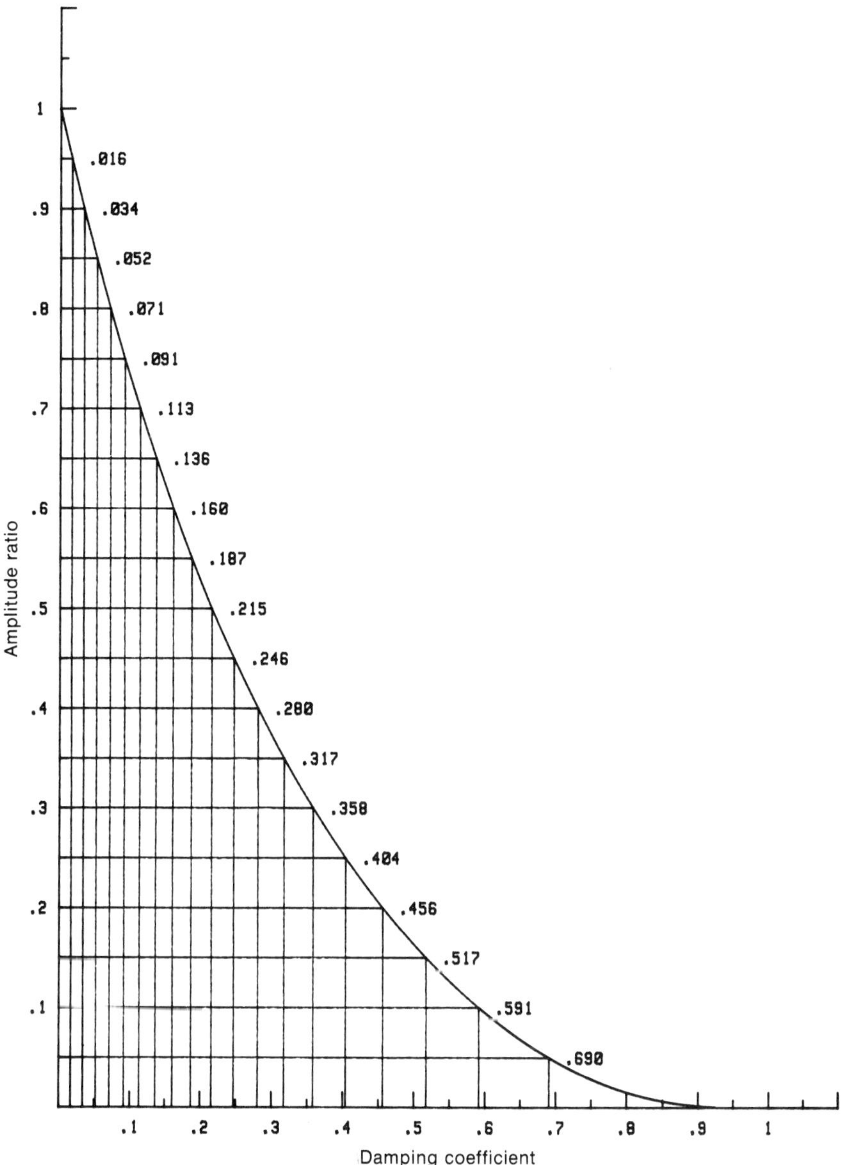

Figure 4-27. To determine the damping coefficient, calculate the ratio D_2/D_1 as shown in Figure 4-26 and apply this nomogram. A 0.5 ratio would give a damping coefficient of 0.215.

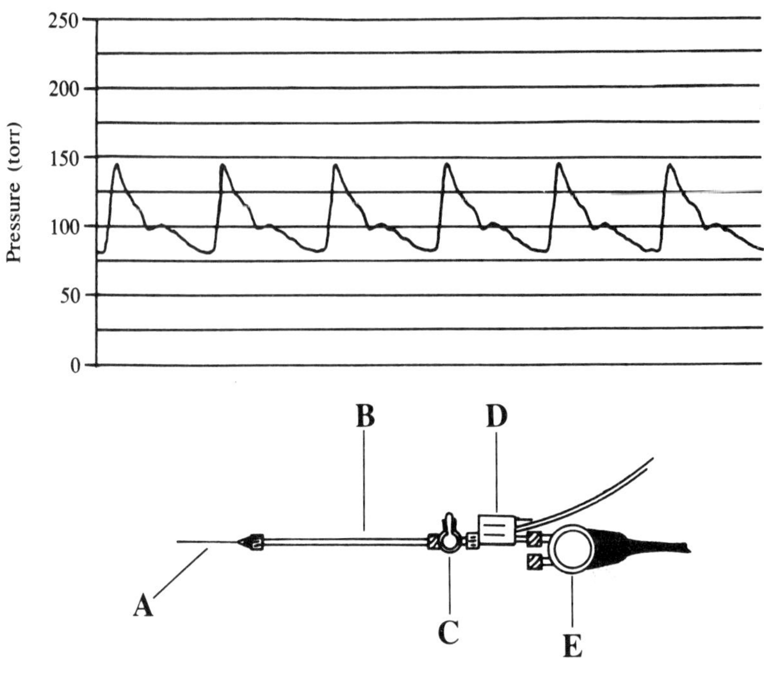
250
200
150
100
50
0
Pressure (torr)
B
D
A
C
E

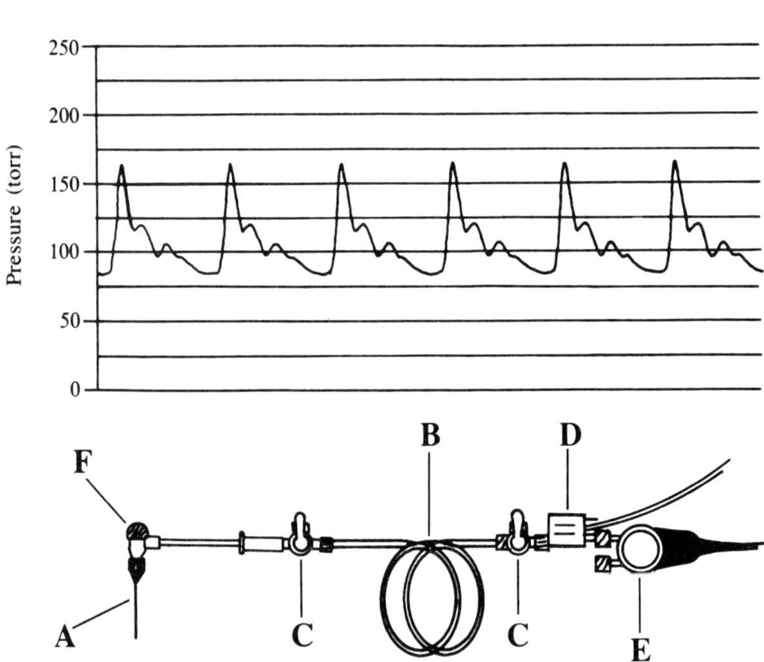
250
200
150
100
50
0
Pressure (torr)
F
B
D
A
C
C
E

rangements of transducers and tubing. Observe how much the pressure is distorted when soft tubing (the T-piece) is added to the system.

WHAT INFLUENCES FREQUENCY AND DAMPING?

BUBBLES There is nothing more common, more difficult to eliminate, and more disturbing to good pressure recording than air bubbles in the system. Bubbles hide in stopcocks, form in tubing, and get trapped in transducers. They damp.

When monitoring continues for hours, the air dissolved in the heparinized saline may come out of the solution and form bubbles. This phenomenon is particularly apt to occur when the saline is pressurized to 300 torr. Air on top of the saline in the plastic bag and in the drip chamber is then forced into the solution. Distal to the low flow valve the pressure drops to that of the patient's blood pressure, and the air comes out of solution and forms little bubbles. At present, there is no satisfactory system to rid the solution of all air. Although an air bubble from the saline bag should be removed, we dare not remove the air from the drip chamber, which should be watched to make sure that a malfunction does not cause heparinized saline to be infused into the artery of the patient. Saline can be degassed by packaging under vacuum, or boiling and packaging without an air bubble. The lines can be flushed with 100% CO_2 gas, which will cause any remaining gas to readily dissolve and vanish. An electric infusion pump can provide the necessary pressure as long as it is nonpulsatile. Only nonpulsatile pumps will serve in this situation. For the average anesthetic, however, most anesthetists use a pressurized bag and nondegassed saline.

TUBING The system is also affected by the properties of tubing. For example, the following formula is used to describe the effects of the in-

←

Figure 4-28. A pressure generator was set to produce a pressure of 145/80 torr. This signal was recorded in two ways. *Top panel*: The system consisted of a 20-gauge catheter (*A*), a 6-inch arterial pressure tube (*B*), a three-way stopcock (*C*), a Sorensen Intraflo device (*D*), and a Hewlett-Packard 1295A quartz pressure transducer (*E*). The system gave a faithful reproduction of the pressure waves. *Bottom panel*: The basic components of the system are the same, but a 36-inch arterial pressure tube, an additional stopcock, and an Abbott extension set with "T" (*F*) were used. This extension set is made of soft tubing and has a rubber cap because it is intended for intravenous, not arterial, use. With these components the pressure was recorded to be 165/85 torr instead of the true 145/80 torr. A false dicrotic notch appeared high on the downslope. The main culprit in this system distorting the blood pressure waveform is probably the extension set, which, though designed for extending intravenous tubing, is often employed for the sake of convenience in arterial systems. Air bubbles produce similar distortions.

ternal diameter of the tubing (D), the density of fluid (ρ), the length of the tubing (L), and the change in volume (ΔV) with a change in pressure (Δp) on the natural frequency of the system (fn).

$$fn = \frac{1}{2\pi}\sqrt{\frac{\pi D^2 \Delta p}{4\rho L \Delta V}}$$

Thus, it is important to keep tubing stiff and use transducers with diaphragms that yield only slightly with pressure change. Tubing for arterial pressure recording comes in different lengths, from 7.5 cm (3 inches) to almost 1 m (3 feet). Since extensions sometimes have to be used in the operating room, keep them short, no longer that 1 m.

Small-bore arterial catheters, in comparison to larger catheters, have a lower natural frequency, a larger damping factor, and less propensity to cause vascular complications. As the lumen of the catheter decreases, the damping coefficient rises more sharply than the natural frequency falls.[46] Small catheters, therefore, often represent true arterial pressures surprisingly faithfully. In infants 24-gauge catheters serve well; in adults 22- or 20-gauge catheters are preferred because they allow more easily the sampling of arterial blood and create less risk of clotting than is true for very small or very long catheters.

Stopcocks are the bane of these systems. They often have lumens narrower than the internal diameter of the tubing. Wide tubing loses its benefit if it is matched with stopcocks with tiny holes. Because the inner surfaces of the stopcocks are complex and contain nooks, bubbles hide there. Therefore, use only as many stopcocks as are essential for good clinical care.

Protocol for Invasive Monitoring

EQUIPMENT

1. A monitor warmed up for use
2. A pressure transducer attached to the monitor
3. A plastic arterial catheter, 20-gauge to 24-gauge, marketed by various companies
4. Extension tubing, 7.6-cm (3-inch), stiff, with Luerlok* connections to go from the catheter to a high-pressure/low-flow infusion device (*e.g.*, Sorenson Intraflo† or an equivalent unit); at times, longer extensions are needed
5. High-pressure/low-flow infusion device (Sorenson Intraflo† or an equivalent device)

* Or equivalent
† Sorenson Co., Salt Lake City, Utah

6. IV tubing from high-pressure/low-flow device to bag with heparinized saline
7. 250 ml saline with 500 units heparin
8. A device to put the saline under 300 torr pressure or a nonpulsatile infusion pump that will deliver 1 ml to 3 ml/hr
9. Stopcock with wide lumen and Luer* fittings between arterial catheter and extension tube to permit sampling of arterial blood; depending on the type of pressure transducer used, additional stopcocks may be needed on the dome of the transducer
10. Iodophore or antibiotic ointment to apply to the junction of skin and catheter
11. Adhesive tape

Disposable pressure transducers often incorporate items 2 to 6 in a single sterile package.

CALIBRATION

Follow the manufacturer's instructions. The first step requires that the system be set to zero.

Calibration of the transducer-monitoring system calls for a mercury manometer, extension tubing, and the transducer filled with sterile saline (Fig. 4-29). Be sure all bubbles are removed. The transducer may have to be tilted and tapped to persuade the last bubble to give up a cherished crevice.

We prefer to set all this up before adjusting to zero, so that the temperature in the transducer can stabilize, and we can record zero with the transducer filled with saline.

An alternative to zeroing with the entire transducer is to use a stopcock that can be opened to air. If it is in a fixed position, we can zero the transducer against it. If the patient is moved so that his heart (or head, if that is what is monitored) is now higher or lower than when the system was adjusted to zero, either the transducer has to be moved by an equal distance as the patient's reference point, or the system has to be zeroed again.

In Figure 4-30A, a transducer that is higher than the reference point is shown. At zero pressure, the diaphragm of the transducer actually is exposed to negative pressure in relation to the atmosphere. This is called an *offset*, and most transducers can handle it without becoming inaccurate. However, there is a limit to the offset that can be tolerated. Since we usually do not bother to test for it,[47] we recommend that any offset be kept to a minimum, and that the transducer be aligned as shown in Figure 4-30B.

Once zero has been established, calibration is accomplished with the mercury manometer. We elevate the mercury column to 200 torr and then

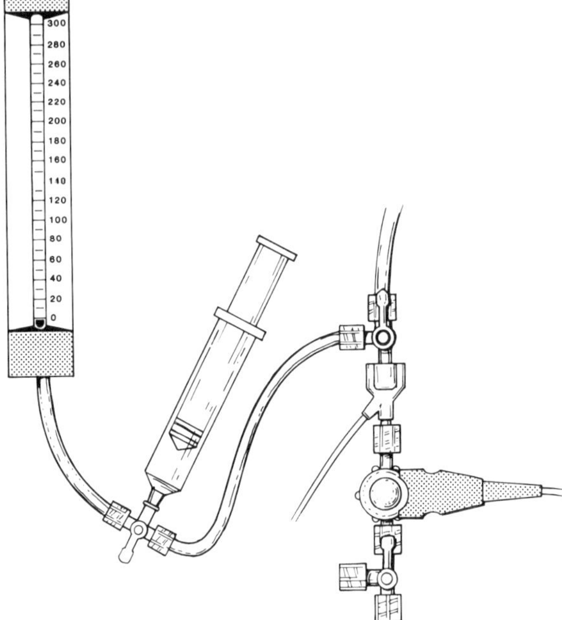

Figure 4-29. For the calibration of an arterial pressure transducer a mercury manometer is attached to the transducer. Pressure is applied with a 20-ml syringe.

bleed the pressure in steps of 50 torr. For most systems, one has to be satisfied with an accuracy within 5% at high pressures and 10% at low pressures.

Most pressure monitors have internal calibration standards that should be rechecked later during the procedure.

When recalibration with the mercury manometer becomes necessary after the patient has been connected to the system, *do not recalibrate until the patient is disconnected from the system.* This precaution guards against a potentially disastrous complication that occurs when the stopcock of the arterial tubing is turned the wrong way, and air shoots into the patient's artery instead of the manometer!

SAFETY MEASURES

In the foregoing procedure, we mentioned Luer connections, which prevent accidental disconnections. When the connections cannot be observed—they are hidden, for example, under drapes—Luer connectors (or their equivalent) are essential to guard against accidental disconnection and the possibility of arterial hemorrhage. When the connections can be watched, friction connectors may be used.

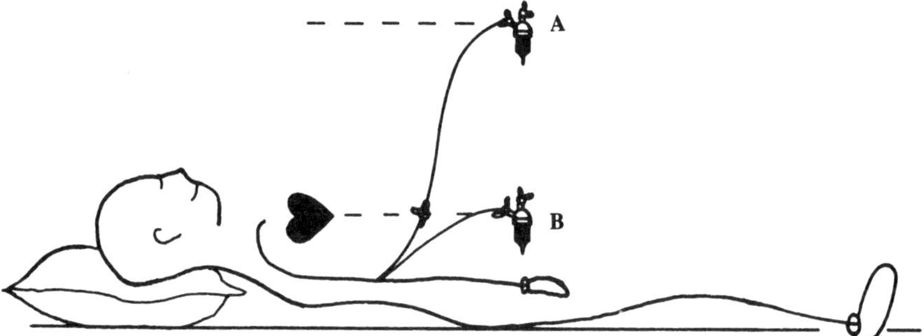

Figure 4-30. To put the transducer at zero pressure, its relationship to the reference point of the body, in this instance the heart, has to be recognized. It is possible to zero the transducer, which is above the body's reference point, by opening a stopcock to air at the level of the reference point (*A*). A preferable method puts the transducer itself at the level of the reference point, in this instance the heart (*B*). By this method, setting the zero value merely requires the opening of one of the ports of the transducer to air or a stopcock that is close by. Most transducers can handle an offset or the difference between *A* and *B*. With very large offsets inaccuracies occur.

Do not inject medications into an arterial tubing or catheter. To prevent possible mistakes, label the tape over arterial and venous tubing so that no one can mistake an arterial for a venous catheter.

Maintain sterile technique. Resist the temptation to use venous tubing or T-pieces to facilitate the sampling of arterial blood by sticking a needle through rubber diaphragms, cuffs, or caps that are found on some venous tubing. These are not easy to clean. After a puncture or two, they tend to leak. They also distort the pressure waveform (Fig. 4-28). Instead, use a stopcock that is kept sterile, with a cap protecting the port when not in use.

After cannulation of the radial or ulnar artery, do not keep the wrist in an excessively hyperextended position.

Do not attach a stopcock directly to the arterial catheter. Operating the stopcock causes the catheter to move back and forth, which may contribute to infection of the puncture site. Also, the stopcocks are bulky and the catheter may be in danger of kinking, particularly in small wrists with superficial arteries.

TROUBLESHOOTING

When using disposable domes, be sure they are sealed properly, without bubbles. Loose domes may give low pressure readings and bubbles cause damping.

If the waveform has more spikes and notches than is natural, if it

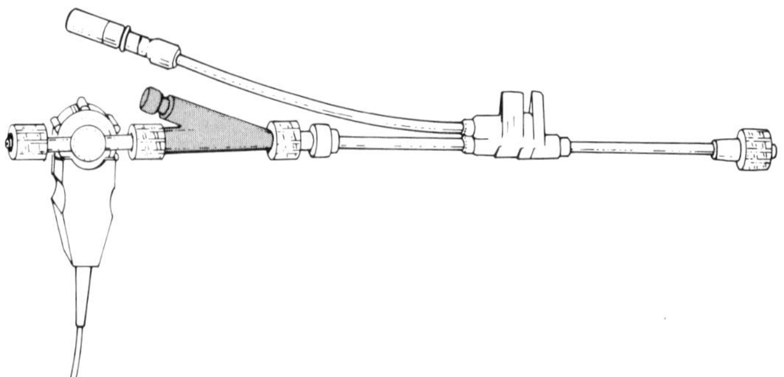

Figure 4-31. Device to increase damping. Shown is one of several commercially available devices that increase the damping of the system, here by an adjustable narrowing of the lumen (*shaded area*) connecting the arterial catheter to the pressure transducer. These devices simultaneously tend to decrease the natural frequency of the system.

looks odd (Fig. 4-28, lower panel), then the system is ringing. The problem may be air bubbles; soft, pliable tubing; excessively long tubing; or low natural frequency and damping factors of the system, including transducer and instrument.

These are common problems, so common in fact that industry now offers sterile, disposable devices designed to reduce the ringing of the system. The idea here is to increase the damping just enough, without decreasing the natural frequency system simultaneously to an unacceptable degree. This damping can be accomplished by inserting a narrow orifice into the system which is adjusted until the desired damping has been attained (Fig. 4-31). Another device allows the user to insert a carefully controlled air bubble into the system, and thus increase the damping. Either device "fights Satan with the Devil." Bubbles and narrowing the tubing can lower the natural frequency while increasing the damping coefficient. The natural frequency in a ringing system is always too low, never too high! Yet, either approach often makes an unacceptable system tolerably acceptable. In a significant paper, Gardner has described how sacrificing on natural frequency while increasing the damping can make for a better recording.[46] Figure 4-32 illustrates this principle. But, before reaching for constrictions or air bubbles, examine the system and see whether there are flaws that can be eliminated, such as excessively long tubing, soft tubing, or, indeed, air bubbles that may account for the observed ringing!

Is there a clot forming at the catheter tip? This is the most common problem of concern. If it occurs, pressures are distorted, probably closer to the mean pressure (Fig. 4-33). If clotting occurs, try to aspirate the

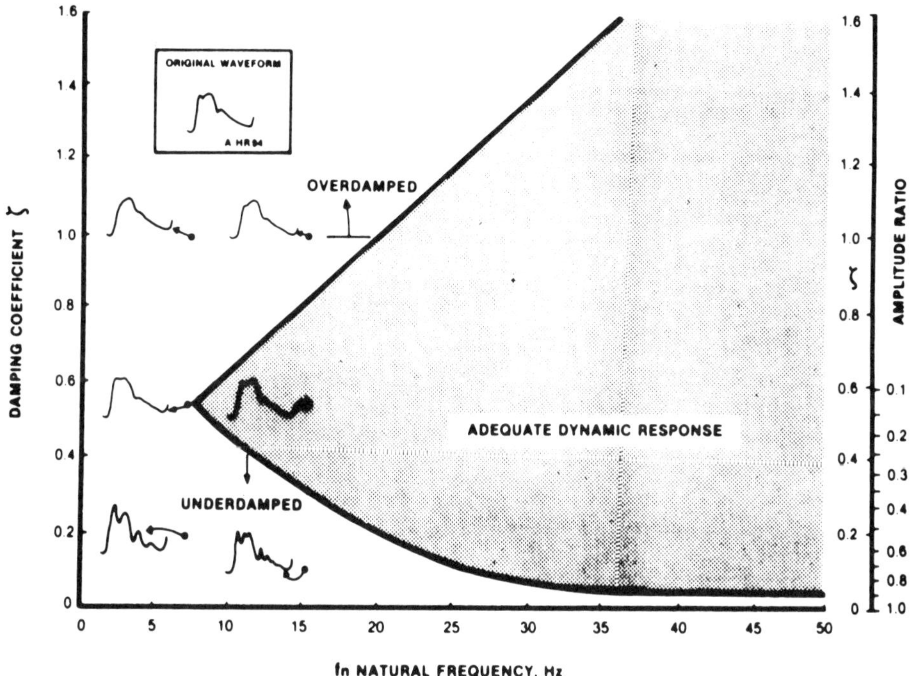

Figure 4-32. This plot shows how damping coefficient and natural frequency may affect the quality of a pressure tracing. The *inset* shows the original waveform. In the shaded area the original waveform is approximated; in the white area it is either overdamped or underdamped. It can be appreciated that increasing the damping coefficient alone may improve or impair the quality of the signal, whereas increasing the natural frequency is likely to improve the quality of the system. Increasing damping, for instance from 0.1 to 0.6, could improve the dynamic response even though the natural frequency of the system might have decreased at the same time from 20 Hz to 15 Hz. The graph shown was plotted for an individual patient. Other patients with different characteristics and different heart rates will have different areas where natural frequency and damping coefficients would conspire to generate a good dynamic response of the pressure waveform. (With permission from Gardner RM: Direct blood pressure measurement—Dynamic response requirements. Anesthesiology 54:227–236, 1981)

clot rather than to flush it in. Many clinicians flush the system to remove a clot. When this is done, the clot flies into the arterial system and may block a small peripheral artery, or, if flushed with too much vigor, may be pushed into the aorta and from there into a vital organ. We recommend continuous, gentle flushing with Intraflo or an equivalent system. This prevents the problem of a damped waveform caused by clotting.

The kinking of lines, partially closed stopcocks, and catheter tips pushed against the arterial wall are other possible occurrences that require

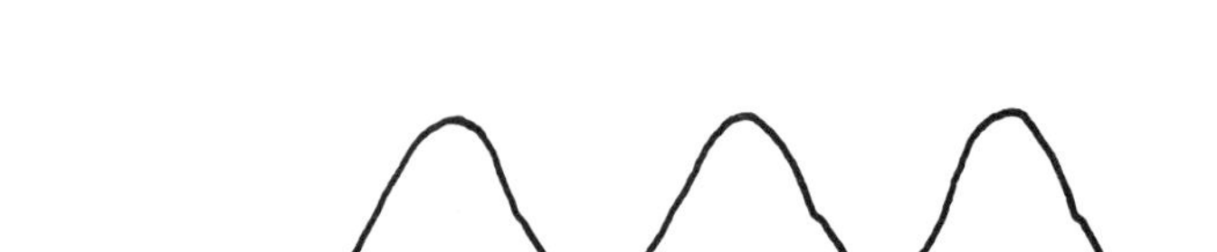

Figure 4-33. A damped waveform has fewer peaks and valleys than designed by nature. The pressure recorded approaches that of the mean pressure. Air bubbles, partial occlusion of the catheter by a clot, kinks, and very narrow orifices in stopcocks may be responsible.

checking. Catheters and stopcocks are quickly checked. Withdrawing the catheter slightly often helps when catheter position is a problem.

If these measures do not correct the "odd waveform," the absence of waveform, or an unusual reading, the system itself may be out of order. Transducers do age and fail, and electronic components do go on the blink. Disconnect the patient and recheck the system against an external manometer. If it cannot be zeroed or calibrated, do not use the system. Do not try to repair a transducer or a unit unless you are an engineer, in which case you will probably not be reading this.

PREVENTION OF INFECTION

Modern tubing and transducer domes come in sterile packages and are disposable. One might, therefore, assume that the danger of infection has been eliminated. This is unfortunately not the case. Buxton and coworkers alerted the profession to the fact that radial arterial catheters may be the route by which bacteria gain access to the blood.[48] In several outbreaks involving over 100 patients, infectious agents transmitted by monitoring devices included *Pseudomonas cepacia*, *P. aeruginosa*, *P. acidovorans* and *Enterobacter cloacae*, *Serratia marcescens*, *P. denitrificans* and *P. maltophila*, *Candida*, and Epstein–Barr virus.[49]

Problems with infection are greater with reusable equipment than with disposable assemblies. It is prudent not to use a transducer and system with disposable components for more than 2 days continuously. If monitoring must be continued for more than 2 days, a fresh, sterile transducer should be used.

If transducers are reused, the following procedure can be employed:

1. Saturate a paper washcloth with a disinfecting solution and wipe down transducer cord.
2. Coil the cord loosely and secure the cord with a twist tie.

3. Pour hydrogen peroxide into a small cup and dip the transducer head into the solution to remove blood. Rinse with sterile water.
4. Rig a transducer holder on a small laboratory stand. Secure the transducer upside down in the clamps. Lower this assembly into a disinfecting solution so that the business end of the transducer is submerged. Do not submerge the entire transducer nor the cord, because rubber is damaged by the solution. Soak the transducer head for 30 minutes.
5. Fill a sterile 12-ml syringe with sterile water, prepare sterile wrappings, and loosen the clamp holding the transducer.
6. Don sterile gloves.
7. Take the transducer out of the clamp, rinse the transducer head with sterile water to remove all disinfecting solution, and let dry.
8. Wrap the transducer in sterile material and label with the appropriate date. The transducer should be used within 28 days or should once again be disinfected as described.

This procedure assures cleanliness, but not sterility.

When the transducer is to be used, unwrap it, and if it has a disposable dome, put a drop of sterile saline on its diaphragm and firmly attach a new, sterile, disposable dome onto the transducer. Do not reuse disposable domes.

Even though no definitive study proves that the application of an antibiotic or povidone–iodine ointment or cream to the skin puncture of an arterial or venous catheter diminishes the incidence or severity of infections, we do apply a dab of such a salve to the skin puncture of every intravascular catheter. It may, indeed, be more a salve to our worry than to the patient's benefit. It must also be remembered that the disinfecting solutions, creams, and ointments may themselves be infected! Craven and co-workers found *P. cepacia* in a povidone–iodine solution.[50] These authors give references to other reports on contaminated disinfecting solutions and hospital supplies.

REFERENCES

1. Gravenstein JS: Essential monitoring seen through different lenses. J Clin Monit 2:22–28, 1986
2. Goldman L, Caldera DL: Risk of general anesthesia and elective operation in the hypertensive patient. Anesthesiology 50:285–292, 1979
3. Berger JJ, Donchin M, Morgan LS, et al: Perioperative changes in blood pressure and heart rate. Anesth Analg 63:647–652, 1984
4. Rasmussen JP, Dauchot PJ, DePalma RG, et al: Cardiac function and hypercarbia. Arch Surg 113:1196, 1978
5. Ream AK: Systolic, diastolic, mean or pulse: Which is the best management of arterial pressure? In Gravenstein JS, Newbower RS, Ream AK, et al (eds):

Essential Noninvasive Monitoring in Anesthesia, pp 53–74, New York, Grune & Stratton, 1980

6. Bruner JMR, Urenis LJ, Munsman JM, et al: Comparison of direct and indirect methods of measuring arterial blood pressure. Part I. Med Instrum 15:11–21, 1981
7. King GE: Selection of blood pressure cuff design. Lancet ii:492–493, 1982
8. Kirkendall EM, Feinleib M, Freis ED, et al: Recommendations for human blood pressure determinations by sphygmomanometers. Circulation 62:1154A–1155A, 1980
9. Sy WP: Ulnar nerve palsy possibly related to use of automatically cycled blood pressure cuff. Anesth Analg 60:687, 1981
10. Schaer HM, Tschirren B: Nervus radialis-Parese infolge automatischer Blutdruckmessung. Anaesthesist 31:151–152, 1982
11. Roy RC, Morgan L, Beamer D: Factitiously low blood pressure from the Dinamap. Anesthesiology 59:258–259, 1983
12. Elseed AM, Shinebourne EA, Joseph MC: Assessment of techniques for measurement of blood pressure in infants and children. Arch Dis Child 48:932, 1973
13. Kimble KJ, Darnell RA, Yelderman M, et al: An automated oscillometric technique for estimating mean arterial pressure in critically ill newborns. Anesthesiology 54:423, 1981
14. Penaz J: Photoelectric measurement of blood pressure, volume and flow in the finger. Digest 10th Int Con Med Biol Engr, Dresden, 1973, 104
15. Gravenstein JS, Paulus DA, Feldman J, et al: Tissue hypoxia distal to a Penaz finger blood pressure cuff. J Clin Monit 1:120–125, 1985
16. Smith, NT, Wesseling KH, de Wit B: Evaluation of two prototype devices producing noninvasive, pulsatile, calibrated blood pressure measurement from a finger. J Clin Monit 1:17–29, 1985
17. Gallagher JD, Moore RA, Nicholas KW, et al: Comparison of radial and femoral arterial pressures in children after cardiopulmonary bypass. J Clin Monit 1:168–171, 1985
18. Allen EV: Thromboangiitis obliterans: Methods of diagnosis of chronic occlusive arterial lesions distal to the wrist with illustrative cases. Am J Med Sci 178:237, 1929
19. Gandhi SK, Reynolds AC: A modification of Allen's test to detect aberrant ulnar collateral circulation. Anesthesiology 59:147–148, 1983
20. Slogoff S, Keats AS, Arlund C: On the safety of radial artery cannulation. Anesthesiology 59:42–47, 1983
21. Bedford RF, Wollman H: Complications of percutaneous radial-artery cannulation: An objective prospective study in man. Anesthesiology 38:228, 1973
22. Bedford RF: Radial arterial function following percutaneous cannulation with 18- and 20-gauge catheters. Anesthesiology 47:37, 1977
23. Bedford RF, Major MC: Percutaneous radial artery cannulation—Increased safety using Teflon catheters. Anesthesiology 42:219, 1975
24. Downs JB, Rackstein AD, Klein EF Jr, et al: Hazards of radial-artery catheterization. Anesthesiology 38:3, 1973
25. Davis FM: Methods of radial artery cannulation and subsequent arterial occlusion. Anesthesiology 56:331, 1982

26. Vender JS, Watts DR: Differential diagnosis of hand ischemia in the presence of an arterial cannula. Anesth Analg 61:465–468, 1982
27. Spaccavento LJ, Hawley HB: Infections associated with intra-arterial lines. Heart Lung 11(2):118–122, 1982
28. FDA Drug Bulletin 12(2):100–111, August 1982
29. Gardner RM, Schwartz R, Wong HC, et al: Percutaneous indwelling radial-artery catheters for monitoring cardiovascular function. N Eng J Med 290:1227, 1974
30. Pyles ST, Scher KS, Vega ET, et al: Cannulation of the dorsal radial artery: A new technique. Anesth Analg 61:876–878, 1982
31. Moorthy SS: Cannulation of the anterior peroneal artery in adults. Anesth Analg 60:360, 1981
32. Gordon LH, Brown M, Brown OE, et al: Alternative sites for continuous arterial monitoring. Southern Med J 77:1498–1500, 1984
33. Waller JL, Zaidan JR, Kaplan JA, et al: Hemodynamic responses to preoperative vascular cannulation in patients with coronary artery disease. Anesthesiology 56:219–221, 1982
34. Morray JP, Branford HG, Barnes LF, et al: Doppler-assisted radial artery cannulation in infants and children. Anesth Analg 63:346–348, 1984
35. Lowenstein E, Little JW III, Lo HH: Prevention of cerebral embolization from flushing radial artery cannulas. N Engl J Med 285:1414, 1971
36. Gardner RM, Bond EL, Clark JS: Safety and efficacy of continuous flush systems for arterial and pulmonary catheters. Ann Thorac Surg 23:534, 1977
37. Bedford RF, Ashford TP: Aspirin pretreatment prevents post-cannulation radial-artery thrombosis. Anesthesiology 51:176, 1979
38. Smith RS: Anesthesia for Infants and Children, p 702. St. Louis, CV Mosby, 1980
39. Shnider SM, Levinson G: Anesthesia for Obstetrics, p 456. Baltimore, Williams & Williams, 1979
40. McMillan JA, Nieburg PI, Oski FA: The Whole Pediatrician Catalog: A Compendium of Clues to Diagnosis and Management, Vol 1, pp 143–144. Philadelphia, WB Saunders, 1977
41. Clark JM, Jun AL: Umbilical artery catheterization by a cutdown procedure. Pediatrics 59:1036, 1977
42. Cole AFD, Rolbin SH: A technique for rapid catheterization of umbilical artery. Anesthesiology 53:254, 1980
43. Houston AB, Garg AK, Maclaurin JC, et al: Ultrasonic positioning of umbilical arterial catheters. Lancet ii:759, 1982
43a. Lesko SM, Mitchell AA, Epstein MF, et al: Heparin use as a risk factor for intraventricular hemorrhage in low-birth-weight infants. N Engl J Med 314:1156–1160, 1986
43b. Hiller JL, Benda GI, Rahatzad M, et al: Benzyl alcohol toxicity: Impact on mortality and intraventricular hemorrhage among very low birth weight infants. Pediatrics 77:500–506, 1986.
44. Fry DL: Physiologic recording by modern instruments with particular reference to pressure recording. Physiol Rev 40:753, 1960
45. Murgo JP, Westerhof N, Giolma JP, et al: Manipulation of ascending aortic

pressure and flow wave reflections with Valsalva maneuver. Relationship to input impedance. Circulation 63:122, 1981

46. Gardner RM: Direct blood pressure measurements. Dynamic response requirements. Anesthesiology 54:227, 1981
47. Wallace JE: The effect of zero offset changes on pressure transducer performance. J Clin Eng 4:221, 1979
48. Buxton AE, Anderson RL, Klimek J, et al: Failure of disposable domes to prevent septicemia acquired from contaminated pressure transducers. Chest 74:508, 1978
49. Retailliau HR: Infection control with invasive pressure monitoring devices. APIC 7:13, 1979
50. Craven DE, Moody B, Connolly MG, et al: Pseudobacteremia caused by povidone–iodine solution contaminated with *Pseudomonas cepacia*. N Engl J Med 305:621, 1981

CHAPTER 5

Cardiac Function

Our primary goal in the treatment of patients with cardiovascular dysfunction is to satisfy the needs of the body for perfusion with the least demands on the heart. Toward this end we measure pressures (in systemic arteries, right atrium, pulmonary artery, and left atrium), cardiac output, and heart rate. Before considering the technical details, we present a brief description of the physiologic principles that govern the cardiovascular variables that we monitor.

PHYSIOLOGIC PRINCIPLES

By measuring pressures in a central vein (close to the right atrium), in the right atrium, and in the left atrium, we approximate preload. By measuring pressures in the pulmonary artery and in a systemic artery, we approximate afterload. By determining cardiac output (CO), we can derive stroke volume. By studying a systemic pressure trace, we learn about contractility. From this, some clinically helpful answers can be given to our clinical management questions. The answers are not fully satisfactory because we can measure neither contractility nor right atrial, left atrial, or ventricular volumes.

Preload

A precise definition of preload accounts for end-diastolic stress in the wall of the ventricle. This is represented as end-diastolic volume—*not* pressure—on Starling's curve. Zero preload, for example, would cause the ventricle to eject nothing; with increased preload, ejection stroke work would increase proportionally but would eventually exceed the ventricle's (usually, the left ventricle's) capability to pump. Because the actual preload cannot be measured, we settle for a clinical compromise: ventricular pressure is used at end-diastole to represent preload. Perhaps we should speak of right and left ventricular end-diastolic pressures, but we do not usually measure them either. We measure right atrial and pulmonary artery pressures, instead. Clinical assessments of "preload," therefore, are at least twice removed from actual preload. We must also remember that compliance of the ventricles is not fixed. This is especially evident early after cardiopulmonary bypass, when high filling pressures are needed initially even though the ventricles are not distended.

Contractility

Much of our worry centers on the function of the heart as a pump. In a famous lecture, Starling proposed a curve in which the preload is plotted against contractility.[1] This relationship has been subjected to uncounted studies. The well-known curve (Fig. 5-1) is sometimes misinterpreted. Ream and Fogdall pointed out that the curve is quite complex and that enlightened cardiovascular management must be based on an appreciation of these complexities.[2] The curve rises almost as a straight line, the slope of which is governed by the contractility of the heart. Contractility is the intrinsic ability of the heart to do work. Clinically, the curve does not possess a descending position, at least not over any length of time. This happens because if the ventricle does not eject as much volume as it did on the previous contraction, the heart "moves" down and to the right on the Starling curve, where once again on the next contraction it ejects less volume. Presumably then, this would lead to cardiac demise in relatively little time. Therefore, it is better to think of the failing heart, in general, as working on the ascending part of the curve, but to the right of an optimal position on the curve, as shown in Figure 5-1.

Even in the laboratory, under experimental conditions, contractility is not easily determined. Clinically, we do not try to measure it, but settle

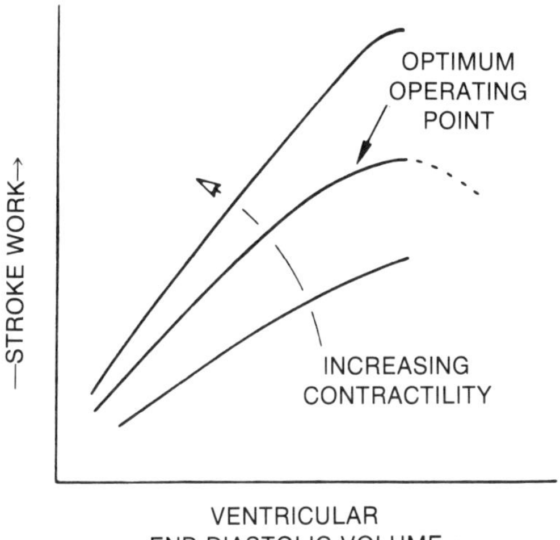

Figure 5-1. Starling's law. The following caveats hold true for understanding this curve. (1) The abscissa is *end-diastolic volume*, not end-diastolic pressure. (2) The ordinate is *stroke work*, not stroke volume or cardiac output. (3) Using a curve requires the assumption that contractility is constant; the slope of the curve varies with contractility. (4) The slope is always positive in the clinically useful range. (5) The concept of the curve bending downward to the right stems from isolated muscle studies, where it is valid. In the intact heart, this part of the curve does not exist. (6) Optimal efficiency appears near the maximal value of stroke work. (Ream AK, Fogdall RP: Acute Cardiovascular Management: Anesthesia & Intensive Care. Philadelphia, JB Lippincott, 1982)

for a qualitative "feel." A lusty, healthy heart pumping vigorously and nearly emptying its ventricles with each beat represents excellent contractility.

A sick, tired heart that cannot empty itself at end-diastole and that has much volume and pressure (preload) remaining in the ventricle, even though it may be pumping against little resistance, would be the picture of poor contractility.[3]

Afterload

Afterload is the impedance to ventricular ejection. It is measured as the ventricular (usually left) pressure, just as the valve (usually aortic) opens in systole. As with preload, a number of factors define afterload. These include, in the absence of valvular stenosis, distensibility of the large arteries, blood inertia, and the resistance offered by the vascular system.

Clinically all of these factors cannot be accounted for. Therefore, we measure arterial pressure and sometimes calculate total peripheral resis-

Table 5-1. NORMAL INTRACARDIAC PRESSURES

Location	Abbreviation	Normal Pressures*	
		Average	Range
Right atrium	RA	3	1–8
Right ventricle, systolic	RV	25	15–30
Right ventricle, diastolic	RV	5	1–8
Pulmonary artery, systolic	PA	23	15–30
Pulmonary artery, diastolic	PA	9	5–15
Pulmonary artery, mean	PA	15	10–20
Pulmonary artery, occlusion pressure	PAOP	10	5–15
Left atrial	LA	8	2–12
Left ventricle, end-diastolic pressure	LVEDP	8	4–12

* Pressure values given in torr.

tance in lieu of afterload. However, pressure measurement is the best approximation to the physiologic parameters of interest, so we use it.

Table 5-1 shows the normal intracardiac pressures. Catheters are put in the central circulation to measure these pressures. A central venous catheter is easily placed in the right atrium. Right ventricular pressure is measured in passing as a balloon-tipped pulmonary artery catheter traverses it on its way into the pulmonary artery. Left atrial and ventricular pressures are seldom measured clinically in the operating room, except during cardiac surgery, when catheters are placed directly into the left atrium and the left ventricle.

Combining the concepts of preload, afterload, compliance, and contractility with Starling's law, the clinician must remember that:

1. Preload pressure is not directly related to end-diastolic volume because, in disease, ventricular compliance changes.
2. The failing heart does not work on a descending part of the Starling curve; the heart moves to a different curve.
3. There is an optimal operating point on the Starling curve. To increase cardiac output when the patient operates to the left of the optimal position on the Starling curve, increase heart rate or add preload, or do both.
4. Afterload is important. It changes the stroke volume for which the stroke work was done.
5. If cardiac performance is still inadequate after preload, afterload, and heart rate have been optimized, getting the patient on "another curve" (increased contractility) may be necessary.

Table 5-2. HEMODYNAMIC PARAMETERS*

Parameter	Symbol	Formula	Units	Normal Values
Mean blood pressure	$\overline{BP}$	$\frac{BP_{sys} + 2(BP_{dia})}{3}$	torr	100 ± 20
Systemic vascular resistance†	SVR	$\frac{\overline{BP} - \overline{CVP}}{CO} \times 80$	$\frac{\text{dynes} \times \text{cm}}{\text{sec}^5}$	1050 ± 350
Stroke volume	SV	$\frac{CO}{HR} \times 1000$	ml/beat	75 ± 15
Cardiac index	CI	$\frac{CO}{BSA}$	$\frac{1}{\text{min} \times \text{m}^2}$	3.2 ± 0.4
Pulmonary vascular resistance†	PVR	$\frac{\overline{PAP} - PAOP}{CO} \times 80$	$\frac{\text{dynes} \times \text{cm}}{\text{sec}^5}$	100 ± 50
Stroke index	SI	$\frac{SV}{BSA}$	$\frac{\text{ml}}{\text{beat} \times \text{m}^2}$	50 ± 10
Left ventricular stroke work index	LVSWI	$\frac{1.36(\overline{BP} - \overline{CVP})}{100} \times SI$	$\frac{\text{g} \times \text{m}}{\text{m}^2}$	50 ± 10
Right ventricular stroke work index	RVSWI	$\frac{1.36\,(\overline{PAP} - PAOP)}{100} \times SI$	$\frac{\text{g} \times \text{m}}{\text{m}^2}$	7.5 ± 2.5
Shunt	$\frac{\dot{Q}_{sp}}{\dot{Q}_T}$	$\frac{C_cO_2 - C_aO_2}{C_cO_2 - C_{\bar{v}}O_2}$	none	<5%
Arteriovenous O_2 content difference	$C(a - \bar{v})O_2$	$C_aO_2 - C_{\bar{v}}O_2$	vol %	4.7 ± 0.8

* BP_{sys} is systolic blood pressure; BP_{dia} is diastolic blood pressure; $\overline{CVP}$ is mean central venous pressure; HR is heart rate; CO is cardiac output; BSA is body surface area (m^2); $\overline{PAP}$ is mean pulmonary artery pressure; PAOP is pulmonary artery occlusion pressure; $\dot{Q}_T$ is total blood flow; $\dot{Q}_{SP}$ is blood flow shunted through the pulmonary circulation; C_cO_2 is pulmonary capillary oxygen content; C_aO_2 is systemic arterial oxygen content; $C_{\bar{v}}O_2$ is mixed venous oxygen content.

† Vascular resistance (R) is expressed in several ways, but fundamentally it is the drop in pressure from one point to another divided by the blood flow through the vascular system being studied. To calculate total peripheral resistance, subtract central venous pressure (CVP) from mean systemic arterial pressure (the "pressure drop" across the vascular system), then divide by cardiac output. CVP is sometimes ignored because it may be low and affect the calculation only a little. We list the most common additional expressions for completeness:

1. Pressure gradient per unit blood flow

$$R = \frac{\text{pressure drop (torr)}}{\text{flow rate (ml/sec)}}$$

2. Peripheral resistance units (PRU)

$$R = PRU = \frac{\text{pressure drop (torr)}}{\text{flow rate (ml/sec)}}$$

3. Aperia's formula (cm × g × sec system)

$$R = 1333 \times PRU = \frac{\text{dynes} \times \text{sec}}{\text{cm}^5}$$

4. Resistance units (RU)

$$R = RU = \frac{\text{pressure drop (torr)}}{\text{flow rate (l/min)}}$$

Derived Variables

Table 5-2 lists hemodynamic and respiratory parameters, both direct and derived, and is used to estimate preload, contractility, and afterload. Mean blood pressure, whether it be systemic (see Chap. 4) or pulmonary arterial, is derived as in Table 5-2. Vascular resistance, systemic or pulmonary, is calculated as shown in Table 5-2. These data help us manage afterload and are the only components of afterload that can actually be manipulated. In order to calculate vascular resistance, cardiac output must be known.

CLINICAL PROCEDURES

Methods of Cannulation

Catheters come in different lengths and in diameters from 10 gauge to 24 gauge. Catheter over needle, needle over catheter, and catheter to be threaded down a guide wire are available. Each has advantages and disadvantages and some have special indications. The most common types are described.

Catheter Over Needle

Because these catheters cannot be longer than the needle, they are used primarily for intravenous therapy, but occasionally for measurements of pressure in the internal or external jugular vein where recordings are not influenced by valves interposed between the vein and the right atrium.

Numerous valves in the upper-extremity veins prevent backflow of blood, particularly when the hand is much below the right atrium. For this reason, venous pressure measurement in the veins of the hand is not clinically useful in this position. In the recumbent patient, the venous pressures in the hand should not be ignored entirely. It is easy to demonstrate distended veins on the back of the hand when the patient is relaxed and the hand is below the level of the right atrium. One can then simply lift the hand and watch the veins collapse as their pressure falls below that of the large central veins or the right atrium. This is a quick and crude, but clinically informative, estimate of right atrial pressure.

The widely used catheter-over-needle assemblies are disposable and usually have radiopaque, tapered-tip catheters that fit snugly onto the needle to ease insertion. We do not recommend the use of catheters that are tapered along their entire lengths and much wider close to the hub than at the tip. These catheters occupy more of the vessel lumen the further they are inserted. Thus, they occlude the vessel and, because their tips are no narrower than those of ordinary catheters of uniform diameter, they do not provide any advantage.

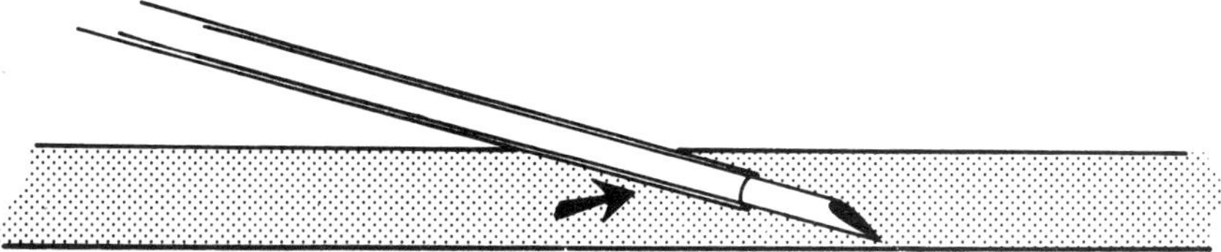

Figure 5-2. Intravenous catheterization. Note catheter entry into vessel lumen before needle is withdrawn.

METHOD OF INSERTION

Prepare the venous site to be cannulated with an iodine-containing preparatory solution, let it dry, and position the patient so that the site is dependent (in other words, below the level of the right atrium). This causes venous engorgement, making identification easy and minimizing the possibility of air embolism. Attach a 3-ml to 5-ml syringe to the catheter and enter the skin at a 30° angle directly above the vessel to be cannulated. Apply constant suction with the syringe while advancing the needle–catheter assembly. Entry into the vessel is heralded by venous blood flowing freely into the syringe. Lower the unit so that it is nearly parallel to the vein and advance slightly to ensure the bevel enters the lumen completely (Fig. 5-2). Hold the needle in position and advance the plastic catheter, rotating it a little, as far as it will go. Withdraw the needle and make sure that blood still flows freely. Sometimes it is necessary to withdraw the catheter a bit while aspirating with the syringe to allow the blood to flow freely.

Needle Over Catheter

With the catheter over a needle, the length of the catheter is limited by the size of the needle. With the needle over a catheter, the needle serves merely to cannulate the vein, and the catheter can be as long as desired. The disposable units are prepackaged in a sterile plastic sheath that makes advancing the catheter into the vein an easy matter once the needle has been placed securely into a suitable vein (Fig. 5-3).

METHOD OF INSERTION

Select the site for venipuncture and position the patient so that the site is dependent, or use a tourniquet. This leads to venous engorgement, which facilitates both locating and catheterizing the vessel. Prepare the skin with antiseptic solution. With the bevel of the needle up and at a 30° angle to the skin, puncture the vein. Once blood returns, lower the hub of the needle to bring it more nearly parallel to the vein and advance the needle a little further so that the entire bevel lies in the venous lumen

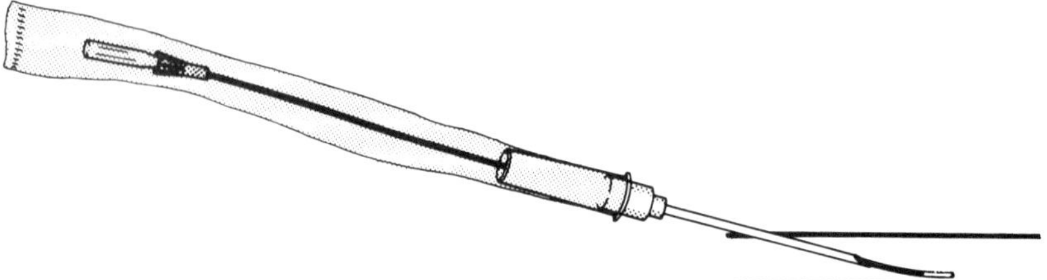

Figure 5-3. Needle-over-catheter intravenous cannulation. Do not shear off catheter by pulling back catheter against needle.

(Fig. 5-4). Remove the syringe and attach the catheter package to the needle hub. Then, advance the catheter into the vein by gently withdrawing blood until the desired position is reached. Most catheters have a thin stylet or wire in the lumen that usually facilitates insertion by giving the plastic catheter more strength. Occasionally, however, an acute angle in the vein can be negotiated more easily by withdrawing the stylet 1 cm ($\frac{1}{4}$ inch) or so, which makes the tip of the catheter more flexible.

A danger in using these catheters must be recognized. The needle's bevel is sharp and can cut off the catheter if the catheter is pulled back. Do not, under any circumstances, pull the catheter back through the needle. Many a catheter has been sheared off with this maneuver, making the catheter tip an embolus in the heart or the pulmonary vascular tree. This is a grave complication that may require a thoracotomy. After an unsuccessful venipuncture, the needle must be withdrawn *before* the catheter is withdrawn, or the two can be withdrawn together, but never may the catheter be withdrawn while the needle is still in place.

After successful cannulation, stabilize the catheter as you pull the needle out to avoid dislodging the catheter. Secure the catheter to the skin with a sterile suture or put a sterile dressing over the site and secure the catheter with tape. Always protect the puncture site with a sterile dressing. We like to apply a dab of iodine-containing ointment to the site. If the catheter crosses a joint, for instance, the elbow, a restraint may be necessary to prevent the catheter from moving in and out across the skin and causing an infection and thrombophlebitis. The needle cannot be removed and must, therefore, be watched lest it injure the patient. Many prepackaged units come with a needle guard for that purpose. After the dressing is applied, once again check for free flow of blood by aspirating with a syringe or by lowering an intravenous solution attached to the catheter.

A modification of this technique has been described. A 22-gauge spinal needle (chosen for its length) is threaded through a larger needle or catheter–needle assembly. The vein (usually the internal jugular vein—

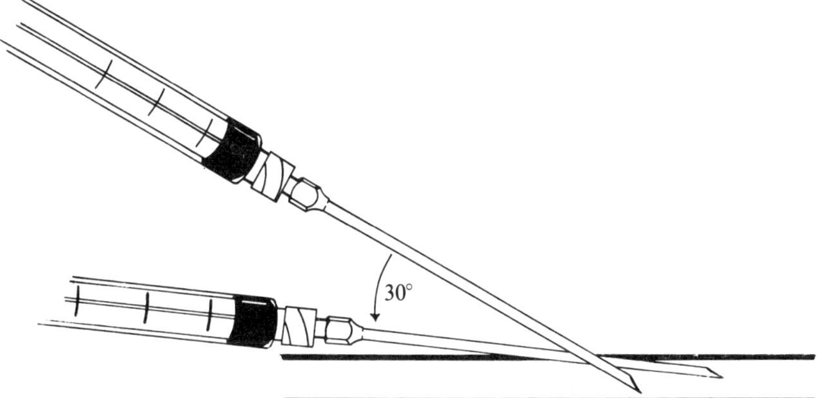

Figure 5-4. After the needle enters the vessel, blood appears in syringe. Lower the needle to advance it into the vessel.

see below) is then entered with the spinal needle. Once that is accomplished, the larger needle or catheter–needle assembly is pushed into the vessel, with the spinal needle serving as a guide. This technique minimizes the damage should one enter an artery (*e.g.*, the carotid) by mistake, because the 22-gauge spinal needle will leave a much smaller hole than the large needle–catheter assemblies used to insert a pulmonary artery catheter. The technique is, however, not without its own risk: the long spinal needle can be pushed in too far and cause a pneumothorax. It is also possible to injure the carotid artery while advancing the larger needle over the spinal needle.[4]

The Seldinger Technique

The Seldinger technique[5] of using a guide wire is frequently helpful in placing catheters. A needle or short catheter is placed into the vein, a guide wire is introduced through this needle or catheter, the needle or catheter is withdrawn, and the monitoring catheter is advanced over the guide wire (Fig. 5-5). The Seldinger technique, therefore, incorporates features of the two previous approaches.

Position the patient so that the desired entry point is dependent, or use a tourniquet. This will cause the vessel to be engorged, and thus, more easily identified and cannulated. Proper positioning also reduces the possibility of venous air embolism. With sterile precautions, prepare the skin, and, after having identified the landmarks, place sterile drapes. Then inject about 1 ml of 1% lidocaine without epinephrine with a 25-gauge needle over the intended puncture site. We frequently locate the vein with

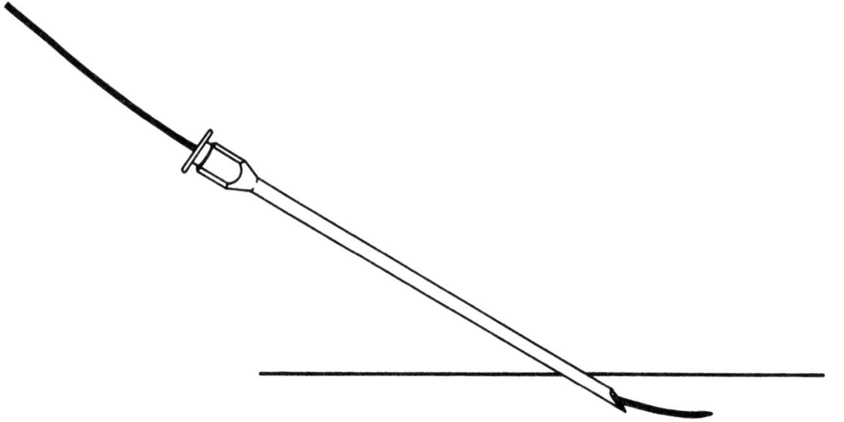

Figure 5-5. A wire is advanced into the vessel. The needle is then withdrawn and a catheter is pushed over the wire.

a 3-ml to 5-ml syringe armed with a 22-gauge needle. Once the vein is located, use the appropriately sized pilot needle or needle–catheter assembly to gain access to the vein. Constantly aspirate as the needle is advanced. As soon as blood flows, stop advancing and lower the assembly so that it is more nearly parallel to the vein. If a catheter over needle is being used, place the catheter into the vein as described before and withdraw the needle. Be sure that blood is flowing freely. Insert the springy guide wire through the needle or catheter. Always push the soft end of the wire in first. For cannulation of the external jugular vein we use a "J" tip (Fig. 5-6) to help negotiate the sharp corner that the external jugular vein makes before it merges with the brachiocephalic vein. The wire should advance easily. The wire must always be visible, even when the pilot needle or the catheter is withdrawn.

If the cannulated vessel lies deep to fascia, as is true for the internal jugular vein, slide a number 11 surgical blade so its back is parallel to the wire to enlarge the fascial opening. Place a suture through the skin and deep to the entry point. This avoids perforating the catheter with a needle later on.

Approximate the length of catheter to be inserted by using external landmarks to locate the desired position of the catheter tip. Slide the catheter over the wire until the wire exits the catheter hub before penetrating the skin with the catheter tip. Always maintain firm control over the guide wire.

Slide the catheter through the skin and into the vessel lumen. If much resistance is felt, withdraw the catheter. Usually this difficulty is brought about by resistance against passing the catheter through skin or fascia

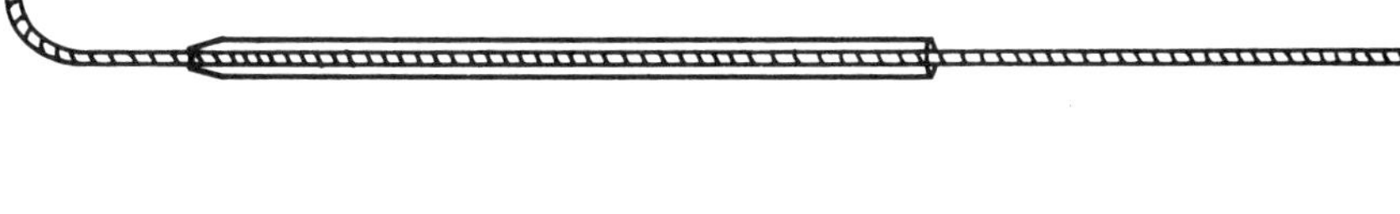

Figure 5-6. A flexible guide wire with a bent tip facilitates the cannulation of tortuous vessels.

and can be resolved by enlarging the access with a number 11 surgical blade. If that does not help, and excessive force is needed to advance the catheter, the wire is probably not in the correct position; to persist with more pressure will bend the wire and damage the catheter tip, which makes both unusable. Advance it as far as necessary to place the tip at the desired position. Usually this requires that the entire catheter be advanced. If a pulmonary artery catheter is to be placed, we often use two concentric catheters (Fig. 5-7), the inner, longer one serving as dilator and the outer, shorter one serving as a sheath to ease the introduction of a pulmonary artery catheter. Advance both catheters, one behind the other, over the guide wire. Withdraw the guide wire and the dilator. Then anchor the catheter with a suture. Check the flow of blood. If the vessel is kinked or perforated, withdraw the sheath a little bit while aspirating, to reestablish the flow of blood. If it fails, start over again. If blood does flow freely, attach the intravenous tubing or introduce the pulmonary artery catheter. Several authors have described complications of guide wires.[6,7] These include knotting of the flexible tip, partial or total separation of a portion of the wire, and, consequently, embolization or displacement of the catheter tip. To minimize the incidence of complications, the investigators suggest the following practices:

- Carefully inspect each wire for defects before its use.
- Treat a guide wire as a delicate instrument.
- When resistance is encountered, reinspect the tip and reposition the needle or catheter so that no resistance to the passage of the wire occurs.
- Make a sufficiently large skin incision to permit smooth insertion of the catheter over the wire.
- When multiple manipulations are required, reinspect the wire and replace if necessary.
- Gently apply traction if the guide wire becomes entrapped in a vein since the vein may be wedged between coils of the wire.
- Always inspect the wire for damage upon removal. Report defects

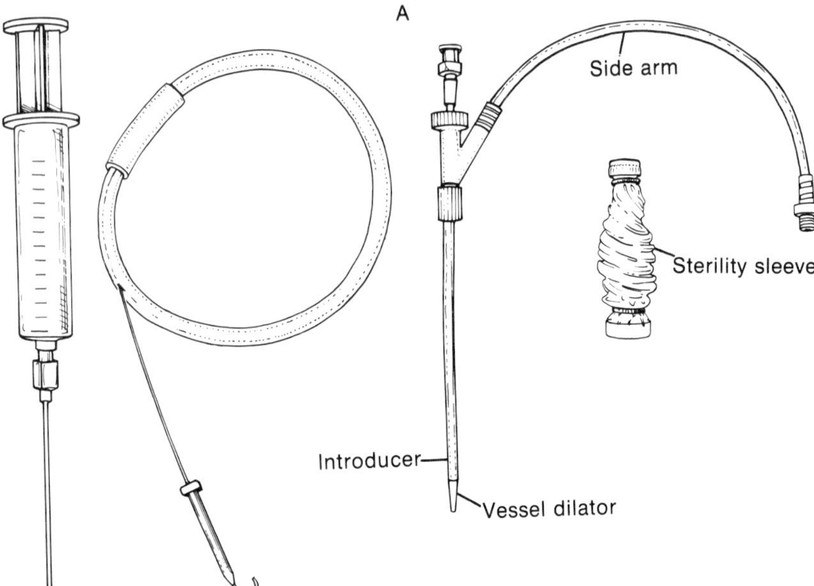

Figure 5-7. Pulmonary artery catheters are available in various lengths and lumen numbers and serve different functions. (*A*) The materials to place the catheter in the pulmonary artery are shown. A needle or catheter–needle assembly is used to gain venous access. Under continuous ECG monitoring the guide wire is advanced through the needle or catheter into the vein. Catheter or needle is then withdrawn. With a number 11 knife blade, skin and fascia are opened. The introducer and vessel dilator are slipped as one over the guide wire and usually advanced as far as possible. The vessel dilator and wire are withdrawn. Blood should flow freely into the side arm. Any air in the side arm is aspirated and then the system is flushed with a physiologic solution. The PA catheter is slipped through the sterility sheath and introducer and advanced into position. The introducer, if it has a hemostatic valve, is secured into position. If it does not have a hemostatic valve, it is withdrawn from the vessel. Two- and three-lumen catheters are available. (*B*) A three-lumen catheter with three hubs marked to identify corresponding catheter lumens. Access to the vessel is through an introducer needle or catheter–needle assembly. The wire is introduced through the needle, to a length such that the wire length barely exceeds that of the CVP catheter length while watching an ECG monitor for arrhythmias. If necessary, the skin and underlying fascia are slit with a number 11 knife blade. The catheter is then slid over the wire and advanced so it does not impinge on the wall of the right atrium. The catheter is secured in place, the wire withdrawn, and, to ensure proper placement, the clinician checks for free flow of blood from the catheter. The proper position of the catheter is demonstrated with a radiogram.

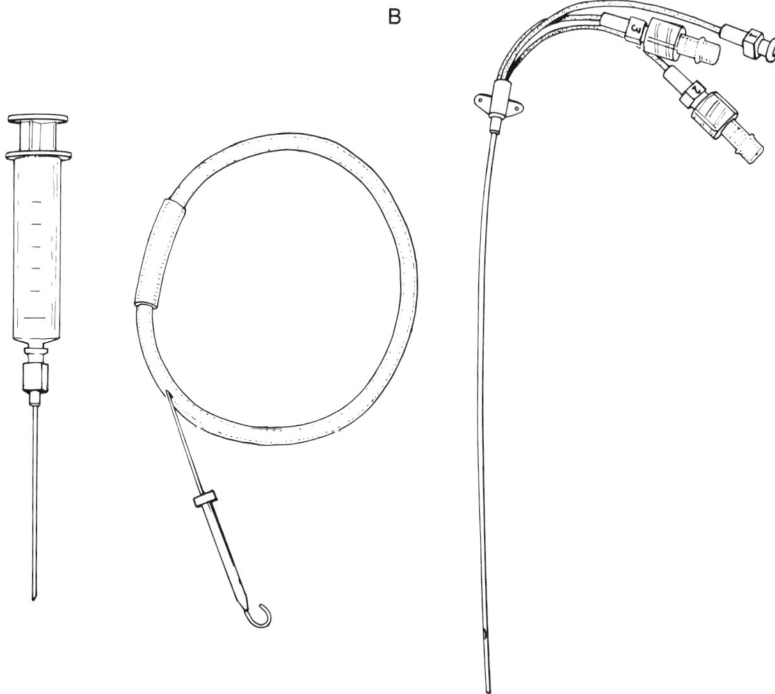

Figure 5-7. (*continued*)

to the manufacturer and consider that the remaining wires from a particular shipment may be defective.

- Do not reuse guide wires.

Cutdown

Select the appropriate site for the cutdown and position the patient so that the site is lower than the level of the right atrium, or apply a tourniquet to engorge the veins to facilitate identification of the vein and to prevent air embolism. Sterilely prepare the area. We use 2 ml of 1% lidocaine without epinephrine to anesthetize the surgical site. Carry an incision perpendicular to the vein in all planes through the skin and underlying fat. With blunt dissection, the vein is isolated, a suture is placed both distally and proximally under the vein (Fig. 5-8), and the distal suture is lifted to occlude the flow without causing the vein to collapse. With a number 11 blade or fine scissors, make a small cut into the vessel. A small hook is sometimes helpful to open up the lumen of the vessel and to facilitate the insertion of the catheter. One can also puncture the vessel

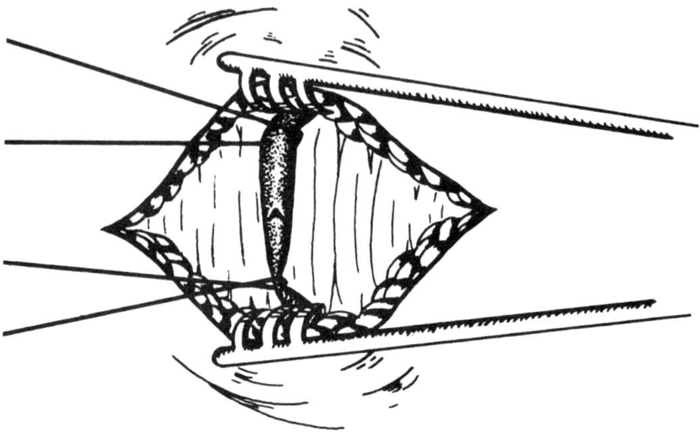

Figure 5-8. Cutdown to vein has been carried through overlying tissue. Sutures are placed distal and proximal to venotomy site.

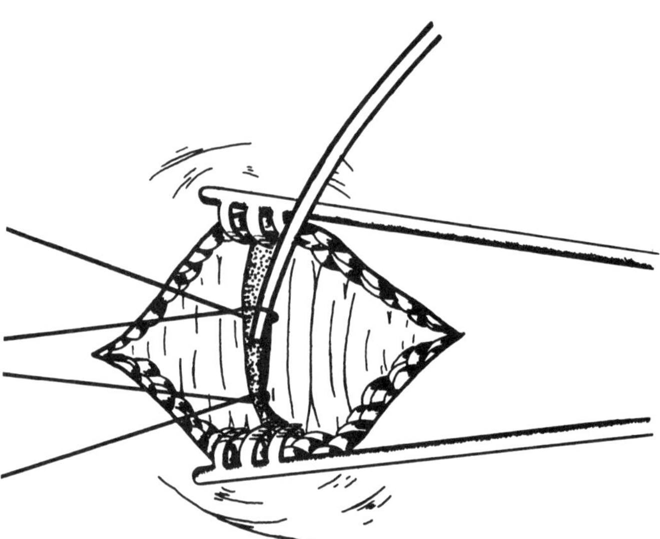

Figure 5-9. A catheter is introduced through a venotomy. Sutures are relaxed to slip the catheter into the vessel.

with a needle through which the catheter is advanced. Lifting the proximal and distal sutures may help also. Release the tourniquet, if one was applied, and tighten the proximal suture over the catheter only if necessary to prevent leakage (Fig. 5-9). Close the skin with two sutures, one of them also encircling the catheter to prevent it from slipping out. Apply sterile dressing.

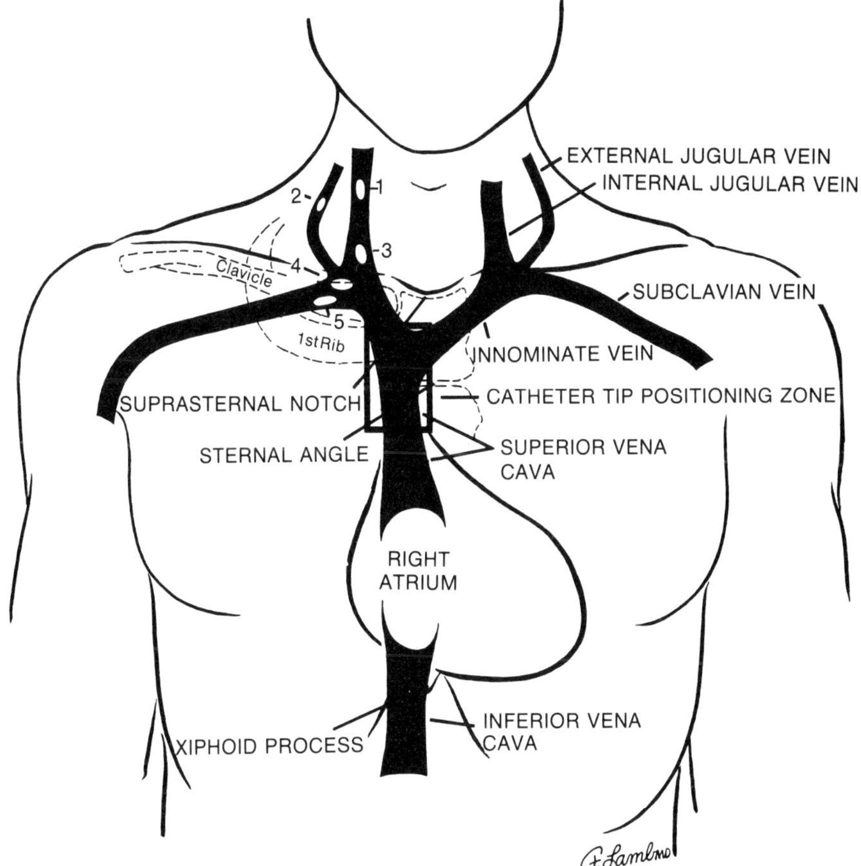

Figure 5-10. Access sites to superior vena cava: (*1*) high internal jugular; (*2*) external jugular; (*3*) low internal jugular; (*4*) supraclavicular; (*5*) subclavian (infraclavicular). (Courtesy of Cook, Inc, and F. Lamb)

Identification and Cannulation of Veins

Multiple sites for central venous access are available. Those about the neck and shoulders are shown in Figure 5-10.

Internal Jugular Vein

We prefer the internal jugular vein for the cannulation of a central vein, the right atrium, or a pulmonary artery. The right internal jugular vein is usually readily accessible even during operation and provides a safer route for cannulation than the subclavian vein.[8] The jugular vein can be used

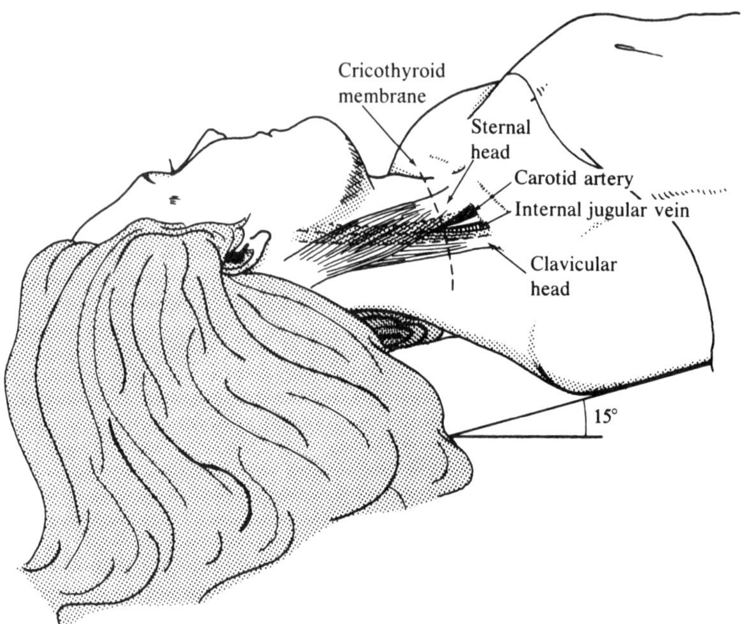

Figure 5-11. The recommended head position is 30° to the contralateral side. A roll under neck or shoulders is helpful, as is a 15° head-down position. A horizontal line drawn from the cricothyroid membrane crosses the apex of the triangle formed by clavicular and sternal heads of the sternocleidomastoid muscle.

for both infants (but watch for high apex of lung) and adults, and has the additional advantage of a relatively straight, short course to the right atrium. The internal jugular vein parallels the clavicular head of the sternocleidomastoid muscle and lies anterolateral to the carotid artery.

CANNULATION

Tilt the supine patient 15° head down to engorge the veins and to prevent air embolism. Ask the patient to lift his head. This maneuver shows the outline of the sternocleidomastoid muscle. Locate the apex of the triangle formed by the clavicular and sternal heads of the muscle. This apex usually lies directly lateral to the cricothyroid membrane (Fig. 5-11), a landmark particularly helpful for obese patients. It helps to identify these structures while the patient is still awake and is able to lift his head, in case cannulation needs to be done during anesthesia. The apex can then be marked with a pen. It also helps to turn the patient's head a little to the side not being cannulated. However, turning the head too much (more than 30°) brings the sternocleidomastoid medial to overlie the internal jugular vein[9] and makes cannulation more difficult.

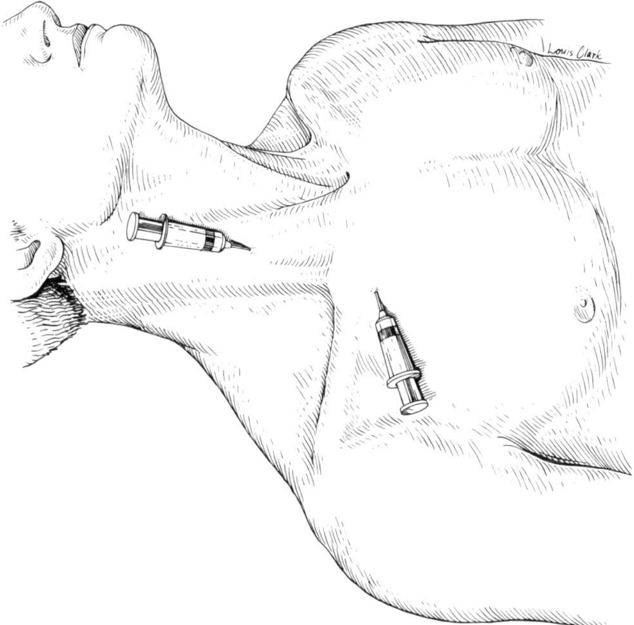

Figure 5-12. The positions for placing the catheters for cannulation of the internal jugular and the subclavian vein on the right. The right internal jugular vein is usually preferred for easy cannulation of central veins and the right atrium; however, the left or right subclavian vein can be used, depending on the circumstances of the operation and the patient.

If the patient is awake, identify the carotid artery by placing a finger close to the cricothyroid membrane and anesthetize the skin. Patients in whom neck landmarks are not identifiable and the carotid artery is not palpable present a particular problem. In this instance, we use a Doppler probe to locate the carotid artery. The most serious complication of cannulation of the internal jugular vein is accidental puncture or laceration of the carotid artery. Continue to palpate the carotid artery and insert a $1\frac{1}{2}$-inch, 22-gauge needle and syringe at the apex of the above-described triangle (Fig. 5-12) and aim for the ipsilateral axilla. Use of a small locating needle will minimize the injury should the carotid artery be hit. With one hand, tighten the skin a little without distorting the underlying anatomy. Advance the needle while maintaining suction with the syringe. Sometimes it is necessary to inject more local anesthetic to keep the patient comfortable. If you do not find the vein within 3 cm of the surface of the skin, aim the needle more medially toward the ipsilateral nipple. Ask the patient to perform a Valsalva maneuver, which will increase the diameter of the jugular vein. After obtaining flow of blood, make sure that the catheter has not entered the carotid artery. If arterial blood flows back during the first or second cannulation, withdraw the small needle, making note of the presumed location of the internal jugular vein, and apply pressure for about 5 minutes. This has to be done carefully because excessive pressure may occlude the carotid artery and cause ischemia of the brain. Pressure on the carotid artery may also trigger vagal reflexes from the carotid sinus.

If the carotid artery has been entered, bleeding may continue for hours, during which time the patient must be checked for a patent airway and neurologic signs. A hematoma may form in the neck and cause respiratory obstruction or may dissect into the thorax and result in hemothorax and respiratory insufficiency. If you are unsure whether the artery rather than the vein has been located, measurement of the intravascular pressure will usually reveal the location.

After cannulation, double-check the flow of blood. Suture the catheter in place and connect it to a monitor, because only then does the danger of air embolism disappear. Take the patient out of the head-down position. Apply sterile dressing and commence monitoring.

If additional access is desired, cannulate the internal jugular vein again just distal or proximal to the initial site using the first guide wire for location.[10]

External Jugular Vein

The external jugular vein offers an appealing access site as it is visible and close to the central circulation. In many patients it appears quite plainly in view as it crosses the sternocleidomastoid muscle. The patient is placed in a slightly head-down position to make the veins stand out or, if this is not possible, pressure is applied with a finger to the supraclavicular fossa to cause the external jugular vein to stand out. After preparation of the skin and administration of local anesthesia, the vein is cannulated under direct vision as is customary for veins of the extremities. Since the vein is embedded in the loose connective tissue of the neck, it is sometimes difficult to catch it with the needle. We find it helpful to put the needle into the skin, to advance it to a position right over the vein, and then, with a quick stabbing motion, to pierce the vein. Since the external jugular vein can join the brachiocephalic or subclavian vein at an acute angle, passage into the superior vena cava is sometimes difficult. We find the Seldinger technique with a J-wire particularly helpful. If obstacles are encountered navigating the wire to the superior vena cava, we can employ several tricks. First, we ascertain that the needle or catheter through which the wire is passed is not too far advanced; it should not impinge on any vascular angle because this will diminish the chance of manipulating the wire around the bend and getting it to traverse the junc-

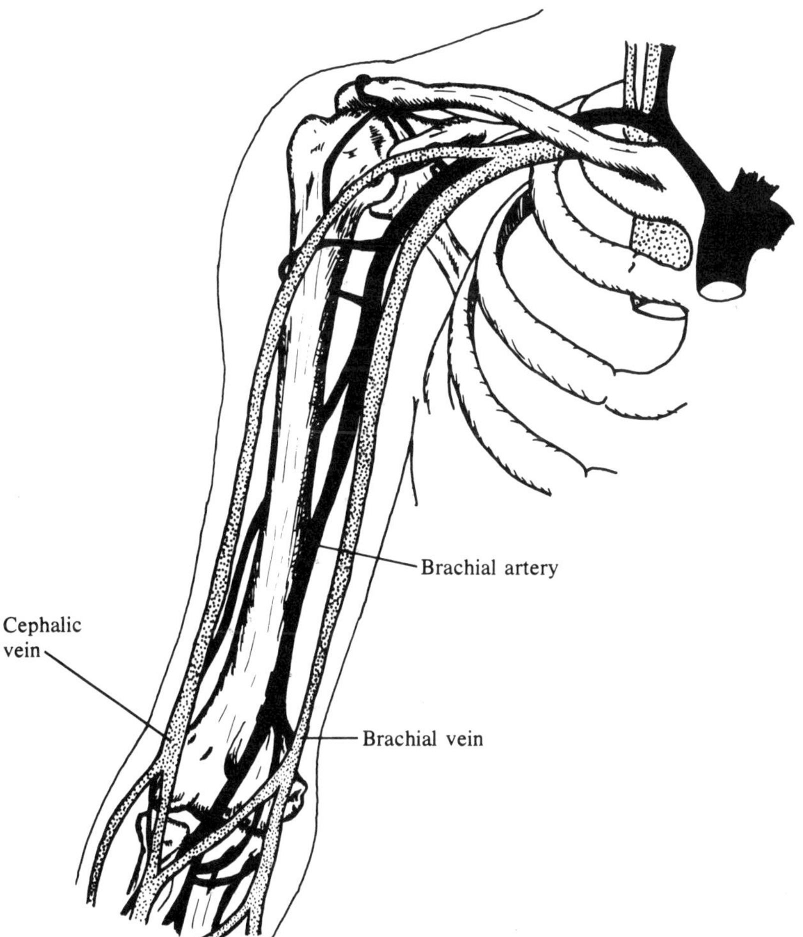

Figure 5-13. Both brachial and cephalic veins empty into the subclavian vein. Note the proximity of the brachial artery to the brachial vein.

tion and reach the superior vena cava. Second, it is helpful to move the patient's ipsilateral arm and shoulder about while manipulating the wire. Lastly, we frequently turn the patient's head to the ipsilateral side. A little patience will usually bear fruit.

Veins of the Arm

When none of the internal, external or subclavian jugular veins are available, we use either the brachial or the cephalic vein (Fig. 5-13). With a long catheter, either of these may be used to gain access to the right

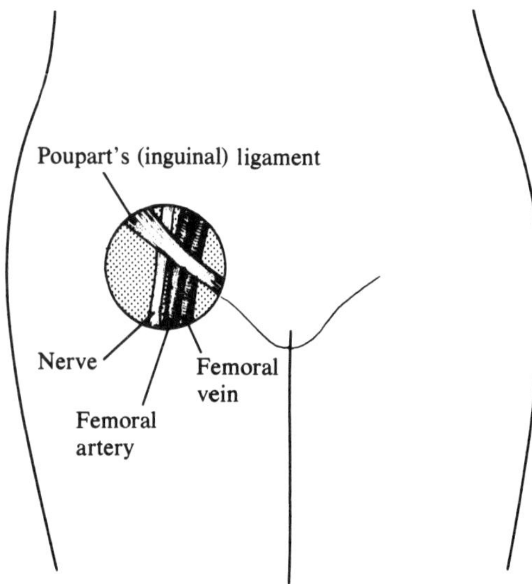

Figure 5-14. Femoral nerve, artery, and vein in close proximity. Cannulate the vessel just caudad to the inguinal ligament.

atrium. However, the success rate is lower than with the veins in the neck. Kellner and Smart[11] and Webre and Arens[12] noted an approximate 25% failure rate with the brachial or cephalic approach. The Seldinger technique improves success dramatically.

When possible, we prefer the right basilic vein over the cephalic vein. Once the vein is cannulated, we ask the patient to turn the head to his side of the cannulated limb and to place his chin on that shoulder. Difficulty is sometimes encountered at the shoulder, but moving the shoulder forward may allow the catheter through. The catheter tip can move significantly with movement of the arm, so we usually use this approach only for short-term access.

Femoral Vein

Palpate the femoral artery. The femoral vein lies directly medial to the artery, but the femoral nerve is lateral to the artery (Fig. 5-14). With obese patients, an assistant may be needed to hold the panniculus out of the way. After preparing the skin, draping the site, and administering local anesthesia, try to retract artery and nerve laterally and to advance the needle into the vein medial to your fingers and to the femoral artery. Puncture the skin and push the needle in the direction of the vein at a 15° angle. As the catheter is advanced in the vein, it sometimes takes a wrong turn and enters the opposite iliac vein. In that case, resistance is soon

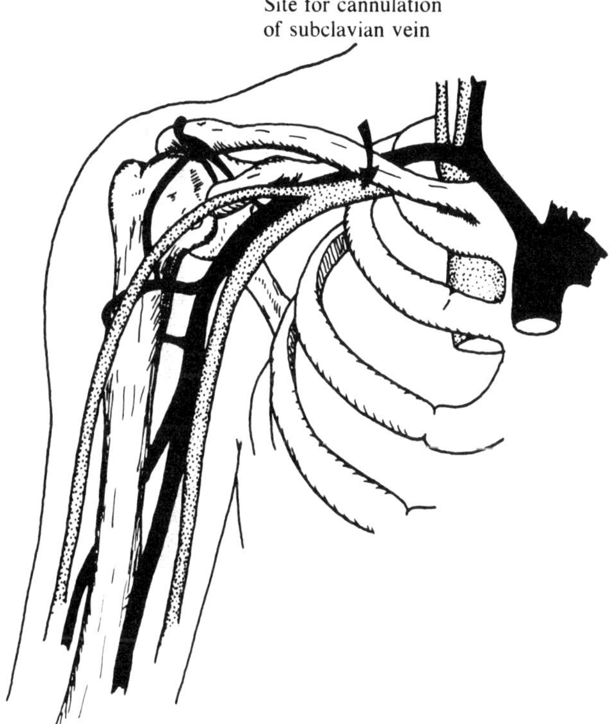

Figure 5-15. The subclavian vein is best cannulated at the junction of the medial and middle third of the clavicle.

met, long before the catheter would have reached the right atrium. Withdraw the catheter, but never through a needle. It may be necessary to start all over again at another site. The femoral vein is more difficult to keep clean and is less accessible during most operations. It is, therefore, not preferred.

Subclavian Vein

Catheterization of the subclavian vein was described by Aubaniac.[13] We rarely use this method because of its higher incidence of major complications. The vein can be catheterized from either the right or the left side.

The patient lies supine with his lands at his sides. Place a support under the shoulder of the side to be cannulated, and tilt the table 15°, head down, to minimize air embolism. Locate the junction between the middle and the medial third of the clavicle and prepare and drape the area sterilely (Fig. 5-15). After local anesthesia with 1% lidocaine without epinephrine, puncture the skin under the clavicle at the junction of the middle to the medial third of the clavicle while aiming the needle at the sternal notch and advancing it close to the clavicle at approximately a 15° angle. Maintaining this angle is not as important as staying close to the clavicle. Although the technique is simple, the potential complications of pneumothorax or hemothorax are more common than with the other methods. Even neurologic damage has been reported: in one case a left-sided paralysis of the phrenic nerve, and in another case a total brachial-plexus paresis that developed after the subclavian artery had been nicked.[14]

When the catheter tip is to be placed in the vena cava it may move cephalad instead toward the right atrium. The patient may complain of an earache, and roentgenologic check may show the tip of the catheter at the level of the mastoid.[15]

Confirmation of the Catheter Tip Location

Electrocardiography

The tip of a central venous catheter (CVC) can be located under electrocardiographic guidance. A modified lead II is used for this, as reported by Richards and Freeman.[16] With the selector switch in the lead II position, the leg and left arm electrodes are left in place and the right arm electrode is modified as follows. Fill the catheter with saline and advance it into the superior vena cava. Then, thread a sterile surgical wire into the CVC so that the wire is in contact with the saline to provide a good electrode. Connect the right arm lead to the wire with an alligator clip. Observe the ECG while the probe is lying in the superior vena cava. By advancing the probe further, a characteristic spiking of the P-wave occurs (Fig. 5-16). Maximal spiking of the P-wave indicates that the probe is in midatrial position; this P-wave may exceed the height of the R-wave. With further advancement, the *P*-wave becomes smaller again and may, in fact, become biphasic. Arrhythmias may occur when the catheter impinges on the ventricular wall. The R-wave is tall when the tip lies in the right ventricle.

Recently Johans[17] has suggested an easier way to obtain electrocardiograph signals through a catheter. As shown in Figure 5-17, a connector is attached to the saline-filled central catheter. The connector consists of a stainless steel, male electrocardiographic nipple, which accepts any female electrode. The saline thus acts as a conductor of the electrocardiographic signal as it travels from the distal catheter lumen to the connector.

This method is convenient but has one potential danger. The catheter can become an active electrode while in the heart; in which case, very little current produces depolarization, an extra systole, or even ventric-

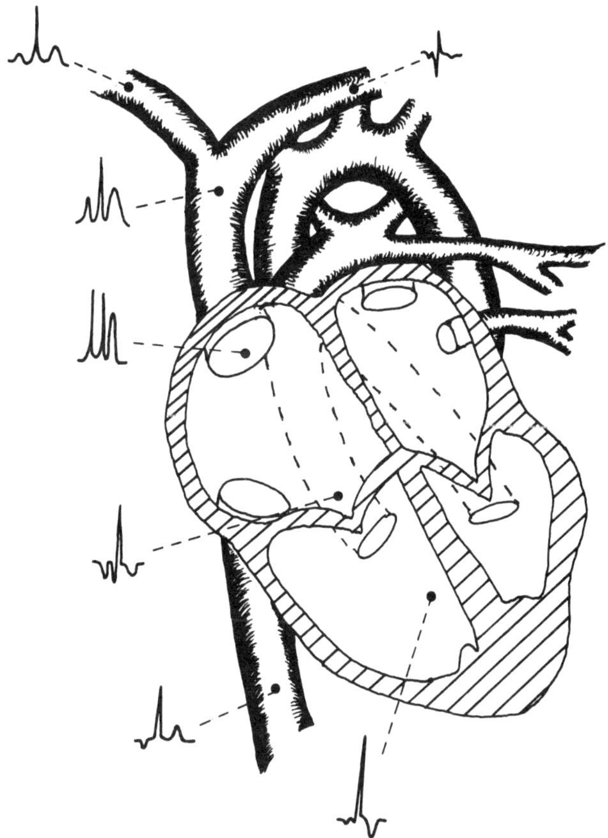

Figure 5-16. The P-wave is the key to proper location of the central venous catheter. Place it where the P-wave amplitude peaks if you wish to place it into the right atrium.

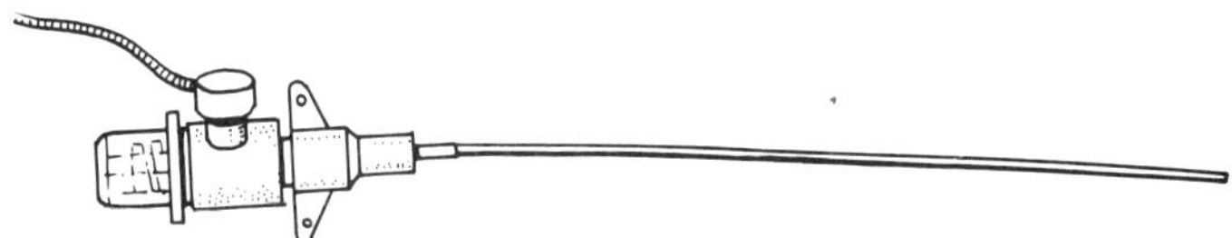

Figure 5-17. Electrocardiograph connection to central vein cannula. A sterile connector inserted between catheter and intravenous tubing allows easy connection of a standard electrocardiograph lead for the recording of an electrocardiogram during advancement of a catheter toward the right atrium.

ular fibrillation. The method should, therefore, be used only if it is known that no electricity can leak into the intracardiac lead (see Chap. 18).

Roentgenography

Location of the catheter tip roentgenographically is sound practice whenever assurance is needed that the catheter tip is properly placed in the vena cava or right atrium or to determine the catheter's location in the pulmonary artery. A chest roentgenogram taken in the operating room before the operation provides this information and much peace of mind. All modern catheters used for cannulation of the right atrium or the pulmonary artery are now radiopaque. A little dye injected into the catheter, for example, Renografin, can strengthen the image of the catheter.

Tocino describes a radiologic sign, a gentle curve at the tip of a central venous catheter, which was a harbinger of superior vena caval perforation in six of nine patients (Fig. 5-18).[18] Appearance of this sign calls for immediate repositioning of the catheter and re-examination by radiograph.

Doppler Technique

As described elsewhere (see Chap. 11), a Doppler probe over the right atrium will give a signal when 1 ml of 100% CO_2 gas is injected into the catheter.

Pressure and Waveforms

Catheters are usually intended for monitoring pressures. Typical waveforms mark the right atrium, right ventricle, and the pulmonary artery (see Fig. 5-19).

Fogarty Catheter Technique

Occasionally, a catheter tip comes to lie in an inappropriate vein, and attempts to reposition it fail. Schaefer suggests a simple and quick method to redirect, for instance, a subclavian catheter that has slipped into the internal jugular vein.[19,20]

With strict aseptic technique, the catheter is freed from sutures and dressings. A balloon-tipped 2-French Fogarty catheter, longer than the mispositioned catheter, is slid through it to a position 2 cm to 3 cm beyond the tip of the mispositioned catheter. The balloon is inflated. Both catheters are then withdrawn until only the Fogarty catheter is intravascular. A light resistance indicates when the balloon reaches the venous entrance. Now, gently advance the Fogarty catheter alone with the balloon inflated. The Fogarty catheter should "float" into the desired position, which can

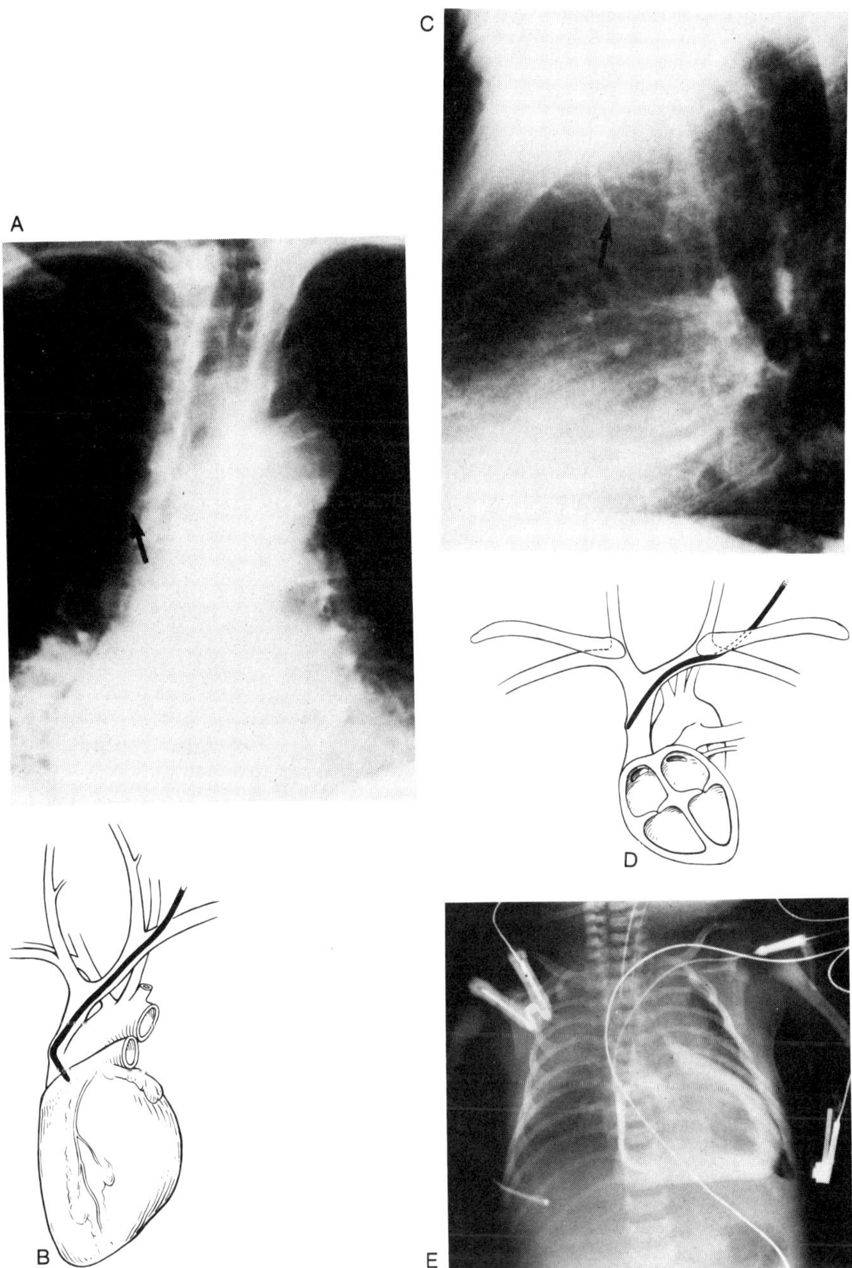

Figure 5-18. Two days after a central venous catheter was inserted, an anteroposterior view showed that the catheter tip appeared to rest against the wall of the superior vena cava (*A* and *B*). A lateral view obtained for further definition showed the bent catheter (*C* and *D*), which eventually perforated the vena cava. *E* shows a similar case, here a child, in whom perforation of an atrium or vena cava with a central catheter was demonstrated with the injection of contrast media that led to opacification of the pericardial space. (Views *A* and *C* courtesy of I.M. Tocino, M.D.)

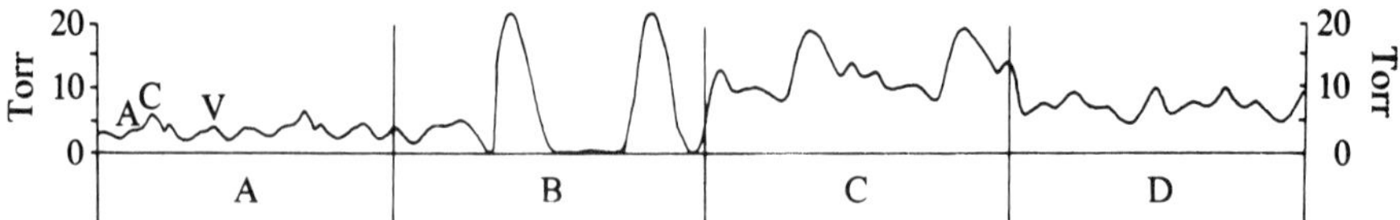

Figure 5-19. Typical pressure waveforms as pulmonary arterial catheter is "floated" into position. *A* is the right atrium. *B* is the right ventricle. *C* is the pulmonary artery. Note the sudden increase in diastolic pressure. *D* is the PA occlusion (wedge). Use the end-diastolic, end-expiratory value when reporting occlusion pressure.

then be confirmed as described above. When the position seems correct, the original catheter is pushed over the Fogarty catheter. The balloon is then deflated and the Fogarty catheter withdrawn.

CARDIAC PRESSURES

Central Venous Pressure

The so-called *central venous pressure* (CVP) is usually measured in the right atrium. The catheter tip may lie in the right atrium close to the tricuspid valve, somewhere else in the right atrium, or in the superior vena cava. Although there are no valves between the tricuspid valve and the vena cava, one must realize that, during diastole, the mean pressure is a little higher in the vena cava than in the right atrium close to the tricuspid valve; otherwise, blood would not flow. If the patient is not supine and horizontal, the hydrostatic pressure between the catheter tip and the right atrium influences the pressure. Pressure in the internal and external jugular veins can be used to approximate right atrial pressure,[21] but if the head is turned toward the side of cannulation, inaccurate readings can result. The patient's position, therefore, has to be taken into account.

Once the catheter is properly placed, it is connected to a monitor, usually a properly calibrated transducer (see Chap. 4). Water manometers are also used, but they respond sluggishly and have, therefore, been criticized.[22] The pressure changes generated by ventilation and cardiac activity can be observed. When these are displayed on paper or on an oscilloscope, three positive waves can be identified. These reflect the pressures of the right atrium shown in Fig. 5-19. The waves are labeled sequentially A, C, and V.

The A-wave represents atrial contraction and, therefore, follows the P-wave on the ECG. If the atrium does not contract, no A-wave is seen. If, however, the right atrium contracts and the tricuspid valve remains closed, then the A-wave rises sharply, as right atrial pressure increases

Table 5-3. CVP AND INFERENCE ABOUT BLOOD VOLUME*

	Assume		Conclude
Measured CVP	**Cardiac Output**	**State of the Heart**	**Effective Blood Volume**
Below normal	Normal	Normal	Low
Below normal	High	Hyperdynamic	Normal
Normal	Normal	Normal	Normal
Normal	High	Hyperdynamic	High
Normal	Low	Depressed	Low
Elevated	High	Normal	High
Elevated	Low	Depressed	Normal

* The table outlines common observations with low, normal, and high CVP. If blood volume is stable, inferences about the state of the heart and cardiac output are made. Note that measuring CVP without matching it with other information can be misleading.

dramatically. After the atrium has contracted and relaxed, the ventricle contracts, which causes the tricuspid valve to bulge and the pressure in the right atrium to increase. This contraction is represented by the C-wave, which follows the QRS complex. The third wave, the V-wave, rises as the right atrium is filled during diastole. The pressure of the V-wave increases because the tricuspid valve remains closed.

Clinical Application

Although measuring CVP may be helpful, it must be interpreted perspicaciously.[23] Common findings are summarized in Table 5-3.

The measurement of CVP is particularly helpful for patients who have no cardiovascular disease. The preload of the right ventricle often corresponds to the preload of the left ventricle. However, if the left ventricle is failing and the right ventricle continues to function adequately, the CVP can remain normal while the left atrial pressure increases. Eventually, the right ventricle, pumping against an increased afterload, will also fail, thereby increasing CVP. Monitoring the CVP of patients with some forms of congenital heart disease, such as atrial septal defects and tricuspid disease, is useful.

Pulmonary Arterial Pressures

Placing the Pulmonary Artery Catheter

Catheterization of the pulmonary artery with a balloon-tipped catheter was popularized by Swan and Ganz. Swan[24] put it this way, "I was watching the sailboats going by one September afternoon on Santa Monica Bay and I thought, Why not put a sail on the end of the catheter?''

Many balloon-tipped catheters are now available. They vary in size, number of lumens, location of pressure ports, and additional features.

Diameter	Length (cm)	Location of Pressure Ports
	Adult Pulmonary Artery Pressure	
5F	110	Tip
6F	110	Tip
7F	110	Tip
	Pediatric Pulmonary Artery Pressure	
4F	60	Tip
5F	60	Tip
	Adult Thermodilution	
7F	110	Tip as well as 30 cm from tip
7F	110	Tip as well as 30 cm from tip—infusion port 31 cm from tip
	Pediatric Thermodilution	
5F	75	Tip as well as 15 cm from tip
	Pacing	
7F	110	Tip as well as 30 cm from tip—two ventricular and three atrial pacing electrodes

Placing a pulmonary arterial (PA) catheter is a highly invasive procedure. Surgical rules of sterility, including preparing the skin, draping, and using sterile gloves, must be obeyed.

We prefer to use the right internal jugular vein for the insertion of a balloon-tipped PA catheter. Other available routes are the right or left subclavian veins; the right and left anticubital fossa, by using the basilic vein; the left internal jugular vein; the left or right external jugular vein; or the right or left femoral veins. We use the Seldinger technique. Insert the guide wire into the chosen vein as suggested. Enlarge the hole by sliding a number 11 blade along the wire. Be sure both skin and underlying fascia are penetrated adequately. Then place over the wire an introducer one French size larger than that of the PA catheter to be used (see Fig. 5-7). The introducer usually consists of two concentric plastic catheters (some units have only one), an inner dilator, and an outer sheath that are

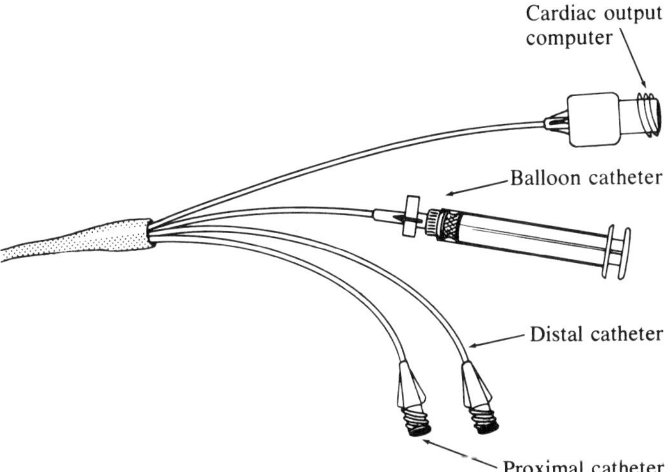

Figure 5-20. Thermodilution pulmonary arterial catheter connections. *Proximal* and *distal* are labeled on the catheter.

used in succession to progressively enlarge the access to the vein through which the PA catheter will be inserted. We prefer to use introducers that have a valved sheath. This reduces blood loss and the risk of air embolism. Advance both catheters simultaneously and briskly into the vein, while at all times holding the guide wire. You will feel a popping as the catheters enter the vein. (When a large catheter in the central veins or the right atrium is open to air, the danger of air aspiration and venous air embolism threatens. A sudden, deep breath might lower the patient's intrathoracic pressure and aspirate air. If the patient is awake during the placement of these catheters, ask him to hold his breath while you are pushing the catheter in. Head-down (Trendelenburg) position and attention to detail are important.) Withdraw the inner catheter as well as the guide wire. Watch for free nonpulsatile blood flow. Place a finger over the outer lumen. Take the looped PA catheter in one hand and give the end of the catheter to an assistant so that it may be connected to a transducer (Fig. 5-20). After the catheter is connected to a transducer, all lumina of the catheter are filled with heparinized saline solution (1 unit of heparin/ml sterile, normal saline), at which time the integrity of the balloon is tested. Check the manufacturer's instructions for the capacity of the balloon. Attach a syringe to the proper lumen to inflate the balloon. Inflate the balloon and carefully note the volume at which the balloon first inflates. You should feel the balloon start to inflate suddenly as you inject air with the syringe. Continue to inflate the balloon to the recommended volume. Some clinicians place the balloon under sterile water to detect small leaks.

Be certain not to inflate the balloon more than is suggested or it may burst. Do not use balloons that inflate eccentrically. If the balloon does not inflate, be certain that the syringe is properly attached and that the gate valve at the hub of the catheter is open. Should the balloon break while in place and 1 ml to 2 ml of air be emitted into the venous circulation, little harm is done. However, as little as 1 ml of air in the arterial circulation causes serious problems. If there is a chance for air to enter the systemic circulation (*e.g.*, by a right-to-left intracardiac shunt or a pulmonary arterial-venous fistula), the balloon should be inflated with carbon dioxide. Carbon dioxide (100%) is 20 times more soluble in serum than air. Remember that 20% to 30% of patients have a potential opening between right and left atria.

The integrity of the balloon may be checked while the catheter is in the patient. After the first measurement is made, release the plunger. It should spring back. If it does not, the balloon may have ruptured. Do not actively aspirate the balloon because this may cause it to rupture.

Once the catheter is inserted through the introducer set and connected to a monitor, a waveform should appear. Slowly and gently advance the catheter and watch the waveform and the ECG. Have 50 mg to 100 mg lidocaine available and give it intravenously should ventricular arrhythmias persist during placement. When the catheter enters the junction of either the superior or the inferior vena cava and the atrium, a respiratory variation in the pressure trace appears (Fig. 5-19) and indicates that the catheter tip is in the thorax. Then, right atrial pressure with the A-, C-, and V-waves will be seen. In the adult, the catheter tip will have been advanced approximately 40 cm from the right or 50 cm from the left antecubital fossa, 15 cm to 20 cm from the jugular vein, or 20 cm from the femoral vein. When the right atrial pressure trace is identified, inflate the balloon to the recommended volume. While watching both the ECG and the continuous pressure monitor, advance the catheter. The right ventricle will shortly be entered and is identified by a marked change in the pressure trace (Fig. 5-19). Systolic and diastolic right ventricle pressures will be prominent. Continue to advance the catheter and eventually you will feel a nibbling sensation on the catheter. This is the pulmonary valve (not a bass).

Once this is passed, the pressure changes (Fig. 5-19). The systolic pressure remains as before, but the diastolic pressure is much higher than in the right ventricle. This identifies the pulmonary artery. If the pulmonary artery is not entered after 20 cm to 30 cm of catheter has been inserted from the first recognition of the right atrial trace, the catheter is not advancing properly. Deflate the balloon by releasing the plunger. If the plunger moves to some extent, but not freely, disconnect the syringe from the catheter to allow the balloon to collapse. (Do not actively withdraw air from the balloon; this may cause it to rupture.)

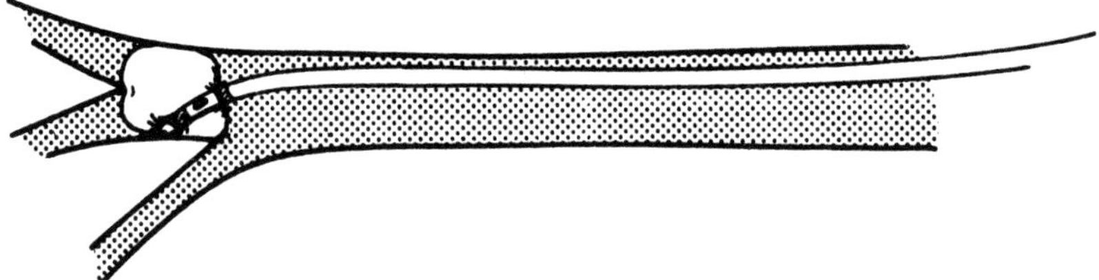

Figure 5-21. Over-wedging. The balloon is overinflated or the inside diameter is asymmetric. The catheter tip pressure port is occluded by the balloon.

In patients with the right atrium or right ventricle enlarged, with low cardiac output or with tricuspid regurgitation, a deep voluntary inspiration will help to advance the catheter (but guard against aspiration of air into the venous system!). Sometimes it is necessary to inject a very small dose of epinephrine to raise cardiac output transiently so that the balloon-tipped catheter will float into the pulmonary artery.

Once the catheter has entered the pulmonary artery, continue to advance the catheter slowly. Suddenly, the systolic pressure will drop substantially and the diastolic pressure will drop a little (Fig. 5-19). This means the tip of the catheter is exposed to the forward (wedge) pressure but no longer to the right ventricular pressures, which are blocked by the balloon. Then, deflate the balloon. This reestablishes the amplitude previously recognized as the pulmonary artery pressure. By reinflating the balloon, the pulmonary capillary wedge pressure is obtained again. Anchor the catheter in place.

A PA pressure trace must be watched continuously because the pulmonary artery may become occluded. Also, the catheter material softens with time, which shortens the transcardiac catheter loop. This allows the catheter tip to migrate into smaller branches of the pulmonary artery and to occlude them. Sudden changes in the patient's blood volume may also contribute to "wedging" of the catheter. If a pulmonary capillary wedge pressure trace is obtained with the balloon deflated, irrigate the catheter. Often, a clot forms on the tip of the catheter and sometimes mimicks pulmonary capillary wedge pressure. Flush the catheter lumen with a few milliliters of heparinized fluid. Even though this releases the clot into the pulmonary arterial system, there is no alternative because the clots cannot be aspirated. If flushing resolves the problem, pull back the catheter 1 cm to 2 cm. A PA trace should be obtained once again.

When convenient, place the PA catheter under fluoroscopy. The catheter is easy to place because its "sail" makes it flow-directed.

Be careful not to inflate the balloon excessively. This may cause overwedging where the opening (Fig. 5-21) of the distal tip of the catheter is compromised, mimicking an elevated pressure. We have seen instances when the recorded pressure exceeded the systolic PA pressure (not a physiologic condition). After each measurement, be certain to deflate the balloon. The normal pressures observed for the various chambers in the heart are shown in Table 5-2.

Physiology of Pulmonary Artery Pressure Measurements

In order to see why PA catheterization is helpful in determining left ventricular preload, we must examine the cardiac cycle.

In early ventricular systole, both the right and left ventricles contract isovolumetrically. This means that the aortic, pulmonary, tricuspid, and mitral valves are closed. This lasts only a short time. Both pulmonic and aortic valves open when the pressure in both the right and left ventricles exceeds the pressures in the pulmonary artery and aorta, respectively. In early diastole, both atria are filled as blood returns to the heart. In late diastole, both atria contract, thereby filling the ventricles. During this period, both the mitral and tricuspid valves are open, but the aortic and pulmonary valves are closed. If we monitor the pressure in the left atrium during the cardiac cycle, we see the three positive waves: A-, C-, and V-waves. The A-wave occurs at the initiation of the QRS complex (Fig. 5-19). The V-wave appears at about the time that the T-wave appears on the electrocardiogram, and the C-wave is seen between the A- and V-waves. The A-wave is caused by atrial contraction during the atrial systole, and the C-wave by pressure generated in the atria by the ventricle (*i.e.*, when the mitral valve bulges back into the atrium during ventricular systole). The V-wave is caused by passive filling during diastole.

The pulmonary arterial and the right ventricular pressures are basically equivalent during systole. However, due to pulmonic valve closure, the diastolic pressure in the right ventricle is considerably less than that in the pulmonary artery. Without obstruction or pulmonary disease, the PA diastolic pressure reflects the end-diastolic pressure of the left atrium. However, in order to isolate the pressure in the left atrium further, consider the following idea.

If a catheter is placed in the pulmonary artery, the pressure at the catheter tip is the pressure in the pulmonary artery at any time. If the balloon that is just proximal to the tip of the PA catheter is inflated so that the pulmonary artery is occluded, the pressure at the tip of the catheter will reflect that in the left atrium. This is the PA occlusion pressure. The value obtained during occlusion is called *PA occlusion pressure* or *pulmonary capillary wedge pressure*. If the artery remains occluded while the mitral valve is open (at the end of left ventricular diastole), thc pressure in the pulmonary artery also reflects that in the left atrium and in the left ventricle. This pressure, the left ventricular end-diastolic pressure, is measured at the end of expiration in order to eliminate distortions from airway pressure. If the balloon is deflated during left ventricular end-diastole, not only PA pressure but also left ventricular end-diastolic pressure (LVEDP) will be recorded. Therefore, PA end-diastole pressure at end-expiration is used many times as an indication of LVEDP or preload.

A few precautions must be taken when using PA end-diastolic pressure or PA occlusion pressure as an indication of LVEDP. First, be certain to zero the transducer to the mid-heart level, which we assume to be at the intersection of the mid-axillary line and the fifth intercostal space. Cross and colleagues suggest a lateral chest roentgenogram to establish a proper reference point—the mid-heart.[25] The same roentgenogram is examined for PA catheter tip location. The course of the superior or inferior vena cava is outlined by the balloon-tipped PA catheter. If the catheter tip lies posterior to the vena cava, the PA occlusion pressure will accurately reflect left atrial pressure, even with positive end-expiratory pressure (PEEP). If the tip is anterior to the vena cava, PA occlusion pressure will reflect airway pressure, particularly with mechanical ventilation and PEEP.[26] Fortunately, most catheter tips are posteriorly located.

During systole, both the tricuspid and the mitral valves are closed. Since the pulmonic valve is open and the balloon is deflated, the pressure measured will be that of PA systole. If the balloon remains inflated during systole, the tip of the catheter is isolated from the pressure generated by right ventricular contraction.

Clinical Application

Often CVP and pulmonary capillary wedge pressure correlate well, particularly when the ejection fraction* is normal or close to normal (*i.e.*, greater than 0.5), and if no angiographically demonstrable ventricular dyssynergy exists.[27,28]

The PA pressure at end-expiration at the end of diastole correlates with LVEDP within 1 torr to 2 torr. However, reliance on this measurement must be tempered. In several clinical situations (*e.g.*, pulmonary hypertension or increased pulmonary vascular resistance), PA wedge pressure or PA end-diastolic pressure does not correlate well with LVEDP. At left atrial pressures of 10 torr or less, PA occlusion pressure and left atrial pressure usually coincide, but, as left atrial pressure increases to 15 torr or more, there is less correlation. When PA occlusion pressure rises over 15 torr, left atrial pressure may be 5 torr higher or lower. Thus, at low left atrial pressure, less than about 5 torr, pulmonary venous pressure and left atrial pressure are independent of each other.

Smith and Butler describe a pulmonary venous "waterfall" effect.[29] Further complicating matters in some clinical situations, LVEDP may not

* The *ejection fraction* is the fraction (also often expressed as a percentage) of the ventricular end-diastolic volume which is pumped into the aorta during systole. A normal ejection fraction should be 0.7; in other words, the ventricle should empty itself about 70% with every systole.

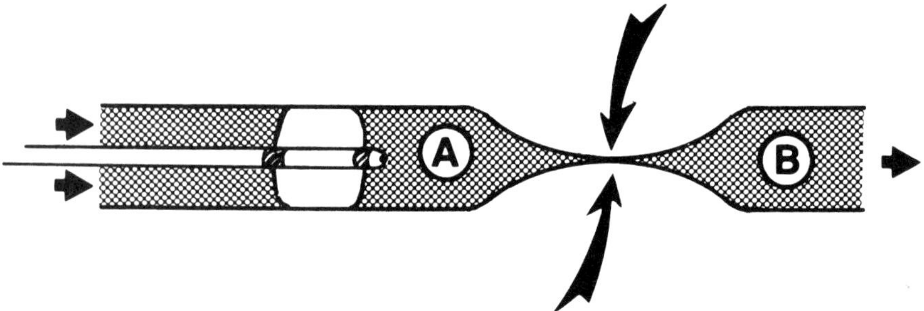

Figure 5-22. The tip of a pulmonary arterial catheter cannot sense left atrial pressure (*area B*) if high airway pressure collapses the vessel. Two conditions favor collapse: an inflated balloon, which blocks systolic pressure from reaching *area A*, and high airway pressures.

be a reflection of the left ventricular end-diastolic volume.[30] For example, Hansen and co-workers found poor correlation between PA wedge pressure and left ventricular end-diastolic volume after coronary artery bypass graft surgery.[31] If a PA catheter with its balloon inflated is positioned in a pulmonary arterial branch with an obstruction distal to the tip of the catheter, the pressures sensed at the tip reflect neither pressures distal to the obstruction (area B in Fig. 5-22) nor diastolic PA pressures. Pulmonary arterial segments may collapse during the inspiratory phases of mechanical ventilation or whenever airway pressure exceeds the pressure distal to the inflated balloon. The PA occlusion pressure then reflects only local conditions (area A in Fig. 5-22).

The decision to monitor invasively with a central venous or PA catheter is still based more on personal beliefs and clinical experiences than on scientifically established data. Furthermore, economic considerations will influence this decision to an ever increasing degree. Several authors have reported on the subject.[28–29,32–35] From these studies and the experience in our and other institutions, we conclude that invasive monitoring is rarely justified—and considerable savings can be realized by avoiding it—in normotensive patients with good ejection fractions. In patients with poor ejection fraction and congestive failure undergoing major surgical interventions, pulmonary arterial monitoring is probably justified. CVP monitoring will reflect, reasonably well, left atrial pressure in some 35% of patients with heart disease. If the clinical course of such patients is benign, one may well limit monitoring to the central venous system, thus saving a considerable amount of money. Should information on output or PA occlusion pressure become important in the course of anesthesia, a PA catheter can be inserted using the already established access route used for the central venous catheter. This can be done by threading a Seldinger wire into the venous catheter, then withdrawing the venous catheter and inserting the PA catheter over the wire, or by placing a large introducer into the internal jugular vein, which can be used as needed either for a central venous or a PA catheter. This approach will often allow the clinician to get by with the least expensive option.

Looking over the last 15 years, the authors are impressed with the changes in attitudes in the medical community. In the mid- to late 1970s, PA catheterization was thought to be indicated in many patients who today are allowed to go through anesthesia—even for cardiac operations—without a PA catheter. Thus, the pendulum is clearly swinging toward less invasive methods. This development speaks perhaps more forcefully than studies in which authors support local customs and beliefs. We are now witnessing the introduction of noninvasive cardiac output measuring devices and intra-operative transesophageal echocardiography. These, in conjunction with pulse oximetry and continuous noninvasive blood pressure monitors, will allow us to to treat more and more patients without invasive monitors. The suggestion that PA pressure monitoring permits early detection of cardiac ischemia requires confirmation. Such confirmation must come from epidemiologic studies that show statistically significant differences rather than anecdotal reports of patients. Abnormal segmental ventricular wall motions and thickness as observed by echocardiography may be the most sensitive indicators of myocardial ischemia.

CARDIAC OUTPUT

The amount of blood pumped by the heart during 1 minute is called the cardiac output (CO). Cardiac output equals heart rate times stroke volume. Stroke volume is the amount of blood that the ventricles eject with each beat. Normal adult CO ranges from about 4 liters to 7 liters per minute. Cardiac index equals CO in liters per minute divided by body surface area in square meters (Fig. 5-23). For children in particular, the cardiac index provides a convenient standard.

Several methods have been used to measure CO. With a balloon-tipped PA catheter, CO is estimated by the thermodilution method. When no PA catheter is in place, the indicator dye dilution or Doppler methods can be used. Because thermodilution determinations of CO are so easy to make, the method is popular.

Thermodilution Method

For the thermodilution method the following equation applies:

$$CO = \frac{1.08 C_T 60 V_I (T_B - T_I)}{\int_0^{\infty} \Delta T_B(t)dt}$$

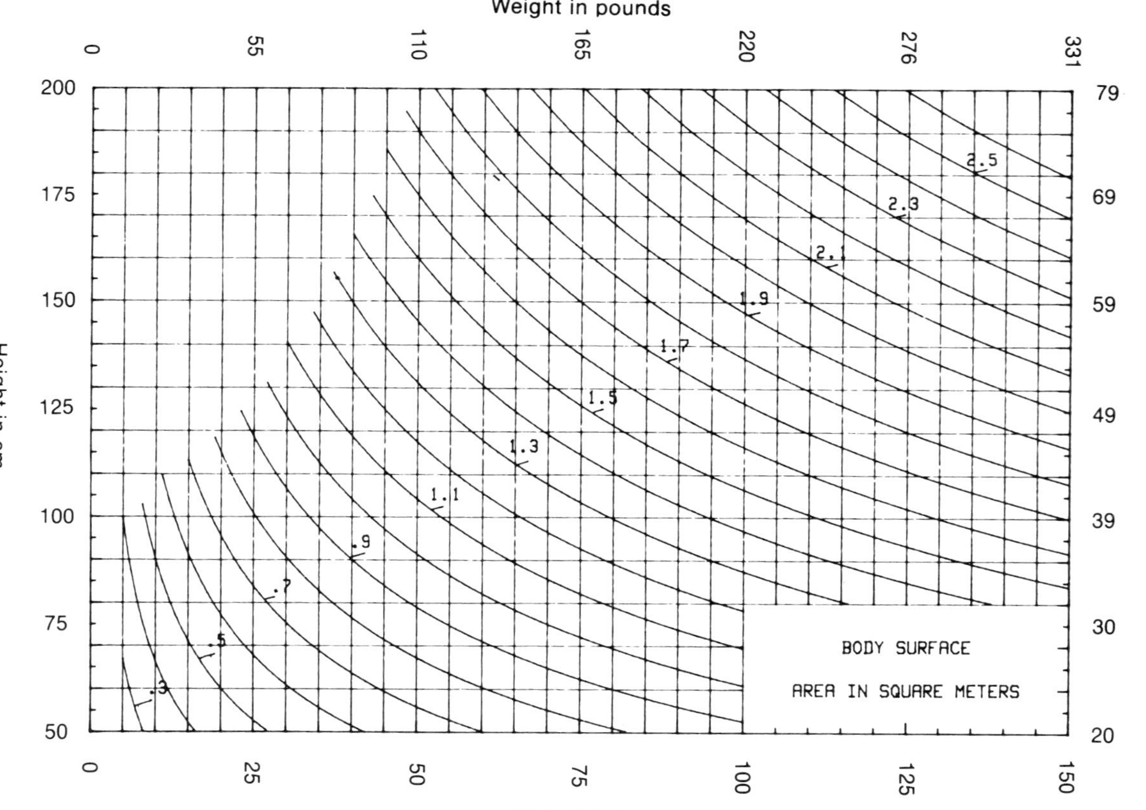

Figure 5-23. Surface area. Based on the formula $WT^{0.425} \times Ht^{0.725} \times 0.007184$ = surface area (m^2), a graph was prepared that allows an estimation of surface area. A patient weighing 60 kg and standing 170 cm tall would have an approximate surface area of 1.7 m^2.

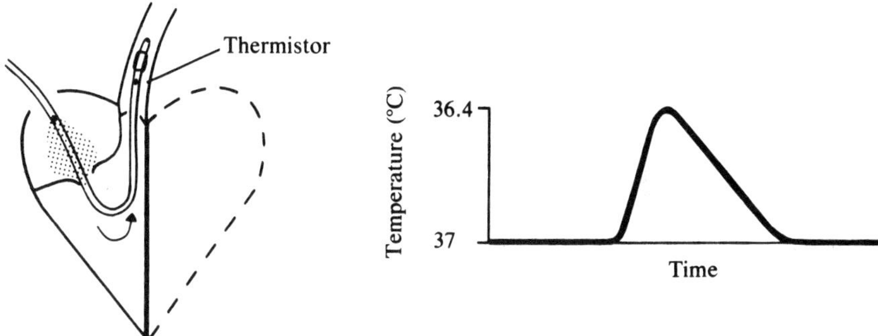

Figure 5-24. A bolus of cold solution is injected mixing with blood (*stippled area*) in the heart chambers. Temperature change is sensed distally by a thermistor.

CO = cardiac output (liters/min)
C_T = correction for the injectate temperature rise
V_I = volume of the injectate (ml)
T_B = initial blood temperature (°C)
T_I = initial injectate temperature (°C)
60 = seconds in 1 minute
1.08 = ρC_p (5% dextrose)/ρC_p (blood)

The equation simply describes the fact that two substances of unequal temperatures are mixed and that the resultant temperature is a function of the previous temperatures of the two substances. If we know the mass of one of the substances (the injected saline), as well as the temperature of the saline and blood, and if we know the specific heat and the density of one, we can calculate the mass (the volume) of the second substance (the blood).

In practice, a known amount of solution is injected through the proximal port of the catheter. After injection, the temperature measured near the tip of the catheter drops much with low flow (the cold lingers) and little with high flow (warm blood sweeps away the cold) (Fig. 5-24). Change in temperature is sensed by a thermistor downstream. The temperature change detected by the thermistor is plotted as a function of time. The curve thus generated is called the *thermodilution curve*. The area determined under the curve becomes a portion of the denominator of the calculation for CO. To estimate CO by the thermodilution method, proceed as follows.

An injectate at room temperature[36] gives an accurate and reproducible CO reading. Ice-cold injectate can lead to bradycardia and, as a result of the mechanism, to an artifactually reduced cardiac output.[37] We use a 10-ml volume for adults and 5 ml for children and keep the injectate at room temperature. Before starting, check computer and all connections and confirm that both the patient's and injectate's temperature readings are reasonable. Enter the proper correction factor. It is entered to account for the volume and temperature of the injectate used. Once the instrument is ready, draw the selected volume into the syringe and attach it to the proximal lumen connector of the catheter. (Note that not all catheters are thermal dilution catheters. Make certain of the type you have before you start.) Activate the computer just before injection. At the end of expiration or peak inspiration, swiftly inject the total amount to be used.[38] Cardiac output is displayed on the instrument. Do this twice more and average the results, if they are all within about 10% of each other. If the results do not make sense, check that the following are true:

- The PA catheter tip is properly placed.
- The correct correction factor has been entered.
- The computer is working properly (see the manufacturer's instruction).
- The battery is charged (if one is used).
- The injection is done smoothly and consistently and at end-expiration or peak inspiration, using the proper temperature injectate.
- The proper lumen is being used for injection and the lumen is placed intravascularly.
- The catheter is connected to the computer.
- The patient is in a reasonably steady state.

Once CO, PA occlusion pressure, mean systemic arterial pressure, and CVP are determined, several hemodynamic and respiratory parameters may be calculated (Table 5-2). Normal intracardiac pressures are shown in Table 5-2.

Dye Dilution Method

The dye dilution technique involves the injection of green dye into the right heart or the pulmonary artery, where the dye mixes well with blood. Poor mixing, for instance, of dye injected into a peripheral vein, produces imprecise estimates. Blood samples are usually taken from the brachial artery through a densitometer that gives rise to an indicator curve similar to that shown for thermodilution (Fig. 5-24). The area under the curve is now usually measured by an automated device employing essentially the following equation:

$$CO = \frac{I \times 60}{ct}$$

CO = cardiac output (liters/min)

I = amount of indicator injected (mg)

60 = seconds in 1 minute

c = average concentration of indicator during primary passage; product of area under extrapolated downslope of dilution curve and calibration factor (mg/liter)

t = passage time (seconds)

Ultrasound

With a Doppler probe we can determine the velocity of blood flowing through a blood vessel. If the diameter of the vessel is also known, the minute volume of blood flowing through the vessel can be calculated. A beam of ultrasound directed at, and reflected from, the blood in the aorta allows us to monitor blood flow in the aorta.[39] Doppler crystals emitting and receiving ultrasound have been incorporated into esophageal probes and positioned to measure blood velocity in the descending aorta. Although positioning the probe and maintaining it there during general anesthesia is relatively easy, calibrating the signal is not. Three approaches can be used:

1. The signal coming from the descending aorta can be accepted as a dimensionless flow value. Changes in flow can then be expressed as percentage deviation from control, permitting the construction of trend data. No statement about total flow in the descending aorta can be made. Nevertheless, such noninvasive trend data would have considerable clinical utility.
2. Cardiac output can be determined by another method, for instance, thermodilution. Simultaneously, the flow in the descending aorta is recorded and then calibrated so as to reflect total cardiac output. If we assume that the ratio of total cardiac output to flow in the descending aorta will remain largely stable even during major systemic cardiovascular changes, we can report the corrected values obtained from the descending aorta as milliliters of CO.
3. The diameter of the ascending aorta can be determined (by ultrasound, radiography, or nomogram) and blood flow in the ascending aorta measured with the Doppler system. This value (ascending aorta), reflecting CO, is then used to calibrate the flow values obtained from the esophageal probe (descending aorta). Theoretically it is possible to measure the diameter and blood velocity in the ascending aorta with the help of a Doppler system applied to the suprasternal notch. However, in some patients anatomical features make that difficult. If aortic diameter changes with hypotension or hypertension, the calculations of blood flow become imprecise.

Once CO is estimated it is an easy matter to calculate cardiac index (cardiac output ÷ surface area) and peripheral resistance if mean arterial blood pressure is known. A new device, the Accucom,* is based on the Doppler principle as here outlined and offers the automated, noninvasive, and continuous estimation of CO, heart rate, cardiac index, and systemic peripheral resistance.[40]

Clinical Application

Abnormal Cardiac Output

During anesthesia, we are often concerned about an inadequate CO. Many healthy organs compensate for a reduced blood flow by extracting an additional amount of oxygen from each milliliter of blood. As more oxygen is removed, the mixed venous blood—normally, and on the average, still about 70% saturated with oxygen—shows a strikingly lower content of oxygen. Simultaneously, the difference between arterial and mixed venous oxygen content ($C(a - \bar{v})O_2$) rises. The average, resting adult consumes about 280 ml oxygen/min or about 4 ml/kg/min. The normal $C(a - \bar{v})O_2$ is 3.5 ml/dl blood. With a lower CO in relation to the demand for oxygen, the $C(a - \bar{v})O_2$ may be 5.5 ml/dl or more.

Mixed venous blood should be drawn from the pulmonary artery. Peripheral venous blood reflects only local conditions, and even right atrial blood may be poorly mixed. Normally, the Po_2 in mixed venous blood is around 35 torr to 40 torr. When it falls below 30 torr, the $C(a - \bar{v})O_2$ should be determined because CO may be inadequate to support the metabolic requirements for oxygen.

Assuming arterial blood is adequately oxygenated, oxygen delivery can be increased by increasing hemoglobin concentration, CO, or both. Increasing hemoglobin concentration raises viscosity and, at 15 g/dl, can compromise microcirculation. Cardiac output can be raised by increasing preload with fluid therapy, by raising contractility and heart rate, or by lowering afterload with drugs.

Abnormal Vascular Resistance and Cardiac Work

The work of the heart is powerfully affected by the vascular resistance against which the heart must pump. Resistance is calculated as shown in Table 5-2. In order to assess cardiac function, we must have some measure of myocardial work. We calculate left and right ventricular stroke work indices. Stroke volume is related to ejection fraction. The severity of

* Datascope, Paramus, New Jersey.

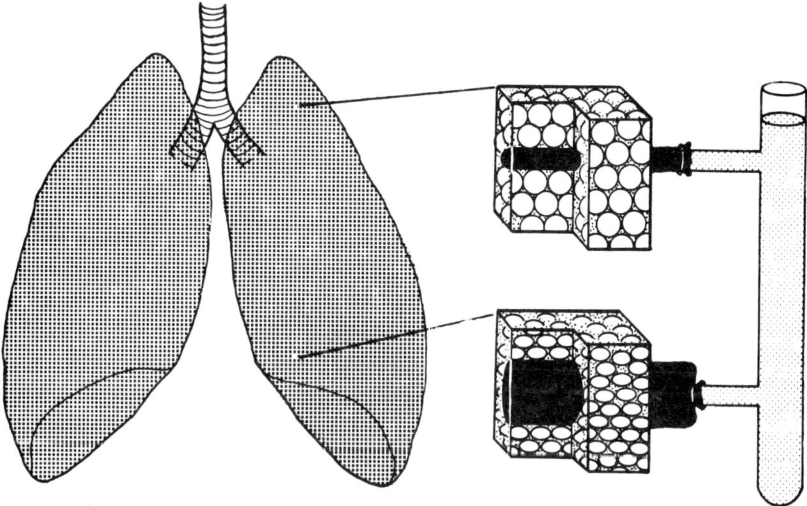

Figure 5-25. Distribution of blood flow and ventilation in the upright subject. Because of hydrostatic forces, the bases of the lungs receive relatively more blood flow than ventilation compared to the apex.

myocardial dysfunction is heavily influenced by the ability of the ventricle to empty itself. These hemodynamic parameters are not routinely monitored in the operating room but provide valuable information in the severely compromised patient.

Shunt

A low CO with a low mixed venous P_{O_2} is particularly worrisome when arterial blood also is not well oxygenated. During anesthesia, when the F_IO_2 is usually high, the arterial blood may not be as well oxygenated as the inspired P_{O_2} suggests. Often, a shunt is the culprit. Shunts may occur when venous blood gains access to the arterial circulation in the heart through intrapulmonary connections between arteries and veins or when ventilation and perfusion are not well matched.

The distribution of blood to the lungs and the ventilation in the lungs is not uniform. The dependent portions of the lung are better perfused and ventilated than the superior portions. The flow varies almost linearly from base to apex in the upright subject (Fig. 5-25). Hydrostatic pressure gradients account for most of the variation in flow. Hypoxic vasoconstriction, quite active in lungs not affected by drugs, reduces blood flow to hypoxic regions of the lung. Acidemia, particularly in conjunction with hypoxia, also causes vasoconstriction.

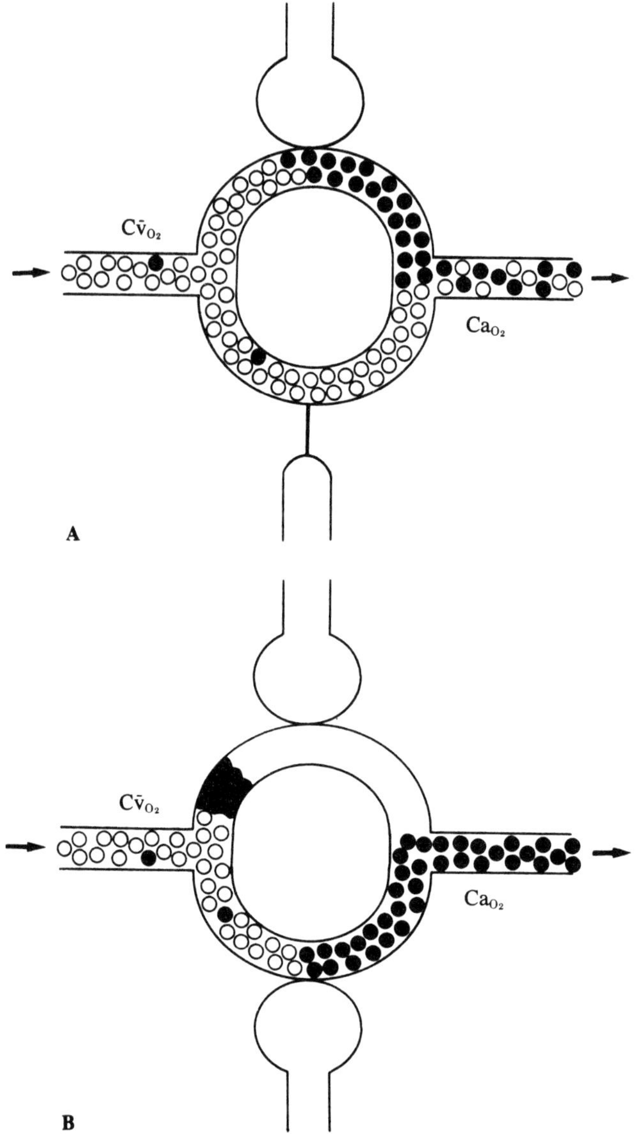

Figure 5-26. (*A*) Ventilation/perfusion mismatch. Blood flowing past ventilated alveoli becomes oxygenated; blood passing unventilated areas does not. (*B*) Ventilation/perfusion mismatch. Ventilation is normal; a part of the lung is ventilated but not perfused. *Black dots* indicate arterialized blood.

Ventilation and perfusion must be balanced for adequate gas exchange in the lungs. Even though the ratios of ventilation to perfusion differ between apex and base (Fig. 5-25), the overall average ratio of ventilation to perfusion (V_A/Q) is usually about 0.8. The variability of ventilation to perfusion is less in children and infants,[41] and during physical exercise. In patients with lung disease, ventilation–perfusion relationships are more disparate. Supine and lateral positions, mechanical ventilation, retractors in the abdomen, thoracotomy, and pulmonary congestion tend to increase the discrepancy between ventilation and perfusion.

We have illustrated a mismatch of ventilation to perfusion in two extreme conditions in Figure 5-26. In one instance (Fig. 5-26A), blood flow is quite normal, but ventilation is not. Some blood will not be oxygenated, regardless of how much more oxygen is provided with ventilation. In the other instance, ventilation is normal, but blood flow is not (Fig. 5-26B). In clinical situations, a mixture of these two extremes is responsible for ventilation–perfusion mismatches that result in a shunt.

To calculate the shunt, we need to determine the total pulmonary blood flow ($\dot{Q}_T$) and the portion that is shunted ($\dot{Q}s$). Pulmonary blood flow can be calculated by the Fick principle. Here, the oxygen content of both pulmonary arterial blood ($C_{\bar{v}}O_2$ = mixed venous O_2 content) and systemic arterial blood (C_aO_2) are determined. Oxygen consumption ($\dot{V}O_2$) is determined by analyzing all the expired gas for volume and the O_2 concentration. The following equation is solved:

$$\text{cardiac output} = \frac{\text{oxygen consumption per minute}}{\text{systemic arterial oxygen content} - \text{pulmonary arterial oxygen content}}$$

which may be written as

$$\dot{Q} = \frac{VO_2}{C_aO_2 - C_vO_2}$$

The shunt itself is estimated by using this formula:

$$\frac{\dot{Q}_S}{\dot{Q}_T} = \frac{C_cO_2 - C_aO_2}{C_cO_2 - C_{\bar{v}}O_2} \simeq 0.05$$

C_cO_2 is the oxygen content in pulmonary capillaries. Since this cannot be determined, used alveolar P_{O_2}. C_aO_2 is the oxygen content in arterial blood. $C_{\bar{v}}O_2$ is the oxygen content in mixed venous blood.

COMPLICATIONS OF CLINICAL PROCEDURES

Perforations

In 1979 Defalque and Campbell reported on the incidence of cardiac tamponade from central venous catheters.[42] This complication has a high mortality and occurs primarily when either the right atrium or the right ventricle is pierced by the catheter.

The diagnosis of this disastrous complication, which may occur within minutes or many hours of insertion of the catheter, must be entertained when suddenly abnormally elevated central venous pressures are observed, respiratory fluctuations disappear, cyanosis sets in, or venous engorgement of face and neck develop. In the conscious patient nausea, dyspnea, retrosternal or epigastric pain, restlessness, confusion, and coma may develop. In other patients few physical signs are detected. Some have died suddenly.

Defalque and Campbell recommend not using central venous catheters for massive infusions when other venous routes exist, and not placing the central venous catheter into the right atrium. The catheters (especially those placed through a vein in the arm) should be securely taped or sutured to the skin so that they cannot be advanced through motion, and the positions of these catheters should be confirmed by x-ray imaging. Their recommendation to keep the catheter tip in the vena cava rather than in the atrium deserves attention. Even the use of "soft" catheters does not prevent this. Delfaque and Campbell claim that atrial placement is rarely necessary.

Once a perforation has occurred, rapid recognition and treatment are important. Diagnosis can be established by echocardiography and roentgenography in conjunction with the slow instillation of 2 ml to 5 ml of radiopaque dye. In the case of a perforation, attempt to aspirate from the central venous catheter to empty the pericardial sac or mediastinum and slowly withdraw the catheter. When aspiration does not yield fluid and clinical signs point to pericardial tamponade, pericardiocentesis is indicated. This can be accomplished by the subxyphoid route or parasternally. If that treatment does not yield fluid and relief, surgical intervention becomes necessary.

Atrial and ventricular perforation are not the only complications caused by a central venous catheter. Several others are not so dramatic and most take time to manifest themselves.

Malposition

Catheters may be malpositioned. For example, a catheter inserted through the subclavian or basilic vein may turn cephalad rather than caudad. Similarly, a catheter introduced through the internal or external jugular vein may find its way into the contralateral neck veins or the ipsilateral arm. A long catheter pushed in too far may result in cannulation of the coronary sinus or the right ventricle.

Catheters may migrate during use. For example, during cardiac surgery the PA catheter tip may migrate several centimeters during sternal retraction. Johnston and co-workers suggest a five-centimeter catheter withdrawal just before cardiopulmonary bypass.[43]

Vascular Injury

Injuries from catheters are generally caused during insertion procedures or by erosion (friction). For example, the internal carotid or subclavian artery can be punctured, particularly during attempts to cannulate the subclavian vein or internal jugular vein. Bleeding from a subclavian artery laceration is difficult to control. Massive blood loss, hemothorax, and respiratory distress, followed by cardiovascular collapse, can occur. We have seen an aortic laceration during attempted placement of a subclavian catheter. A carotid artery puncture can cause hematoma formation with respiratory embarrassment. After such an injury one must try to still the bleeding with pressure, but this has to be done carefully; the carotid might be occluded by external pressure or carotid sinus reflexes triggered. Surgical exploration of the neck sometimes becomes necessary. Rarely an internal mammary artery or pulmonary artery will get injured during subclavian vein catheter insertion. We have seen an attempted subclavian vein catheterization result in a catheter being threaded into the pericardial sac. Injuries to both artery and vein at the same time can cause an arteriovenous fistula. Lastly, the thoracic duct may be damaged. A very rare but devastating complication is catheterization of the coronary sinus with resultant thrombosis. A hydrothorax is not uncommon and develops when the tip of the catheter comes to rest outside the vessel. We have observed over a liter of intravenous fluid in the chest cavity following such an occurrence.

Nerve Injuries

Brachial plexus, phrenic, and recurrent laryngeal nerves have been injured during both internal jugular and subclavian vein cannulation.

Respiratory

Pneumothorax is most commonly seen from an attempted subclavian vein catheterization. This injury may take days to become clinically or radiologically evident. For this reason, the normal appearance of lung fields on a chest radiograph immediately post-procedure does not rule out a developing pneumothorax.

We have seen perforation of an endotracheal tube cuff during attempted subclavian vein cannulation, which led to hypoventilation and hypoxia.

Embolism

Both air and catheter embolisms have been reported. The incidence of catheter tip embolism diminished markedly in our hospital with adoption of the Seldinger technique. This complication occurred when a catheter was withdrawn through the needle and the tip of the catheter was sheared off by the sharp facet of the needle tip. Air embolism can result whenever atmospheric pressure exceeds intravascular pressure and an open path exists between the two. It is the most lethal complication of central venous catheterization, with a 50% mortality rate.[44] Its occurrence may be much more subtle than other complications and therefore more difficult to diagnose. To prevent this complication the patient should be placed in a head-down position and should not take a deep breath or cough during insertion of the catheter. It is difficult always to maintain occlusion of the catheter, needle, or introducer during insertion, but one should try. Always attach a syringe and forcibly inject heparinized fluid through all catheter lumens to remove air and assure patency. Also, closely inspect the catheter for fluid leaks. They occur most often at the catheter hub and junctions of catheter and hub. Air may be aspirated through such breaks. When removing catheters be certain the patient is head down. After removal of the catheter, cover the entry site with an occlusive dressing. Catheter tracks can be a cause for considerable air aspiration. Patients who suddenly take a "turn for the worse" often are found to have central venous catheter–induced air embolus. This problem and its treatment are discussed in Chap. 11.

Infection

Infections related to catheters are of particular concern when catheters have to stay in place for extended times. Meticulous attention to sterile technique during all phases of catheter insertion and use is mandatory. Not only may the catheter become a nidus for infection leading to bacteremia, but reports of osteomyelitis in adjacent bone have been recorded. If infection of a catheter is suspected, a Gram stain of the distal catheter tip is a helpful and quick test.[45] Unfortunately, infective endocarditis as a consequence of catheter-induced myocardial damage may not be suspected clinically. Rowley and colleagues[46] suggest that right-sided infective endocarditis should be anticipated in bacteremic patients whose central vein or pulmonary artery has been catheterized.[37]

Clots

Thrombi form at the tip of most PA catheters and invariably cause emboli when the catheter is withdrawn. Most are benign unless they are large or become infected.

Kim and co-workers reported that, in patients with a PA catheter in place, the platelet count declined as long as the catheter was not removed and recovered once the catheter had been pulled out.[47] The difference in platelet count between patients with a PA catheter and those with a central venous catheter was statistically significant and amounted to approximately 80,000 platelets/mm^3. Platelet consumption triggered by PA catheters is, therefore, not trivial. Platelet consumption, of course, means clot formation, which may occur within a couple of hours or less after catheter placement. In order to prevent this very undesirable side-effect of PA catheterization, heparin bonding to the PA catheter has been recommended.[48]

Knots

Catheters may form knots, particularly with undue advancement of the catheter when the tip is still in the right atrium or ventricle. Should a knot be suspected, the catheter should be viewed by using fluoroscopy. First check that the balloon is deflated, then gradually withdraw the catheter. It has been reported that the use of a guide wire may resolve the problem; if not, the catheter may be gradually withdrawn until the knot tightens. Continue to pull the catheter gently. Eventually the venous segment will enlarge, which will allow the catheter to be removed. Always use heparinized saline in order to keep the lumina patent. Whenever the catheter is withdrawn, be certain that the balloon is deflated. We have seen one case in which a PA catheter and central venous pressure catheter became entangled. Only surgical exposure may be able to extricate the tangle.

Cardiac Injury

Lesions of the right side of the heart by both PA catheters and central venous catheters are quite common. Of 141 consecutive autopsy cases in which a central catheter had been used, Ducatman and colleagues found mural thrombi in 33% of the patients.[49] Rowley and co-workers had similar findings, as shown in Figure 5-27.[46] The authors found lesions on the pulmonic valve, the tricuspid valve, and the right atrium and ventricle, as well as the main pulmonary artery. Interestingly, damage was not a function of duration of catheterization, but was observed in 53% of catheterized patients.

INTRAOPERATIVE ECHOCARDIOGRAPHY

Cardiologists have employed echocardiography for several years in the diagnosis of cardiac lesions and functional disturbances. Recently, echo-

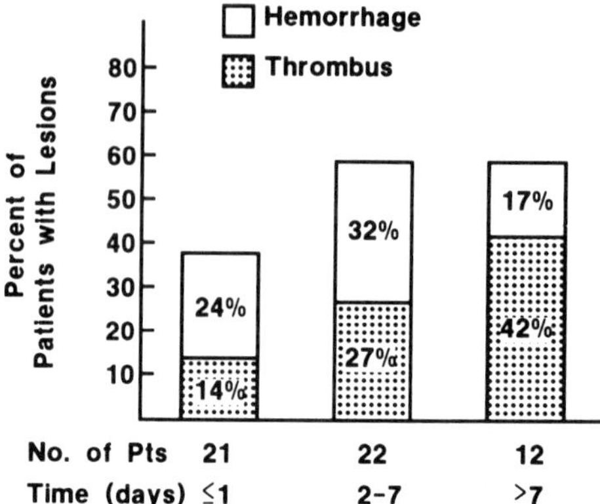

Figure 5-27. Relation of the length of time of pulmonary artery catheter placement to the frequency of observation of endocardial lesions. There were no statistically significant differences among the three groups of patients in the overall frequency of lesions or in the percentage of lesions that were thrombi. (Rowley KM et al: Right-sided infective endocarditis as a consequence of flow-directed pulmonary-artery catheterization. N Engl J Med 311:1156, 1984. Reprinted by permission of the New England Journal of Medicine.)

cardiography has been introduced into the operating room, primarily for monitoring ventricular function.

As the term "echocardiography" suggests, the structures of the heart are visualized with the help of a beam of inaudible sound that is directed at the heart and is then bounced back much as an echo in the audible range would be returned from a canyon wall. The energy used for echocardiography is in the range of 3 to 4 megahertz (MHz) which equals 3,000,000 to 4,000,000 cycles per second; audible sound lies below 20,000 cycles per second or 20 kHz.

A rapidly vibrating piezoelectric element produces short bursts (in the range of milliseconds) of ultrasound; when the instrument does not transmit it functions as a receiver, usually for hundreds of milliseconds so that there is enough time to catch the echos returning from distant structures.

The higher the frequency of the ultrasound, the better the resolution of the reflected image; unfortunately, the higher the frequency, the poorer the penetration of tissue. A frequency in the range of 3 MHz to 4 MHz offers a useful compromise between resolution (in the range of 1 mm to 2 mm) and penetration.

Echocardiographers distinguish an A mode (A for amplitude), a B mode (B for brightness), and an M mode (M or motion). A signal that returns from distant structures is attenuated and has a lower amplitude; the amplitude of the returning signal therefore reflects the distance of the structure from which the signal is returned. When the varying amplitudes returning from a moving structure are converted into brightness of different degrees, one can recognize stronger signals by their greater brightness on an oscilloscope screen. In the familiar pictures in which an echocardiogram is matched with an electrocardiogram, the oscilloscope usually sweeps from left to right and the physician can monitor in the M mode the excursions and the rate of motion of cardiac structures together with the electrocardiogram.

An additional refinement is a two-dimensional echocardiogram which relies on swiveling the ultrasonic beam rapidly back and forth so that a pie-shaped picture of cardiac structures results.

A number of investigators have now placed the ultrasonic transmitter and receiver element into the esophagus of anesthetized patients and have obtained two-dimensional echocardiograms during anesthesia. The position of the probe in the esophagus has two advantages: it reduces the distance from probe to heart and thus enhances the chances of obtaining images of excellent resolution, and it allows the application of echocardiography even during operations in which an external probe would interfere with the surgeon's work.[50]

Intraoperative transesophageal echocardiography may permit the early detection of changes of the left ventricle that occur with ischemia. Particularly wall thickness and segmental wall motion abnormalities of the left ventricle are monitored. These may develop before ST segment changes appear in the electrocardiogram.[51]

Transesophageal echocardiography is not yet widely available. It may offer significant advantages in cardiac monitoring of patients with heart disease.

CARDIAC OUTPUT BY IMPEDANCE

Since Kubicek and co-workers[52] demonstrated reproducibility of stroke volume determination by impedance cardiography in astronauts, attempts have been made to apply their work to a more heterogenous population, as is found in patients in operating rooms and intensive care units. Srameck and associates[53] and Bernstein[54] have applied modifications to Kubicek's equations that have been used to determine CO in patients.

The principle that applies is that flow in the descending aorta can be predicted from the change in electrical impedance (resistance to alternating current) in the thorax. By cleverly subtracting changes in thoracic impedance caused by respiration, motion, and diastolic filling, stroke volume can be predicted and CO calculated. Pairs of electrodes are placed along the frontal plane, bilaterally on the neck and lateral to the xiphoid process. Low-amperage, high-frequency current is applied to the most distal electrodes and voltage is measured at the more central electrodes.

The voltage changes as impedance varies with the phases of the cardiac cycle and respiration.

Clinical studies to compare CO determined by impedance and by thermodilution indicate that about 80% of the readings are within 20% of each other. This method is a noninvasive measurement technique that depends on precise and diligent electrode placement and adherence. It does present difficulties in the face of electrocautery, low CO, and dysrhythmias, as well as extremes of body habitus.[55,56]

REFERENCES

1. Larnoff SJ, Berglund E: Ventricular function. I. Starling's law of the heart studied by means of simultaneous right and left ventricular function curves in the dog. Circulation 9:706–718, 1954
2. Ream AK, Fogdall RP (eds): Acute Cardiovascular Management, Anesthesia and Intensive Care, pp 31–34. Philadelphia, JB Lippincott, 1982
3. Chambers DA: Anesthesia for the patient with acquired valvular heart disease. In Kaplan JA (ed): Cardiac Anesthesia, pp 198–199. New York, Grune & Stratton, 1979
4. Ellison N, Jobes DR, Schwartz AJ: Cannulation of the internal jugular vein: A cautionary note. Anesthesiology 55:336, 1981
5. Seldinger SI: Catheter replacement of needle in percutaneous arteriography: A new technique. Acta Radiol 39:368, 1953
6. Schwartz AJ, Horrow JC, Jobes DR, et al: Guide wires—A caution. Crit Care Med 9:347, 1981
7. Hay NTP, Mahood JHS, Pietak SP: A complication of external jugular cannulation. Anesthesiology 64:836–837, 1986
8. Kaplan JA (ed): Cardiac Anesthesia, p 80. New York, Grune & Stratton, 1979
9. Bazaral M, Harlan S: Ultrasonographic anatomy of the internal jugular vein relevant to percutaneous cannulation. Crit Care Med 9:307, 1981
10. Fabian JA, Jesudian MCS, Rah KH: Double internal jugular vein cannulation in pediatric and adult cardiac surgery patients: An easy and convenient technique. Anesth Analg 65:419–420, 1986
11. Kellner GA, Smart JF: Percutaneous placement of catheters to monitor "central venous pressure." Anesthesiology 36:515, 1972
12. Webre DR, Arens JF: Use of cephalic and basilic veins for introduction of central venous catheters. Anesthesiology 38:389, 1973
13. Aubaniac R: Une nouvelle voie d'injection ou de ponction veineuse: La voie sous-claviculaire (veine-sous claviére, tronc brachio-céphalique). Sem Hop Paris 28:3445, 1952
14. Janda A: Neurologische Komplikationen beim Vena subclavia–Katheterismus. Anaesthesist 30:148, 1981
15. Cozanitis DA: Earache following caval catheterization. Anaesthesist 30:150, 1981
16. Richards CC, Freeman A: Intra-atrial catheter placement under electrocardiographic guidance. Anesthesiology 25:388, 1964

17. Johans TG: Right atrial electrocardiography for the placement of multi-orificed catheters. Anesthesiology 64:411, 1986
18. Tocino IM, Watanbe A: Impending catheter perforation of superior vena cava: Radiographic recognition. Am J Roentgenol 146:487–490, 1986
19. Schaefer CJ, Geelhoed GW: Redirection of misplaced central venous catheters. Arch Surg 115:789, 1980
20. Schaefer CJ: Personal communication. June, 1980
21. Reynolds AD, Cross R, Latto IP: Comparison of internal jugular and central venous pressure measurements. Br J Anaesth 56:267–269, 1984
22. Civetta JM: Invasive catheterization. Crit Care 1:1(B), 1980
23. Toussaint GPM, Burgess JH, Hampson LG: Central venous pressure and pulmonary wedge pressure in critical surgical illness. Arch Surg 109:265, 1974
24. Swan HJC: Personal communication, 1978
25. Cross CJ, Cain HD, Deaton WJ, et al: Vertical relationships of the pulmonary artery catheter tip and transducer reference point in estimation of the left atrium. Am Rev Respir Dis (Part 2) 117:105, 1978
26. Kronbert GM, Quan SF, Scholbohm RM, et al: Anatomic locations of the tips of pulmonary-artery catheters in supine patients. Anesthesiology 51:467, 1979
27. Lowenstein E, Teplick R: To (PA) catheterize or not to (PA) catheterize—That is the question. Anesthesiology 53:361, 1980
28. Mangano DT: Monitoring pulmonary arterial pressure in coronary-artery disease. Anesthesiology 53:364, 1980
29. Smith HC, Butler J: Pulmonary venous waterfall and perivenous pressure in the living dog. J Appl Physiol 38:304, 1975
30. Alderman EL, Glantz SA: Acute hemodynamic interventions shift the diastolic pressure-volume curve in man. Circulation 54:662–671, 1976
31. Hansen RM, Vigverat CE, Matthay MA, et al: Poor correlation between pulmonary artery wedge pressure and left ventricular end-diastolic volume after coronary artery bypass graft surgery. Anesthesiology 64:764–770, 1986
32. Walker JG, Johnson SP, Kaplan JA: Usefulness of pulmonary artery catheters during aortocoronary bypass surgery (abstr). Anesth Analg 61:221–222, 1982
33. Kaplan JA, Wells PH: Early diagnosis of myocardial ischemia using the pulmonary artery catheter. Anesth Analg 60:789–793, 1981
34. Bashien G, Johnson PW, Davis KB, et al: Elective coronary bypass surgery without pulmonary artery catheter monitoring. Anesthesiology 63:451–454, 1985
35. Liban BJ, Davies DM: Elective coronary bypass surgery with pulmonary artery catheter monitoring. Anesthesiology 64:664–665, 1986
36. Elkayam U, Berkley R, Azen S, et al: Cardiac output by thermodilution technique. Effect of injectate's volume and temperature on accuracy and reproducibility in the critically ill patient. Chest 84:418–422, 1983
37. Harris AP, Miller CF, Beattie C, et al: The slowing of sinus rhythm during thermodilution cardiac output determination and effect of altering injectable temperature. Anethesiology 63:540–541, 1981
38. Stevens JH, Raffin TA, Mihm FG, et al: Thermodilution cardiac output measurement: Effects of the respiratory cycle on its reproducibility. JAMA 253:2240–2242, 1985

39. Chandraratma PA, Nunn M, McKay C, et al: Determination of cardiac output by transcutaneous continuous-wave ultrasound Doppler computer. Am J Cardiol 53:234–237, 1984
40. Mark JB, Steinbrook RA, Gugino LD, et al: Continuous noninvasive monitoring of cardiac output with esophageal Doppler ultrasound during cardiac surgery. Anesth Analg 65:1013–1020, 1986
41. Smith RM: Anesthesia for Infants and Children, 4th ed, pp 64–67. St. Louis, CV Mosby, 1980
42. Delfaque RJ, Campbell C: Cardiac tamponade from central venous catheters. Anesthesiology 50:249, 1979
43. Johnston WE, Royster RL, Choplin RH, et al: Pulmonary artery catheter migration during cardiac surgery. Anesthesiology 64:258–262, 1986
44. Kashuk JL, Penn I: Air embolism after central venous catheterization. Surg Gynecol Obstet 159:249–252, 1984
45. Cooper GL, Hopkins CC: Rapid diagnosis of intravascular catheter-associated infection by direct Gram staining of catheter segments. N Engl J Med 312:1142–1147, 1985
46. Rowley KM, Clubb KS, Smith GJW, et al: Right-sided infective endocarditis as a consequence of flow-directed pulmonary-artery catheterization. N Engl J Med 311:1152–1156, 1984
47. Kim YL, Richard KA, Marshall BE: Thrombocytopenia associated with Swan–Ganz catheterization in patients. Anesthesiology 53:261, 1960
48. Hoar PF, Wilson RM, Mangano DT, et al: Heparin bonding reduces thrombogenicity of pulmonary-artery catheters. N Engl J Med 305:993, 1981
49. Ducatman BS, McMichan JC, Edwards WD: Catheter-induced lesions of the right side of the heart. JAMA 253:791, 1985
50. Schluter M, Hinrichs A, Thier W, et al: Transesophageal two-dimensional echocardiography: Comparison of ultrasonic and anatomic sections. Am J Cardiol 53:1173–1178, 1984
51. Beauppe PN, Kremer P, Cahalan MK, et al: Intraoperative detection of changes in left ventricular segmental wall motion by transesophageal two-dimensional echocardiography. Am Heart J 107:1021, 1984
52. Kubicek WG, Karnegis JN, Patterson RP, et al: Development and evaluation of an impedance cardiac output system. Aerospace Med 1:208, 1966
53. Sramek BB, Rose DM, Miyamoto A: Stroke volume equation with a linear base impedance model and its accuracy as compared to thermodilution and magnetic flow meter techniques in humans and animals. Proceedings of the Sixth International Conference on Electrical Bioimpedance, Zadar, Yugoslavia, 1983, p 38
54. Bernstein DP: A new stroke volume equation for thoracic electrical bioimpedance: Theory and rationale. Crit Care Med 14:904–909, 1986
55. Appel PL, Kram HB, Mackabee J, Fleming AW, Shoemaker WC: Comparison of measurements of cardiac output by bioimpedance and thermodilution in severely ill patients. Crit Care Med 14:933–935, 1986
56. Donovan KD, Dobb GJ, Woods WPD, Hockings BE: Comparison of transthoracic electrical impedance and thermodilution methods for measuring cardiac output. Crit Care Med 14:1038–1044, 1986

CHAPTER 6

Monitoring Ventilation and Gases

VENTILATION

Problems associated with inadequate ventilation contribute significantly to the risk of anesthesia. In an analysis of "critical incidents" during anesthesia, Newbower and colleagues found that disconnected breathing circuits, incorrect gas, and inappropriate airway maintenance contributed to 37% of the critical incidents.[1] Ventilators that become disconnected are also the bane of patients dependent on mechanical ventilation in the intensive care unit. Finally, inadequate uptake or distribution of oxygen to brain, heart, and kidneys can cause devastating damage. Monitoring ventilation and the delivery and concentration of gases therefore has become a most important aspect of the care of patients in operating and recovery rooms and intensive care units. We start out with a brief summary of physiologic concepts.

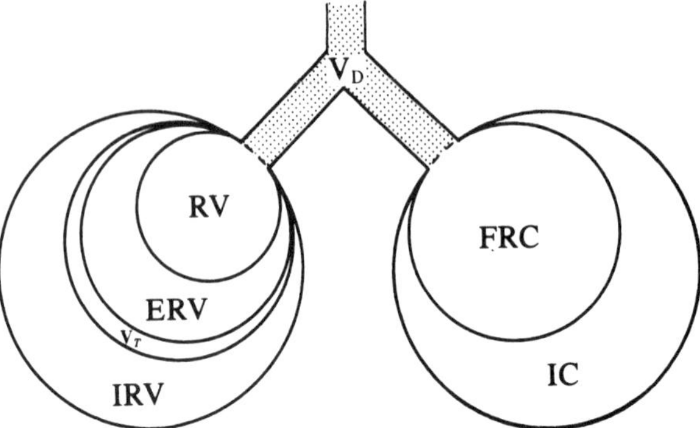

Figure 6-1. Lung volumes and capacities. V_D = dead space; *RV* = residual volume; *ERV* = expiratory reserve volume; V_T = tidal volume; IRV = inspiratory reserve volume; *FRC* = functional residual capacity; *IC* = inspiratory capacity. Vital capacity is ERV + V_T + IRV. During anesthesia V_T is often measured. FRC may decrease during anesthesia; it increases with age. Dead space may increase with faulty valves or an exhausted CO_2 absorber in the anesthesia circuit and may decrease with tracheostomy or tracheal intubation. The ratio of V_D/V_T should be around 0.3.

Physiologic Concepts

Lung Volumes

Total lung capacity is the maximal volume the lungs can contain in full inspiration. It is divided into four portions: the inspiratory reserve volume (IRV), tidal volume (V_T), expiratory reserve volume (ERV), and residual volume (RV) (Fig. 6-1).

Pressures, Compliance, and Resistance

When patients are breathing spontaneously while attached to a ventilator or anesthesia breathing circuit, the needle of the pressure gauge does little more than tremble. During assisted ventilation, 5 cm to 20 cm of H_2O peak inspiratory pressure or more may develop (see Table 4-2 for conversion of centimeters of H_2O to torr). With mechanical ventilation, pressures may peak at 30 cm to 50 cm H_2O, sometimes more. With positive end-expiratory pressure (PEEP), 5 cm to 15 cm H_2O may be imposed during the exhalation.

A healthy, conscious adult can generate an expiratory pressure of about 120 torr by straining mightily. In most healthy persons, this is a safe exercise because the lungs are compressed by the contraction of abdominal and thoracic muscles. This pressure cannot be sustained for more than a few seconds, however, because it compresses the vessels in the thorax, so that arterial blood pressure and cardiac output fall substantially. The diagnostic Valsalva maneuver used to test cardiovascular responses also involves the generation of high intrathoracic pressures, but by forcefully exhaling against resistance. We limit maximal exertion usually to less than 10 seconds and to pressures under 40 cm of H_2O. When raising airway pressure in a paralyzed patient by the same amount, with the help of an external source of power (*i.e.*, gas under pressure from a ventilator, or from a compressed gas tank, or squeezed from the breathing bag of the anesthesia circuit), much less pressure is tolerated for these reasons:

- When airway pressure is raised during anesthesia, compensatory autonomic cardiovascular reflexes may be depressed and profound hypotension may supervene.
- Pressure is supplied to the lumen of the bronchial tree (instead of the lungs being compressed from the outside by the contraction of muscles), and an airway may rupture and lead to pneumothorax, mediastinal emphysema, or both.

Elastance describes elasticity and *compliance* is its reciprocal. Compliance (C) is expressed as a change in volume (ΔV) divided by a change in pressure (ΔP).

$$C = \frac{\Delta V}{\Delta P}$$

Edematous, boggy, or stiff lungs have low compliance.

Resistance is the opposition to flow. Where R is the resistance, ΔP is the pressure change, and $\dot{Q}$ is the gas flow,

$$R = \frac{\Delta P}{\dot{Q}}$$

About two-thirds of the airway resistance in humans resides in the upper airway between the nose or mouth and the trachea. Most of the remainder occurs in the large central airways.

Resistance (R) for nonturbulent, laminar flow is expressed by Poiseuille's law:

$$R = \frac{8l\eta}{\pi r^4}$$

l = length

r = radius of tube

η = viscosity of gas

For turbulent flow, resistance is inversely proportional to r^5. Even with laminar flow, infants are particularly at risk when edema decreases their airway lumen. For instance, if edema reduces an infant's airway by 1 mm, from 2 mm to 1 mm in diameter, resistance increases by a factor of 16. Compare this to an adult's airway 6 mm in diameter, edema also reduces the diameter by 1 mm to 5 mm, but resistance increases only by a factor of 2. For their weight, infants consume much oxygen in relation to normal adults. Therefore, they tolerate respiratory obstruction poorly, and their airways require meticulous attention.

Diffusion and Oxygenation

Blood passes through an alveolar capillary in about 0.75 seconds. This time, brief as it is, amply allows CO_2 to leave the blood and oxygen to enter. In a healthy lung, O_2 accomplishes this in about 0.25 seconds. Carbon dioxide takes as long, even though its partial pressure gradient is only about 5 torr (45 torr venous to 40 torr arterial) versus 40 torr (90 torr arterial to 50 torr venous) for oxygen, but the solubility of carbon dioxide is 20 times that of oxygen.

In order to estimate the amount of oxygen in an alveolus, the ideal alveolar oxygen tension is calculated using this formula:

$$P_AO_2 = (P_B - P_{H_2O})F_IO_2 - \frac{P_aCO_2}{R}$$

P_AO_2 = alveolar oxygen tension

P_B = barometric pressure

P_{H_2O} = water vapor tension at the alveolus at 37°C.

F_IO_2 = fraction inspired oxygen

P_aCO_2 = arterial carbon dioxide tension

R = respiratory quotient (0.8); not measured during clinical monitoring, we use 0.8 as a reasonable estimate of this variable.

For example, a patient breathing room air at sea level should have an alveolar oxygen tension of

$$P_AO_2 = (760 - 47) \times (0.21) - \frac{40}{0.8} = 99.7 \text{ torr}$$

This important formula makes a point often overlooked. A patient breathing room air (F_IO_2 of 0.21) may appear to do well, maintaining an

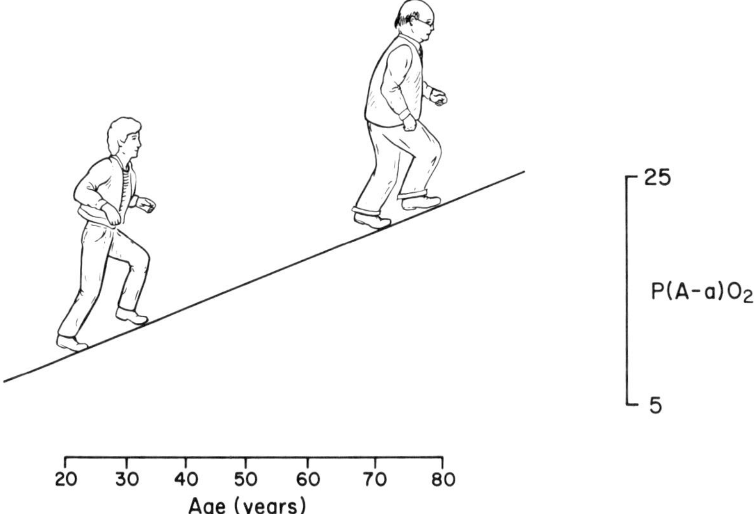

Figure 6-2. $P(A - a)O_2$ and age. The difference between alveolar and arterial oxygen tension $P(A - a)O_2$ increases with advancing age. This is reflected in lower arterial oxygen tension in old as compared to young adults. Lung disease, more common in advanced age, contributes to the falling P_aO_2 and rising $P(A - a)O_2$ in the aged. Some old patients in good health have P_aO_2 levels similar to those of young adults.

arterial Po_2 (P_aO_2) of 85 torr. If his P_aCO_2 were 45 torr, the difference between alveolar and arterial $P(A - a)O_2$ would be as follows:

$$\left[(760 - 47) \times (0.21) - \frac{45}{0.8}\right] - 85 \text{ torr} \qquad = 8.5 \text{ torr}$$

$$(\text{alveolar } Po_2) \qquad - (\text{arterial } Po_2) = P(A - a)O_2$$

However, if the arterial Pco_2 were 20 torr instead, in other words, if the patient were hyperventilating, perhaps in response to a metabolic acidosis, the figures would look much worse:

$$\left[(760 - 47) \times (0.21) - \frac{20}{0.8}\right] - 85 \text{ torr} \qquad = 39.7 \text{ torr}$$

$$(\text{alveolar } Po_2) \qquad - (\text{arterial } Po_2) = P(A - a)O_2$$

Large Aa gradients are common in anesthesia (see below). The gradients also increase with advancing age (Fig. 6-2).

Once we know the arterial pressure of oxygen, how much oxygen the hemoglobin can carry can be calculated. The sigmoid oxyhemoglobin dissociation curve describes the relationship of the saturation in hemoglobin

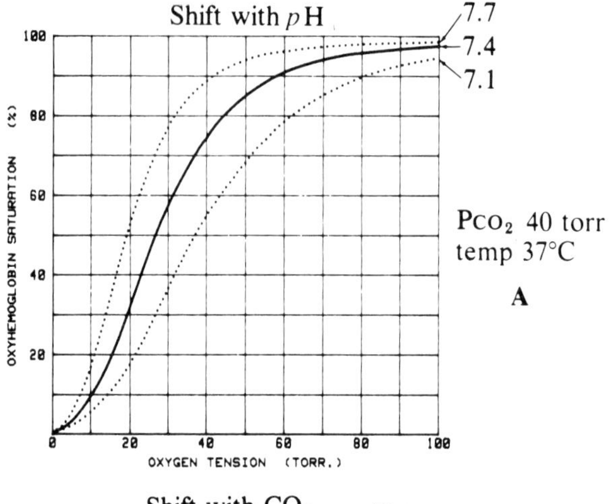

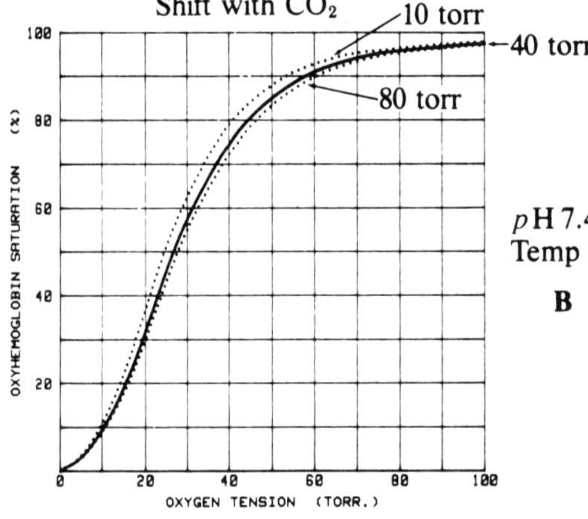

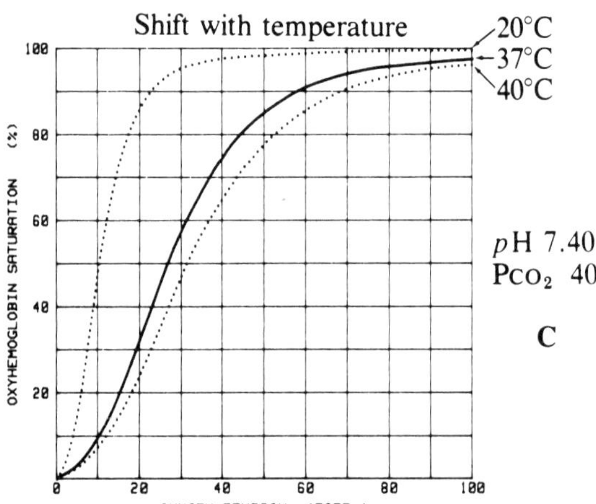

Figure 6-3. Saturation of hemoglobin with oxygen. The typical S-shaped dissociation curve can be shifted to the left (with loss of H^+ ions; temperature; 2,3-DPG) and to the right (with gain of H^+ ions; temperature; 2,3-DPG). Observe that CO_2 affects the position of the curve only a little provided that the pH is constant. Usually, pH shifts with changes in P_{CO_2}, and thus, the dissociation curve also shifts. Only the effects of pH (*A*), P_{CO_2} (*B*), and temperature (*C*) are shown because these are purposefully manipulated during anesthesia; however, 2,3-DPG is not.

to the partial pressure of oxygen (Fig. 6-3). The curve shifts as the affinity of hemoglobin for oxygen changes.

A shift to the right (decreased affinity for oxygen) helps release oxygen into tissue. A shift to the left (increased affinity for oxygen) causes less oxygen to be available to tissue.

The curve can be shifted by changing hydrogen ion concentration, temperature, carbon dioxide tension, or 2,3-diphosphoglycerate (2,3-DPG). Decreasing any or all of these variables shifts the curve to the left; increasing them shifts it to the right. An easy mnemonic device is: "right with height" (of temperature, 2,3-DPG, hydrogen ions) and "left with theft."

We can determine total oxygen content by measuring the oxygen that can be driven out of blood (a laboratory procedure) or by estimating the oxygen that is bound to hemoglobin and dissolved in plasma.

The amount dissolved in plasma is influenced by temperature (the higher the temperature is, the less soluble the gas). The formula to estimate total oxygen content in arterial blood (C_aO_2) follows:

$$C_aO_2 = (0.003 \times P_aO_2) + 1.34 \times \text{Hgb} \times O_2 \text{ sat}$$

$0.003 \times P_aO_2$ = dissolved O_2

$1.34 \times \text{Hgb} \times O_2$ sat = oxygen bound to hemoglobin

P_aO_2 = partial pressure of oxygen in arterial blood at 37°C

O_2 sat = saturation of hemoglobin as determined from Figure 6-3.

Compliance

Physiologists distinguish between static and dynamic compliance. *Static compliance* refers to a measurement at which no gas flows and pressure and volume are kept constant. *Dynamic compliance* is obtained at the moment when inspiration changes to expiration or vice versa, that is, when flow momentarily ceases. Under ideal circumstances these two expressions of compliance yield similar data. However, when some of the gas flow is impeded, for instance, by kinks of the endotracheal tube or narrowed airways, dynamic compliance is more and more affected by the resistance to flow and less and less reflects true static compliance of the lung. Nevertheless, during anesthesia, effective dynamic compliance is often assessed in the paralyzed patient whose lungs are mechanically ventilated.

We measure compliance by dividing expired tidal volume by inspiratory pressure. Sudden changes in compliance call for an immediate investigation because they almost always signify problems that require attention, such as a kinked endotracheal tube or an endotracheal tube that has slipped into one bronchus, pulmonary edema, or a pneumothorax, to name a few common examples.

Effective static compliance can be measured with a giant syringe—not a routine procedure for the operating room.

V_D/V_T Ratio

For efficient gas exchange in healthy persons, tidal volume exceeds dead space by a ratio of about 500:150. In pulmonary disease, however, physiologic dead space often increases. The ratio of dead space (V_D) to tidal volume (V_T)—normally about 0.3—is, therefore, often estimated. For this we use the formula

$$\frac{V_D}{V_T} = \frac{P_aCO_2 - P_ECO_2}{P_aCO_2}$$

V_D = dead space

V_T = tidal volume

P_aCO_2 = arterial CO_2 partial pressure (torr)

P_ECO_2 = mixed-expired CO_2 partial pressure (torr)

Clinical Monitoring of Ventilation

In the early days of anesthesia, when most anesthetized patients breathed spontaneously, ventilation was monitored by inspecting the patient's chest and neck, where evidence for unusual efforts to move gas in and out of the lungs could be observed. The color of the blood and skin was watched for evidence of inadequate oxygenation as manifested by cyanosis, and heart rate and blood pressure were monitored to detect tachycardia and hypertension with a wide pulse pressure, which were taken as an expression of CO_2 retention, particularly when occurring together with sweating. These time-honored clinical signs should still be appreciated by the clinician who is called to a patient in an emergency. Although these clinical signs are discussed in Chapter 2, and even though some of them are repeated in Chapter 8, because of their importance a brief recapitulation is in order.

During normal spontaneous inspiration, chest and abdomen should rise with little effort, the neck and the floor of the mouth should be still, the nostrils should not move, and the tongue should be relaxed. During expiration the abdomen should be flaccid, and the chest and abdomen should return to their resting positions in a smoothly coordinated, easy relaxation of the muscles responsible for inspiration. That is the normal state. Contrast that with agonal breathing—the extreme of respiratory inadequacy. During agonal inspiration, air enters the chest with a gasp, the upper chest falls, the abdomen rises, the nostrils dilate, the larynx moves down, the floor of the mouth tightens, the lips spring open, and the tongue is pulled.

Clinicians have occasion to observe all stages that lie between adequate and agonal breathing. The most subtle and most common physical expression of respiratory inadequacy is the inspiratory downward excursion of the larynx. This slight tracheal tug is found in many people with chronic lung disease who have not yet decompensated and who are up and about doing their job. In obese patients, the tracheal tug may be obscured under a layer of fat, but a gentle hand resting on the patient's larynx can detect the laryngeal motion. In children in mild respiratory distress, one of the earliest signs is the flaring of nostrils, so common, for instance, during pneumonia. The anesthesiologist should examine every patient before inducing anesthesia to look for evidence of respiratory insufficiency, such as a tracheal tug or flaring nostrils. If none could be found before, but it is manifest after anesthesia, lingering muscle weakness, airway obstruction, atelectasis or aspiration must be considered.

Tightening of abdominal muscles with expiration is a sign of light anesthesia or pain (often with phonation in patients without an endotracheal tube), or respiratory distress such as brought about by bronchospasm.

CO_2 retention stimulates the sympathetic system (as long as it is not blocked by drugs or excessive levels of CO_2) and with it comes perspiration, tachycardia, and an elevated blood pressure with a wide pulse pressure. In vascular beds devoid of sympathetic innervation (*e.g.*, with a sympathetic block), CO_2 causes vasodilatation, as it does in the brain.

In addition to observing the patient, the adequacy of ventilation is monitored by listening for breath sounds through the precordial or esophageal stethoscope, observing the breathing bag or ventilator bellows, and watching spirometers, pressure gauges in the breathing tubes, inspired and expired gases, and blood and tissue gases.

The Precordial or Esophageal Stethoscope

Some rank this simple and reliable device among the essentials of monitoring. It does not depend on electricity or circuitry, and is almost immune to malfunction. Only when the diaphragm in the stethoscope bell is missing or damaged, or with an esophageal stethoscope, the balloon is broken, will the listening device fail to perform well. When it is used for monitoring ventilation, it is placed in the esophagus where it conveys both heart and breath sounds, or over the chest where again both sounds can be monitored, or over the jugular notch where often only breath sounds can be heard. In this last position the sounds are harsh, wheezes (evidence of bronchoconstriction) are not detected early, but the presence of inspiration and expiration as well as leaks around the inflated cuff of the endotracheal tube can be readily detected. In pediatric anesthesia placing the stethoscope over the jugular notch is advisable when an uncuffed tube is used: if the tube fits snugly, inspiratory and expiratory sounds will be almost equal (depending on the flow rates), and a small leak around the tube during mechanical inspiration will generate a typical "bubbling/blowing" sound. The bigger this leak, the more pronounced the noise, and the less air that returns during expiration. In the extreme case, it is possible to spill most inspired air through the leak, resulting in hypoventilation of the patient. A decrease in lung compliance will cause a small leak to become unacceptably large. A jugular stethoscope helps to detect this problem. It also assists in adjusting the volume of air in the cuff of the endotracheal tube. One should inflate the cuff only enough to barely stop the inspiratory leak. Excessive pressure damages the cilia of the trachea. Remember that the level of anesthesia may affect the diameter of the trachea (larger with deeper general anesthesia) and that nitrous oxide can diffuse into the balloon and increase its volume and, thus, the pressure on the trachea. Repeatedly adjusting the pressure in the cuff as described prevents unnecessary complications brought about by a cuff being over- or underinflated. A further advantage of a stethoscope over the jugular notch is that a change in sounds may be early evidence of either a kinked endotracheal tube or one that is becoming obstructed with secretions.

Pressure Gauges

Modern anesthesia systems and ventilators have pressure gauges. These important devices allow the anesthesiologist to gauge the pressure needed to deliver the desired tidal volume. During mechanical ventilation, patients with stiff lungs (low compliance) may require a peak inspiratory pressure of 40 cm or even 50 cm of H_2O, whereas patients with normal compliance can maintain large tidal volumes with 15 cm to 20 cm of H_2O pressure. Monitoring peak airway pressures generated during mechanical inspiration is important, as excessive pressures can rupture small bronchi or alveoli and cause pneumothorax and mediastinal emphysema. Once gas under pressure gains access to the mediastinum, emphysema may reach the subcutaneous tissue of neck and face. Gas may dissect along the mediastinum into the abdomen, where it can spread along the mesentery to envelop the bowels, and it can break into the peritoneal cavity to cause pneumoperitoneum.

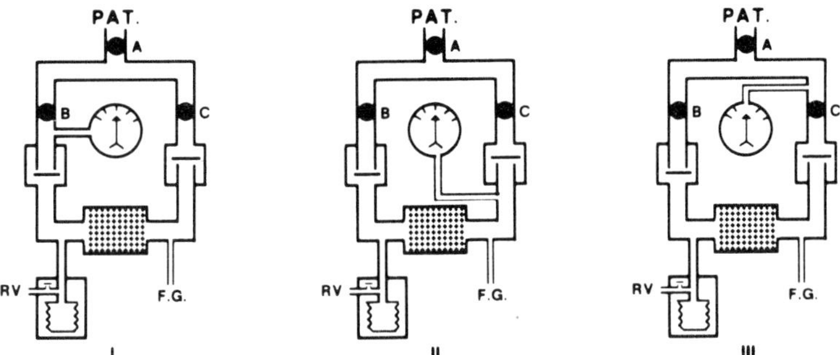

Figure 6-4. The position of the pressure gauge influences its ability to detect obstructions. Diagrams of a typical circle system are shown with obstructions: *A* between Y-piece and patient (for instance in the endotracheal tube); *B* between Y-piece and expiratory valve; (*C*) between Y piece and inspiratory valve. The pressure gauge is pictured in position I (between patient and expiratory valve); in position II (between the valves and communicating with the ventilator or breathing bag); and in position III (between inspiratory valve and the patient). See Table 6-1 for consequences of positioning the gauge at different sites.

With partial obstruction of the breathing tubes of the respirator or the anesthesia system (*e.g.*, with a malfunctioning bacterial filter), or of the endotracheal tube (e.g., a kink or, particularly in the endotracheal tubes of small diameter used in infants, a mucous plug or a blood clot), or of the bronchial tree (*e.g.*, bronchospasm), more than normal pressure is required to move the gas. However, the pressure gauge will show abnormal pressures only if the site of obstruction and the position of the pressure gauge make that possible. With manual ventilation, the position of the pressure relief ("pop-off") valve also influences the outcome of an obstruction. With mechanical ventilation, the pressure relief valve is incorporated into the ventilator and gas is spilled only during expiration.

From all of this it becomes obvious that—paradoxically—the pressure gauge cannot be relied on to alert the anesthesiologist to all problems relating to excessive pressures in the system. This important point is illustrated with the help of Figure 6-4 and Table 6-1.

Three positions for the pressure gauge are shown in Fig. 6-4 for a typical arrangement of a circle system with CO_2 absorber, one-way valves, and a ventilator. In all diagrams the same obstructions are shown, namely in the patient's endotracheal tube or airway (A), in the expiratory (B), or in the inspiratory limb or valve (C) of the anesthesia breathing circuit. When we make the assumption that in each case only one of the obstructions exists, and that the gauge shows zero pressure during normal expiration, the pressure readings shown in Table 6-1 can be expected during the delivery of a normal tidal volume by a mechanical ventilator.

Table 6-1. PRESSURE ON GAUGE IS DEPENDENT ON POSITION*

	Position of Gauge		
	I	II	III
Obstruction A			
Inspiration	AH	AH	AH
Expiration	N	N	N
Obstruction B			
Inspiration	AL	N	N
Expiration	N	N	AH
Obstruction C			
Inspiration	AL	AH	AL
Expiration	N	N	N

* Positions of gauge refers to Figure 6-4. N = normal; AH = abnormally high; AL = abnormally low.

With mechanical ventilation, all excess gas escapes during expiration. The pressure gauge will show abnormal values during expiration only when outflow is obstructed and pressure is measured between lung and obstruction (obstruction B, gauge position III). With manual ventilation, the findings would be different, because excess gas escapes during inspiration; the pressure gauge under these circumstances shows the pressure generated before and after the "pop-off" valve opens. The diagram could be expanded for spontaneous ventilation where gas also escapes during expiration and negative pressures can be generated during inspiration, and by other locations of obstructions and positions for the pressure gauge. The presentation shows why the pressure gauge is not the first line of defense against obstruction; too many circumstances of serious obstruction may go unnoticed by watching only the pressure gauge. As soon as the pressure gauge is monitored in combination with gas flows, the sensitivity of the method improves considerably.

It is clear the pressure gauge should be as close to the patient as possible; however, to put it close to the mask or endotracheal tube is not convenient (inexpensive gauges are bulky): it would be difficult to clean the gauges, and sensitivity to water vapor would threaten the gauge's performance. Pressure gauges are therefore incorporated in the hardware of the anesthesia machine and ventilators.

Disconnect Monitoring

The pressure gauge will also show abnormally low values when the patient becomes disconnected from the ventilator, regardless of where the pressure gauge is positioned or where the disconnect occurs, as long as it does not occur simultaneously with an obstruction. Because disconnect accidents are so common, so-called "disconnect alarms" have been incorporated in many ventilators. Typically, they are set to sense an inappropriately low pressure during the inspiratory phase of the ventilator. However, it is conceivable that no alarm is sounded if the patient has very compliant lungs and a relatively small tidal volume requiring only low inspiratory pressures (*e.g.*, 15 cm H_2O); and if the low pressure alarm is set too far below the peak inspiratory pressure (*e.g.*, an alarm threshold set at 7 cm of H_2O instead of close to the 15 cm of H_2O of the peak inspiratory pressure); and if the ventilator bellows descends during expiration. Under such conditions the alarm might not sound when the patient becomes disconnected from the ventilator. In this case, during expiration the bellows will descend by its own gravity and will aspirate air through the disconnect. Once the bellows is filled, the ventilator will empty it with its next inspiratory stroke (that is one reason why modern ventilators have bellows that descend during inspiration and rise during expiration). If the valves, tubings, and connectors of the system offer little resistance and if the inspiratory time is short, resulting in rapid flows and correspondingly high pressures, 7 cm of H_2O may be exceeded during inspiration and no alarm may sound. Watching the pressure gauge will not help either, nor can any clinician maintain such vigilance over every monitor for hours on end. But watching the patient's chest and listening to the lungs will help to discover a disconnect before a disaster occurs.

There are also several back-up systems that assist the anesthesiologist in the discovery of disconnects. These include devices incorporated in modern ventilators that monitor the tidal volumes of gas delivered (which work only in ventilators with bellows that cannot fill by gravity) with each respiratory cycle. The alarm algorithm calls for a comparison of the volumes dialed by the clinician and the tidal volumes actually delivered. Two other safeguards are the capnograph and the oximeter. CO_2 monitors will sound an alarm when CO_2 is not detected. Pulse oximeters sound an alarm when oxygen saturation of hemoglobin falls below a critical level. This will happen later than a "no CO_2" signal by the capnograph and, depending on the oxygen concentration in the patient's lungs, may cause an alarm after a few, or many, futile ventilator strokes.

Spirometry

In addition to observing the variables that give information about pressure and disconnect, a spirometer will show the volume of gas flowing through the tube in which the device is positioned. Because we are primarily concerned about the tidal volume of gas reaching the patient's lungs, the spirometer is usually incorporated in the *ex*piratory limb of the breathing system. A spirometer in the inspiratory limb will show the volume of gas being propelled toward the patient, but not how much of it reaches the patient. In the case of a disconnect, for instance, a spirometer in the inspired limb would indicate normal delivery of gas, but the gas may all escape through the disconnected tubing, never reaching the patient. A spirometer in the expiratory limb would show gas returning from the patient; in the case of a disconnect nothing would return as nothing had been pushed into the patient's airway. However, even a spirometer in the expiratory limb can show an adequate tidal volume, particularly in children, and yet no, or at least less, gas than shown by the spirometer actually reached the patient's lungs. This dangerously erroneous spirometer reading is likely to occur when three conditions are met:

1. Relatively high inspiratory pressures are used because the patient's lungs are not compliant or some obstruction has to be overcome.
2. The breathing system is compliant (about 1 ml/cm H_2O for rubber tubing and 0.3 ml/cm H_2O for disposable tubing), thus the corrugated breathing tubes expand during inspiration and store gas.
3. The circle system of the anesthesia machine has a large volume, as is the case when extension tubes are used or when capacious humidifiers are incorporated into the system. The larger the internal volume of the breathing system, the easier to store gas by compression during inspiration.

When these three factors coincide, a considerable volume of gas can be stored in the breathing system during inspiration, and can then be released during expiration when the pressure in the system drops; the compressed gases reexpand; and the distended, elastic, corrugated tubing returns to its resting state. The gas thus mobilized can only move forward toward the expiratory valve, as the inspiratory valve closes behind it. It passes through the spirometer, which registers what looks like a tidal volume, even though the patient may have benefited little or not at all from it.

MONITORING THE BREATHING BAG AND VENTILATOR BELLOWS

One can also be deceived by the ventilator's stroke volume or breathing bag during spontaneous or manually controlled ventilation. The tidal volume of the ventilator may, for instance, be set to deliver 800 ml. Assuming that its calibration is correct, the ventilator will indeed deliver 800 ml into the circuit with each inspiration, much of which will be forced into the patient's airway, while some of it will expand the corrugated tubing. But during the inspiration phase of the ventilator, the fresh gas from the anesthesia machine will continue to flow and, having nowhere else to go, it too will enter the patient's airway. A simple calculation shows that a fresh gas flow of 5 liters will add 2.5 liters/min to the minute volume of the ventilator if the ratio of inspiration to expiration of the ventilator is 1:1. For a respiratory rate of 10 breaths per minute, the tidal volume will be increased approximately from 800 to about 1050 ml. An inspiratory to expiratory ratio of 1:2 will allow less time for fresh gas to flow into the patient's lungs; higher fresh gas flows more. The lesson is that the calibration of ventilator bellows or inspection (or "the feel") of the breathing bag must be interpreted in the light of the fresh gas flow.

While one tends to underestimate tidal volumes with high fresh gas flows, leaks in the system can cause serious overestimation of tidal volumes in the absence of a spirometer in the expiratory limb of the breathing system. We use a mechanical or electronic respirometer in the expiratory limb of the breathing tubes. Mechanical respirometers contain a lightweight vane connected through gears to an indicator needle. They tend to underestimate at low, and overestimate at high, gas flows.[2]

Few anesthesia circuits do not leak. A leak of 200 ml/min is not considered excessive, yet it may consume, depending on the patient's size, several percent of the minute volume. Many leaks are much larger and may cause considerable error in estimating the volumes of gas given to the patient.

Gas may be removed from the anesthesia circuit for analysis. Some analyzers aspirate 200 ml to 300 ml of gas per minute. Some units recirculate this gas; others vent it through a scavenging system.

MONITORING GASES

The partial pressure in torr or the concentration in volume percent of gases can be monitored in the inspired or expired gas mixture as it enters or leaves the patient. Gases, in particular oxygen and CO_2, can also be measured as they diffuse through the skin or in arterial or venous blood.

Oxygen

Since tissue hypoxia cannot only stop the machine, but can also wreck it in a short time, concentrations of inspired oxygen are now often—if not yet universally—monitored in the breathing circuit. Low concentrations of inspired oxygen may arise for the reasons cited below:

- One cause is faulty central gas supply from the hospital. Many accidents in new operating rooms have been reported when it was found too late that an oxygen pipe had been connected to a nitrous oxide source. Sometimes the fail-safe systems are bypassed, or pin indexes and other provisions to avoid giving the wrong gas are disabled. A fault in the machine can cause oxygen to leak through a crack and, thus, insufficient concentrations of oxygen reach the patient.

- Another cause is incorrect flow-meter settings. For instance, a flow-meter is misread and 200 ml of oxygen is administered instead of 2000 ml together with 2000 ml of nitrous oxide.

Attempts have been made to prevent these problems by redesigning the system. However, many old systems are still in operation. A series of coincidences or mistakes may lead to disaster: oxygen analyzers help guard against these.

Many anesthesia machines now come equipped with small, self-contained oxygen analyzers. This highly desirable development makes it less likely that gas concentrations containing less than 21% oxygen are given or that premature newborns at risk of retrolental fibroplasia receive high concentrations of oxygen without anyone being aware of it. Most self-contained oxygen analyzers respond relatively slowly; that is, many seconds pass before these instruments indicate the actual concentration of oxygen in the sample. This makes it impossible to get accurate breath-to-breath data on oxygen, but allows us to monitor slowly changing concentrations of oxygen in the gas mixture. The electrode of the analyzer is usually placed in the inspiratory limb of the circuit, where gases tend to be dry. With this location, one can see whether the inspired mixture contains the proper concentration of oxygen, but not whether enough of the proper mixture is being given. For example, to flow into a circle system 25 ml oxygen and 75 ml nitrous oxide per minute means giving a concentration of more than 21% oxygen, but not enough volume of oxygen to satisfy the oxygen consumption of a normothermic adult patient. Putting the analyzer into the expired limb might make this less likely, because the expired gas in this example would contain less than 21% oxygen, but to discover hypoxia by this route would be slower than picking up indications of inadequate oxygenation by pulse oximetry. Also, some analyzers are sensitive to moisture and, therefore, may perform more reliably in the inspiratory than the expiratory limb. Several methods are employed by these dedicated (one to each ventilator or anesthesia machine) oxygen analyzers.

Polarographic Method

The polarographic analyzer is based on the principle of the Clark electrode. Oxygen diffuses through a membrane that covers a charged metal electrode at which the oxygen is reduced. The current generated by this reaction is proportional to the oxygen reaching the metal, which in turn is proportional to the partial pressure of oxygen over the membrane. The device depends on a battery, and the electrode has a limited life expectancy; regular preventive maintenance is therefore important. Many electrodes require replacement every 3 to 4 months. Every day, before use, the electrode should be calibrated against room air and 100% oxygen. A malfunctioning oxygen analyzer is worse than no analyzer at all. Because of the slow response time, do not rush the calibration. It will take several minutes to do it properly.

The Fuel Cell Method

The term "fuel cell" has established itself, yet some prefer to speak of self-polarizing electrodes because the principle of their operation resembles that of the polarographic method, except that a reference metal in the electrode will generate a small current, obviating the help of a battery. What has been said about the polarographic method applies for the fuel cell as well, namely limited life expectancy and daily calibration.

Paramagnetic Method

This ingenious principle was described by Linus Pauling and exploits the fact that oxygen is attracted by a magnetic field. In the analyzer, oxygen displaces a reference gas and the degree of displacement is calibrated in percentage of oxygen present.

Hot Zirconium Oxide Method

At high temperatures, oxygen in contact with platinum ionizes, and the zirconium oxide functions as an ion-selective electrode. The method is fast and can be accurate.

The Raman Method

In the Raman method, the gas to be analyzed is passed through a cavity and exposed to monochromatic light generated by a laser.[3] Gas molecules that scatter the incident light can be identified because these frequency shifts are species specific. The method is rapid and can be quite accurate.

The Mass Spectrometer Method

The gas sample is ionized in a vacuum chamber and exposed to a magnetic field in which the ions travel along a curvilinear path that is a function of the ion's charge-to-mass ratio. For each ion species the trajectory is highly predictable. This makes it possible to position collecting plates where specific ions are known to impact and to "count the hits," the total of which are assumed to constitute 100% of the gas sample. (Hence the mass spectrometer may give erroneous results when gases not anticipated—and therefore not detected—are represented in the sample.)

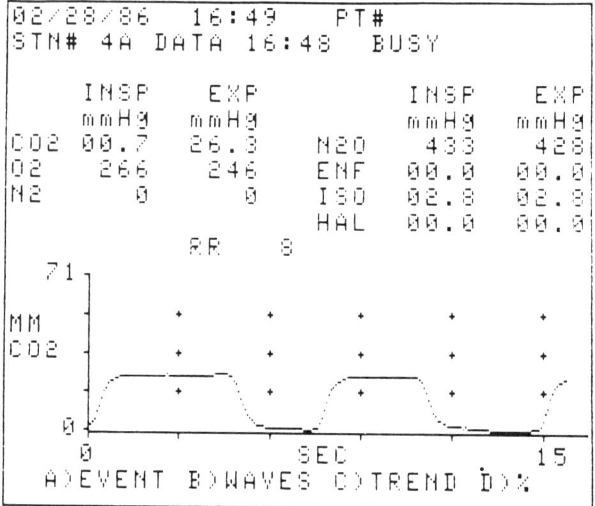

Figure 6-5. Typical display of mass spectrometer. The data were taken from a Perkin-Elmer (Norwalk, CT) mass spectrometer in clinical use in an operating room where a patient received isoflurane in oxygen and nitrous oxide. The top line identifies the patient (not active here); the second line, the station and time of sampling and the date; the third line identifies the columns as inspiratory and expiratory; the fourth line gives the units of measurement; and the fifth line shows the gases being analyzed. *RR* stands for respiratory rate. The display shows a 15-second capnogram, with options for different types of displays at the bottom.

The fraction derived by dividing the number of hits at each target by the total number of hits, multiplied by 100, equals the percentage of each gas. The results are expressed in percent or, once the barometric pressure is known, can be converted and reported in torr. The data are then displayed on a cathode ray tube (CRT), together with a calculation of respiratory rate in some units (Fig. 6-5).

A mass spectrometer system, as it is generally used in the medical environment, consists of sampling tubing, a set of valves, a vacuum pump (either an ion pump or an oil-diffusion pump, both of which have good records of performance), a suction pump, an ionizing chamber, collecting plates, a small computer, and a display. The components are shown in Fig. 6-6. The response time of the mass spectrometer is rapid enough to allow construction of curves that depict the changes in gas (typically done for CO_2—see below) concentration during inspiration and expiration. Mass spectrometers are also quite accurate and precise, but, because they are so expensive, a single unit usually serves multiple locations sequentially. Small-bore sampling tubes collect gases as close to the patient's

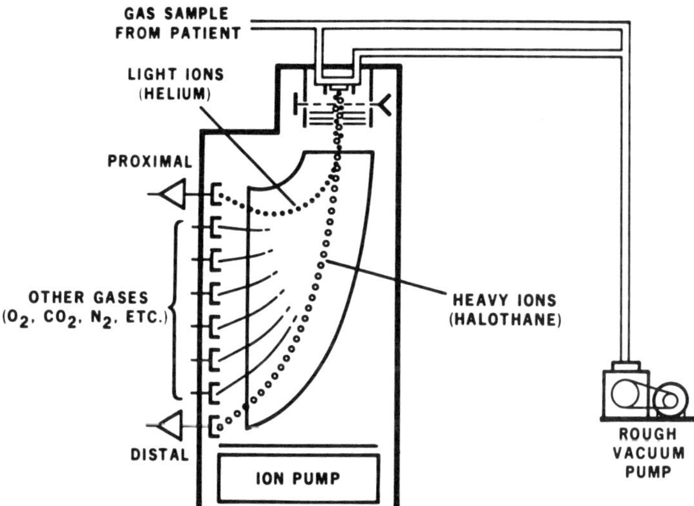

Figure 6-6. Mass spectrometer. A block diagram of the operation of a magnetic sector mass spectrometer is shown. Gas is drawn by a vacuum system. Only a small amount of this gas is allowed to leak into the analyzer, where a low pressure is maintained by the evacuation pump, and into the ion source. Here, the gas molecules are bombarded by an electron beam, and the gas molecules become positively ionized. Electrostatic fields accelerate and focus these ions into an ion beam. When these ions experience the magnetic field of the analyzer, they are deflected. Their circular trajectory has a radius proportional to their mass-to-charge ratio. The ion beam entering the magnetic field is dispersed into several different beams, each having a specific mass-to-charge ratio. After leaving the magnet, each different beam is collected by an individual collector and amplified to the appropriate level for the output device(s). The remaining nonionized gas molecules are evacuated from the analyzer by the evacuation pump.

mouth as possible. Continuous suction removes gas and delivers it to a centrally located valve, or set of valves, that, like a traffic policeman, allows gas from one patient after another to enter the spectrometer for analysis. In older systems, sampling was not continuous, and only when the valve turned to the next patient did gas begin to flow. It was, therefore, necessary to clear the "old" gas sitting in the tube before an analysis of fresh gas could be carried out. Continuous sampling significantly decreased delays between sampling. With continuous sampling, gases from each of ten patients can be analyzed every 150 seconds if the mass spectrometer returns to each patient for 15 seconds.

By their nature, mass spectrometers can only analyze the gases that are presented to them. Should a gas for which no collector plate has been prepared be presented to the mass spectrometer, one of two things can happen:

1. The mass spectrometer does not detect the extra gas and reports the concentration of the other gases as if they made up 100% of the sample. Thus, the mass spectrometer will overestimate the concentration of all the gases it detects.
2. The extra gas overlaps in its physical properties with one or more of the gases for which the mass spectrometer is programmed. For instance, when we administered a metered bronchodilator during anesthesia to an asthmatic patient, the propellant of the bronchodilator was not discovered, but the mass spectrometer reported a high concentration of one of the halogenated anesthetics because the spectral components of the propellant overlapped those of the anesthetic.[4]

Helium is not easily ionized. It cannot be evacuated quickly from the analyzer's high vacuum chamber by the ion pump. This will lead to erroneous measurements of gases not only of the patient who contributed the helium to the mixture to be analyzed, but also to several of the subsequent patients.

Water presents another problem for mass spectrometers, as it does for infrared CO_2 analyzers. First, the tubing may become clogged with condensed water because water vapor cools on its way from patient to tubing. Secondly, in a circle system the inspired gas is dry, but the expired gas is saturated with water. Yet, the mass spectrometer does not measure water vapor and, therefore, cannot recognize the volume difference introduced by water vapor. Assume, at sea level, a total pressure of 760 torr, which equals 100% of the gas, the inspired gas being dry and thus measured correctly. In the expired gas, vapor pressure for water would rise to 47 torr, that is about 6% of the total pressure. Most users, therefore, set their mass spectrometer to 713 torr (760 torr − 47 torr) to reflect the composition of alveolar gases. The values reported, therefore, are correct for alveolar but not for dry, inspired gases. The result is shown in Table 6-2.

Because the mass spectrometer can follow the changes during inspiration and expiration of oxygen and CO_2, it is possible to obtain the mean of the inspired and expired concentrations of these two gases. The difference between the inspired-to-expired mean, multiplied by the patient's minute ventilation, will generate a measure of oxygen consumption or CO_2 production per minute.

The mass spectrometer's advantage over other gas analyzers is that it can analyze not only oxygen but several other physiologic gases and anesthetics as well.

Cutaneous Oxygen Monitoring

Probes applied to the skin to detect gases are sometimes referred to as *transcutaneous sensors*. We prefer the term *cutaneous* because the gases measured are those of the skin and its blood vessels.

Table 6-2. CORRECTION FOR WATER VAPOR

	N_2O	O_2	CO_2	H_2O
Inspired gas %	70	30	0	0
Barometric pressure = 760 torr	532	228	0	0
But the mass spectrometer is set at 713 torr and therefore reports as follows:				
Pressure set in mass spectrometer = 713 torr	499	214	0	0
In the alveoli oxygen will be taken up and CO_2 added. If the RQ is 0.8, about 20% more oxygen will disappear than CO_2 will be excreted. The figures might, therefore, look as follows:				
Alveolar gas %	65	24	5	6
Barometric pressure = 760 torr	493	181	39	47
and be reported as below by the mass spectrometer, which ignores water vapor and is set at 713 torr:				
Pressure set in mass spectrometer = 713 torr	493	181	39	0

Since we are more interested in what the gas values in the patient's lungs might be, compensating for water vapor pressure seems reasonable.

In 1951, Baumberger and Goodfriend demonstrated that a finger placed in a 45°C phosphate buffer would cause the Po_2 of the buffer to approach arterial Po_2 in 15 minutes to 60 minutes.[5] Unfortunately, many years passed before this observation could be applied clinically. Under normal conditions, the Po_2 of the surface of the skin is close to zero. By heating the skin, blood flow, and with it the Po_2 of the skin, increase markedly. With the development of the Clark polarographic electrode and the addition of the heating element, Huch and coworkers began to measure cutaneous oxygen in 1973.[6] They recognized that cutaneous Po_2 was not equivalent to arterial Po_2, but that they correlated very well ($r = 0.95$). Heating the capillaries of the skin to 43°C or above shifts the oxyhemoglobin dissociation curve to the right. This decreases the solubility of oxygen in blood and increases the Po_2 in capillary blood. But, because metabolism increases at the same time, the divergent effects of decreased solubility and increased consumption of oxygen tend to cancel, and cutaneous Po_2 (Tc Po_2) generally reflects arterial Po_2.

Cutaneous oxygen measurements change with blood flow to the skin. Ideally, both cutaneous oxygen and blood flow to the area under the electrode should be known.[7] Unfortunately, this information is rarely available. Transcutaneous monitoring of oxygen therefore requires much clinical acumen. Low oxygen tensions under the transcutaneous electrode may mean arterial hypoxemia or poor blood flow under the electrode. Either condition requires additional assessment of the patient. Thus, normal gas tensions under the electrode are reassuring; both arterial Po_2 and flow must be adequate. However, in the premature newborn, where the clinician has to guard against hyperoxia, the interpretation of cutaneous oxygen values can be difficult. A "normal" Po_2 may be the result of reduced blood flow in the face of high arterial Po_2 values. When in doubt, other methods must be recruited, such as analysis of arterial blood samples for blood gases.

The electrode of the cutaneous monitor is usually placed on the chest or the inner aspect of the arm. First, the skin is cleansed with alcohol. Then it is debrided with surgical or cellophane tape—although it hurts—by repeatedly applying and pulling off the tape. The electrode is then placed on the skin and held in place with tape. Because the heat of the electrode causes mild burns or irritations, its location is changed approximately every 2 hours to 4 hours. A coin-shaped erythema marks the previous location. It may persist for a day or two. The monitor is zeroed and calibrated according to the manufacturer's specifications. Some drift is to be expected. After the electrode is placed, the initial Tc Po_2 drops significantly because the Po_2 of unheated skin is under 10 torr. Gradually the Po_2 rises as the capillaries dilate and as oxygen diffuses through the outer layer of the skin. Within 15 minutes to 20 minutes in neonates and 30 minutes to 45 minutes in an adult, a plateau is reached that correlates with the level of arterial oxygen.

Monitoring cutaneous Po_2 has been found to be quite useful in neonatology when cannulation of the vessels is difficult and continuous monitoring is necessary. Lofgren studied 15 adults and found a good correlation between cutaneous and arterial oxygen measurements.[8] In obese patients, cutaneous readings were considerably lower than the arterial ones, but, nevertheless, they were parallel.

Cutaneous oxygen monitors are not (yet) common in operating rooms. There are several reasons for this. In the older units, the initial starting time is slow. The polarographic Clark electrode may be sensitive to anesthetic agents.[9] Check the monitor and electrode before use in the operating room for interference with anesthetic agents.

Pulse Oximetry

Noninvasive methods for determining the saturation of hemoglobin have been available for many years. But only recently have clinically popular pulse oximeters become widely accepted. Small sensors applied to fingers, ears, and toes have helped to overcome the problems of the past, which were associated with strapping a bulky sensor to the ear.

The principle of pulse oximetry is based on the fact that reduced hemoglobin absorbs different wavelengths of light than does oxyhemoglobin. By shining the light of two distinct wavelengths (650 nm and 805 nm, or 660 nm and 940 nm) through the fingertip and sensing the absorption, one can calculate the ratio of reduced hemoglobin to oxyhemoglobin, and report saturation in percent. Modern clinical pulse oximeters ignore methemoglobin and carboxyhemoglobin. Thus, should there be large concentrations of methemoglobin, the pulse oximeter will overestimate saturation of hemoglobin with oxygen. In patients suspected of having carboxy- or methemoglobinemia, traditional laboratory analyses with blood samples are indicated.

In order to measure arterial blood saturation, the fingertip is assumed to consist of two compartments: the "blood" compartment and the "nonblood" compartment. The blood compartment comprises arterial and venous blood, and the nonblood compartment bone, muscle, skin, and other tissues. Some of the incident light is attenuated by the nonblood compartment, which stays constant, as does that contributed by venous blood, whereas the attenuation caused by the arterial blood varies with each heartbeat. By subtracting one from the other, the background attenuation (constant) can be removed and the signal from the arterial blood analyzed.

Initial results with arterial saturation were quite satisfactory, except that values were overestimated when saturation fell below 90%. Recognition of the effect of multiple scattering of incident light by the blood and tissue led to refinements of the calculations; current pulse oximeters show good correlation with invasively obtained measurements of saturation. The method becomes less reliable with very low saturation, decreased circulation, decreased temperature, extreme vasoconstriction, and vital dyes.[10,11,12] Many clinical studies with pulse oximeters have shown that hypoxia and poor circulation are relatively common. Thus, hypoxia was diagnosed quickly and easily by pulse oximetry in patients during one-lung anesthesia, during postoperative transport, in the recovery room, with pulmonary disease in the intensive care unit, undergoing shunt procedures for congenital heart disease, and during dental procedures under sedation. The device also proved useful in detecting local ischemia—or evidence of good perfusion—during the reimplantation of severed fingers.

However, pulse oximeters can give misleading data when the patient shivers or moves, during use of the electrosurgical unit, or with direct exposure to excessive ambient light—including infrared heat lamps. The features, benefits, and pitfalls of cutaneous and pulse oximetry are shown in Table 6-3.[7,13] In using pulse oximeters it is important to use other monitors and one's clinical observations to add additional insight to the measurement. A comparison of three different oximeters shows significant differences among them in the estimation of oxygen saturation values.[14] Pulse oximeters and cutaneous oxygen monitors measure different variables and so are also likely to report different oxygen levels.[15]

Table 6-3. COMPARISON OF PULSE OXIMETER AND CUTANEOUS OXYGEN TENSION MONITOR

Pulse Oximeter	Cutaneous Oxygen Tension Monitor
Advantages	
Continuous arterial oxygen saturation	Continuous oxygen tension
No warm-up	Low cutaneous blood flow detection (indirect)
Multiple site choices	Noninvasive
Noninvasive	
No tissue injury	
Direct reading of signal strength	
No calibration	
Easy sensor application	
Heart rate gives indication of signal quality	
Disadvantages	
Ambient light can affect	Low cutaneous blood flow mars correlation with arterial O_2
No trend of P_aO_2 until low (70 torr)	Warm-up required
Calibration not available	Burns skin
Electrocautery causes errors	Requires membrane changes
Motion artifact	Requires calibration
Pulsatile signal needed	Requires site changes
May fail with anemia	Sensor application not easy
Dyes may affect	No signal strength indication
Need nonpulsatile venous pressure	

(Barker, Tremper: Transcutaneous oxygen tension: Physiologic variables for monitoring oxygenation. Journal of Clinical Monitoring 1:130–134, 1985)

Mixed Venous Oxygen Saturation

The noninvasive pulse oximeter measures arterial saturation continuously, but tells nothing about oxygen consumption. According to Fick's formula ($CO = \dot{Q}O_2/(C_aO_2 - C_{\bar{v}}O_2)$, which relates cardiac output (CO) to oxygen consumption $\dot{Q}O_2$, and the difference between arterial (C_aO_2) and mixed venous ($C_{\bar{v}}O_2$) oxygen content, an assessment of mixed venous oxygen can guide the clinician. The lower this value, the more oxygen has been extracted by the body per liter of blood pumped by the heart. Thus, low mixed venous O_2 content is often an expression of low cardiac output. By monitoring the oxygen saturation in venous blood where it is truly mixed, namely in the pulmonary artery, one can gain a useful variable to assess the overall supply of the body with oxygen, which is going to be influenced by

1. The concentration of oxygen offered in the inspired gas (*percent oxygen in inspired gas*)

Table 6-4. MIXED VENOUS OXYGEN SATURATION IN CERTAIN CLINICAL CONDITIONS

$S_{\bar{v}}O_2$ (%)	$P_{\bar{v}}O_2$	Clinical Condition
		F_IO_2 = 1.0
>77	>42	Sepsis
		Left-to-right shunt
		Excess exogenous inotropic agent
		Hypothermia
		Cell poisoning
		Sample taken from wedged catheter (arteriolized sample)
60–77	30–42	Normal
<60	<30	Cardiac decompensation
		Lactic acidosis
		Cerebral depression
		Permanent cellular damage

2. The amount of oxygen delivered to the lungs with ventilation (*minute volume*)
3. The amount of oxygen carried by blood (carrying capacity is a function of hemoglobin content)
4. The amount of oxygen delivered to the tissues with circulation (cardiac output and tissue perfusion)
5. The amount of oxygen consumed by the tissue (*state of peripheral tissue*)

Normally, the mixed venous blood is about 75% saturated, with a Po_2 of 40 torr to 50 torr. The potential utility of such a measurement is summarized in Table 6-4.[7]

The relationship between hemoglobin saturation and the partial pressure of oxygen is shown in Figure 6-3, the oxyhemoglobin dissociation curve. The saturation remains at 95 ± 2% over the normal range of P_aO_2. The "steep part" of the curve represents venous blood with a partial pressure of oxygen around 40 torr, corresponding to an $S_{\bar{v}}O_2$ of about 75%. About 70 times as much oxygen makes its way to organs in the lap of hemoglobin molecules than is true for oxygen carried in solution in plasma.

To demonstrate the utility of monitoring mixed venous oxygen saturation, take as an example a patient with a hemoglobin concentration (Hb) of 14 g/dl, an arterial O_2 saturation (S_aO_2) of 97%, and a mixed venous O_2 saturation ($S_{\bar{v}}O_2$) of 75%. We wish to calculate the arterial oxygen (C_aO_2) and mixed venous oxygen ($C_{\bar{v}}O_2$) contents respectively:

$$
\begin{aligned}
C_aO_2 &= 0.003\ (P_aO_2) + 1.34\ (Hb)\ (S_aO_2) \\
&= 0.003\ (100) + 1.34\ (14)\ (0.97) \\
&= 0.31 + 18.2 \\
&= 18.51 \text{ ml } O_2/\text{dl blood} \\
C_{\bar{v}}O_2 &= 0.003\ (40) + 1.34\ (14)\ (0.75) \\
&= 0.12 + 14.07 \\
&= 14.19 \text{ ml } O_2/\text{dl blood}
\end{aligned}
$$

By subtracting $C_{\bar{v}}O_2$ from C_aO_2 we can calculate the oxygen consumption of the patient (VO_2) (in milliliters of oxygen per deciliter of blood):

$$
\begin{aligned}
VO_2 &= C_aO_2 - C_{\bar{v}}O_2\ (= a - \bar{v}DO_2). \\
&= 18.51 - 14.19 \\
&= 4.32 \text{ ml } O_2/\text{dl blood}
\end{aligned}
$$

To measure milliliters of oxygen per deciliter of blood is not of any great clinical use; the patient's cardiac output (CO) is therefore calculated. If we multiply C_aO_2 by CO, we obtain the total volume of oxygen flowing to the organs, or by doing the same calculation for the venous side, the total volume of oxygen being returned to the lungs:

$$O_2 \text{ transported to tissue } (O_2 \text{ in}) = CO \times C_aO_2$$

$$O_2 \text{ not used by tissue } (O_2 \text{ out}) = CO \times C_{\bar{v}}O_2$$

Assuming our patient has a cardiac output of 6 l/min:

$$
\begin{aligned}
O_2 \text{ in} &= (6 \text{ l/min}) \left(18.51 \times \frac{\text{ml } O_2}{\text{dl blood}}\right)\left(10\ \frac{\text{dl}}{1}\right) \\
&= 1111 \times \frac{\text{ml } O_2}{\text{min}} \\
O_2 \text{ out} &= (6 \text{ l/min}) \left(14.19 \times \frac{\text{ml } O_2}{\text{dl blood}}\right)\left(10\ \frac{\text{dl}}{1}\right) \\
&= 851.1 \times \frac{\text{ml } O_2}{\text{min}} \\
O_2 \text{ consumption} &= O_2 \text{ in} - O_2 \text{ out}
\end{aligned}
$$

therefore

$$O_2 \text{ consumption} = 1111 - 851.1 = 259.9 \text{ ml/min}$$

If oxygen demand cannot be met, anaerobic metabolism will supervene and the blood lactate level will rise. To avoid this, the patient will preferentially increase cardiac output. (Atheletes can pentuple theirs and extract more oxygen from blood (tripling $a - \bar{v}DO_2$) as it passes through the tissue.)

If we once again take our patient as an example, to find the maximum oxygen consumption, assuming that cardiac output is now 15 l/min (up from 6 l/min), and that he has an $a - \bar{v}DO_2$ of 12 ml O_2/100 ml blood, then the maximum O_2 consumption is

$$VO_2 \text{ (max)} = (15 \text{ l/min}) \times 120 \text{ ml } O_2/\text{l}$$
$$= 1800 \text{ ml/min}$$

If arterial oxygen tension (which influences arterial O_2 content), *p*H, temperature (which influences the binding of oxygen to the hemoglobin), and oxygen consumption remain stable, monitoring venous oxygen saturation allows us to assess changes in cardiac output. Neglecting oxygen in solution, the Fick equation can be rearranged to solve for mixed venous oxygen saturation ($S_{\bar{v}}O_2 = S_aO_2 - VO_2/[(CO)\ (Hb)\ (1.34)]$). We can see that $S_{\bar{v}}O_2$ will drop in the face of hypoxia, increased oxygen consumption, decreased cardiac output, and anemia. Although it lacks specificity, it can alert us to review the patient's status. Also, as long as venous oxygen saturation remains high, organ perfusion can be assumed to be satisfactory (unless poisoning of enzymes in the tissue has interfered with oxygen uptake; see Table 6-4).

At low output states, small changes in cardiac output will cause large changes in $a - \bar{v}DO_2$. Similarly, the oxygen and ventilatory requirements of patients in respiratory distress can be assessed more easily when continuous data on $S_{\bar{v}}O_2$ are available. But, remember that all interpretations of venous oxygen saturation must proceed with the awareness that several variables (Hb concentration, pH, temperature, output, respiration) can be responsible for changes in oxygen in mixed venous blood.

Principles of Operation

Pulmonary artery oximetry has become much more useful recently since a better understanding has been achieved of the problems associated with calibration, catheter stiffness, vessel wall artifact, and relationships to other variables. The theory of operation is similar to that of the pulse oximeter, except that pulse oximetry usually makes use of a system in which the light enters one side of the finger and exits on the other, whereas the pulmonary artery catheter for $S_{\bar{v}}O_2$ uses reflectance. The *in vivo* oximetry instruments use reflection spectrophotometry. A light source is used to shine light through a fiberoptic device to where the distal tip is located in a flowing blood stream. The light to be analyzed is reflected back to a set of receiving fibers, which transmit it to a photodetector. Proper sampling of mixed venous blood is necessary; for example, the catheter should not be in a wedged position.

Carbon Dioxide

The effective alveolar ventilation is usually monitored by determining the levels of CO_2 in expired gas or arterial blood. Arterial CO_2 (P_aCO_2) at sea level should be about 40 torr. While end-expired concentrations of CO_2 are said to reflect the concentration of CO_2 in arterial blood, a gradient between alveolar and arterial concentration of CO_2 is common, usually causing the alveolar to be 4 torr to 6 torr lower than the arterial.

Factors other than ventilation and perfusion can affect end-expired P_{CO_2}. When acids gain entrance to the body, bicarbonate is converted into CO_2 (see Chap. 12), and when bicarbonate is injected, some CO_2 is liberated. The formed gas depends on transport to the lung, and elimination by the lungs. Monitoring CO_2 therefore allows inferences about metabolism, blood flow to the lungs, and ventilation. Finally, just checking whether CO_2 appears in the expired gas after intubation of the trachea gives the reassuring confirmation that, indeed, the trachea rather than the esophagus has been intubated.

When patients rebreathe the gas they have inhaled, as is customary during inhalation anesthesia, the CO_2 must be removed from the expired gas in order to render it fit for reinhalation. CO_2 appearing in the inspired gas under these circumstances means either that the CO_2 absorber no longer functions properly or that the valves directing the flow of gases are incompetent.

CO_2 powerfully affects cerebral blood flow (see Chap. 9). This fact is exploited during some craniotomies, in which the volume of the brain is to be reduced and the patient's lungs are hyperventilated until the end-expired CO_2 falls from the normal 40 torr to less than 30 torr.

During cardiac arrest, of course, no blood flows through the lungs, no CO_2 is delivered, and none appears in expired air. CO_2 thus gives some information about pulmonary blood flow; with pulmonary embolism (air or clot) and with a fall in cardiac output for other reasons, less CO_2 will appear in the expired gas.

When metabolism decreases, as during hypothermia, or increases, as with fever (*e.g.*, during malignant hyperpyrexia), more CO_2 will be collected in the expired gas. The diagnostic changes of CO_2 in expired gas must be interpreted with the awareness that hyperventilation will cause more, and hypoventilation less, CO_2 to be exhaled. But, hypoventilation will lead to an accumulation of CO_2 in pulmonary blood and soon this will be reflected in higher end-expired levels. Changes in pulmonary blood flow and metabolic rate can, therefore, only be detected with confidence when the alveolar ventilation of the patient has remained steady.

Cutaneous CO_2

The factors regulating the diffusion of CO_2 through the skin are similar to those discussed for oxygen. The cutaneous CO_2 electrodes either employ the technology used in blood gas analyzers (several manufacturers) or tiny infrared detectors.* CO_2 skin electrodes have a reputation of drifting and of being difficult to calibrate. Their response times are slow. Heating the skin affects CO_2 production, for which mathematical corrections have to be introduced. Cutaneous partial pressures of CO_2 thus corrected are reported as $PsCO_2$ values.

Prolonged Hyperventilation

After anesthesia, another condition may produce normal CO_2 levels, and yet, inadequate ventilatory exchange results in inadequate oxygenation. Assume that a patient's lungs were hyperventilated for hours. The arterial and the tissue levels of dissolved CO_2 were thereby lowered markedly. When at last we allow the patient to breathe spontaneously, he requires relatively small minute volumes to maintain a normal $PaCO_2$ (40 torr or less) because much of the metabolically produced CO_2 will not be exhaled but, instead, will be soaked up by the tissue until the levels of CO_2 in the tissue are replenished and are in equilibrium with the level of CO_2 in the blood. Thus, ventilation that is reduced but sufficient to maintain a normal level of CO_2 in blood and in expired air may disguise the fact that minute ventilation and, with it, oxygen uptake are reduced (Fig. 6-7).

With modern equipment one can obtain a curve describing the concentration of CO_2 in the expired and inspired gas as it passes a point close to the patient's mouth. These so-called *capnograms* should be inspected by the clinician to ascertain that the instrument measuring CO_2 is not fooled by an abnormal waveform.

CO_2 Waveform Analysis

To analyze the CO_2 waveform, we suggest a process similar to that used to evaluate electrocardiograms, where several elements of the curve allow diagnostic inferences.

* Hewlett-Packard, Waltham, Massachusetts.

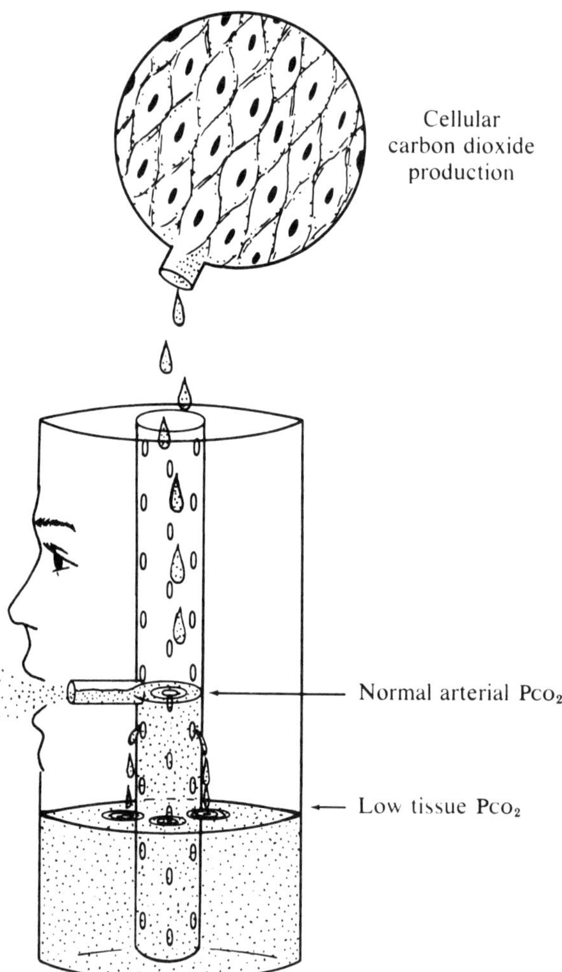

Figure 6-7. CO_2 arterial and tissue levels. Normally, tissue and arterial levels of CO_2 are in equilibrium. After prolonged hyperventilation, both fall. After such hyperventilation, a little ventilation suffices to maintain normal levels of arterial P_{CO_2} because much of the CO_2 produced is absorbed by the tissue. This figure represents the state after hyperventilation. The arterial P_{CO_2} fed by cellular CO_2 production is at the normal level shown here at the height of the mouth. Tissue levels should be equally high. After prolonged ventilation, they are, as shown, low. Some CO_2 replenishes tissue storage. Once the two compartments are in equilibrium, ventilation needs to increase to normal levels to excrete all metabolically produced CO_2.

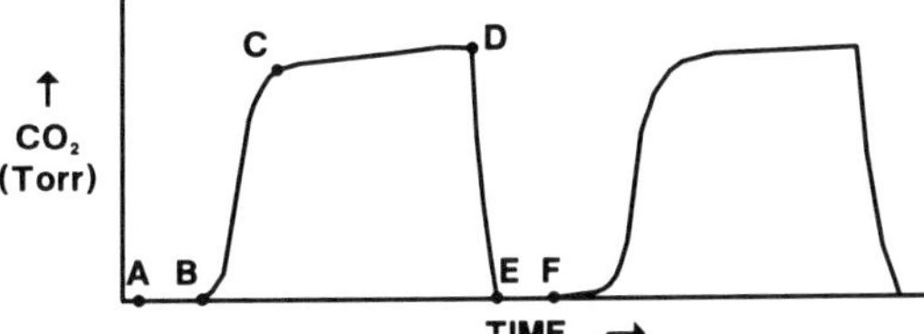

Figure 6-8. A normal capnogram. Gas is sampled continuously close to the patient's mouth. An ideal capnogram allows the identification of points *B*, *C*, *D*, and *E*, but not *A* and *F*. *A* = expiration begins, but dead space must be cleared before CO_2 appears under the sensor. *B* = first gas containing expired CO_2 appears under the sensor. *C* = alveolar gas appears, but because of uneven emptying of alveoli, the slope from *C* to *D* continues to rise gently. *D* = end-expired or alveolar CO_2 is recognized and inspiration begins to replace alveolar gas. E = inspiration has replaced all aveolar gas. This does not necessarily coincide with the end of inspiration. F = inspiration stops and the respiratory pause commences.

RATE

The respiratory rate is easily approximated from the capnogram either by taking the product of the sweep speed and the number of breaths per unit distance across the display, or by timing the breaths. Generally, CO_2 monitors display respiratory rate. If this rate differs considerably from the respiratory rate counted by the observer, all data reported by the capnograph may be in error.

RHYTHM

When spontaneous breaths intervene during mechanically controlled ventilation, then the rhythm will be irregular and the end-tidal CO_2 presentation may be in error. This can also happen if the patient is "fighting the ventilator." Such interposed spontaneous breaths bespeak either very light or no anesthesia (*e.g.*, in the intensive care unit), or inadequate ventilation (respiratory or metabolic acidosis?), or pain. In the operating room, giving a muscle relaxant to arrest attempts at spontaneous ventilation must be carefully considered; often it is not a relaxant that is missing, but adequate anesthesia or sufficient ventilation. Hiccups and external compression of the chest (*e.g.*, by a surgical elbow) also will generate dips in the plateau.

BASELINE

The baseline portion of the capnogram indicates whether rebreathing occurs. Figure 6-8 displays a regular capnogram without rebreathing. During inspiration no CO_2 is sensed. CO_2 frequently appears during inspiration when non-rebreathing systems are used. These valveless breathing

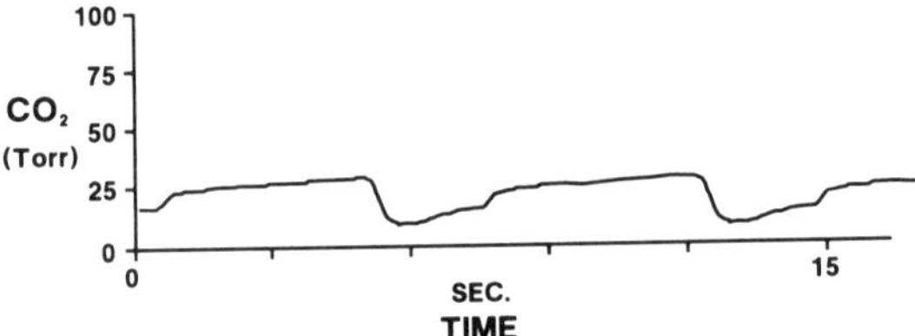

Figure 6-9. Capnogram with valveless (Bain) circuit. The elevated baseline demonstrates rebreathing.

systems, such as the Bain circuit, present special difficulties to capnography. For one, fresh gas may be introduced close to the site at which CO_2 is measured or sampled. The fresh gas may dilute the gas sample and lead to artificially low end-expired CO_2 readings.[16] For another, rebreathing typically occurs when the patient's peak inspiratory flow rate exceeds the fresh gas flow rate. Thus, the capnogram will show CO_2 in the inspired gas. This may be associated with normal or abnormal alveolar P_{CO_2} values, depending on the many factors that influence gas exchange when valveless systems are used.[17] Figure 6-9 shows a capnogram obtained when the Bain system was used. This need not cause an elevation of the patient's arterial P_{CO_2}, provided that dead space is not too large and minute ventilation large enough. However, there are limits to the amount of rebreathing for which one can compensate with increased minute volumes. Incompetent valves in the breathing circuit (*i.e.*, valves stuck in the open position) generate typical capnograms. Figures 6-10 and 6-11 show examples. When the expiratory valve stays open, rebreathing of exhaled gas causes the baseline to be elevated. An incompetent inspiratory valve may look similar or may show first rebreathed, expired gas and then fresh gas.

CONTOUR

As shown in Figure 6-8, a capnogram consists of a baseline and an ascending or expiratory portion, followed by a plateau, the final part of which is said to represent alveolar gas. Capnograms without a plateau are diagnostic only of inadequate and unreliable measurements. They are typically seen with rapid ventilation, which does not give the instrument enough time to reach a plateau. (For an example, see Fig. 6-12, which shows a normal breath followed by panting.) Most capnographs take 100 msec to 200 msec to reach 96% of their full excursion. With high-frequency ventilation, where the respiratory rate may be 100 breaths per minute and the inspiratory time only 20%, the capnogram typically shows sine waves, the extremes of which reflect neither the patient's lowest inspiratory, nor his highest expiratory, concentration of CO_2. In order to obtain inspired

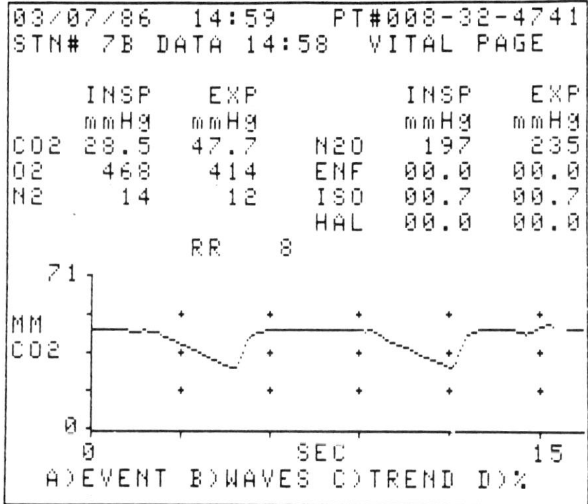

Figure 6-10. Capnogram showing rebreathing. The expiratory valve was stuck, and during inspiration this expired gas was reinhaled.

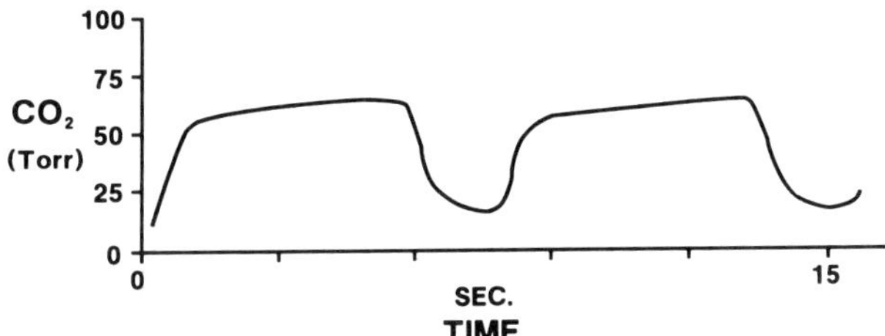

Figure 6-11. Capnogram showing rebreathing. The inspiratory valve was stuck and during inspiration some of the expired gas was reinhaled.

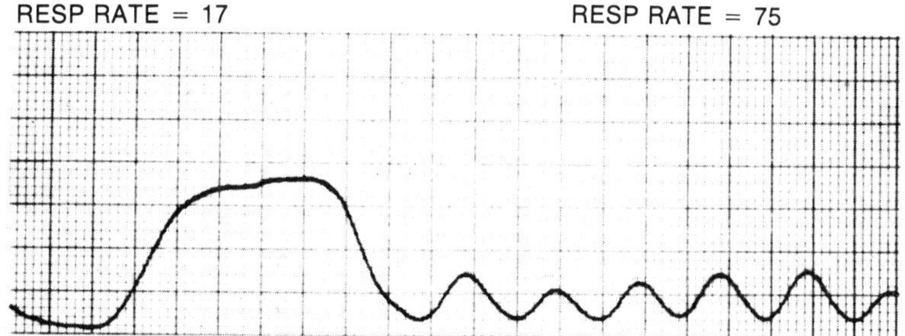

Figure 6-12. The subject took a normal breath and then panted. Observe that the end-expired CO_2 values during panting do not reflect aveolar gas.

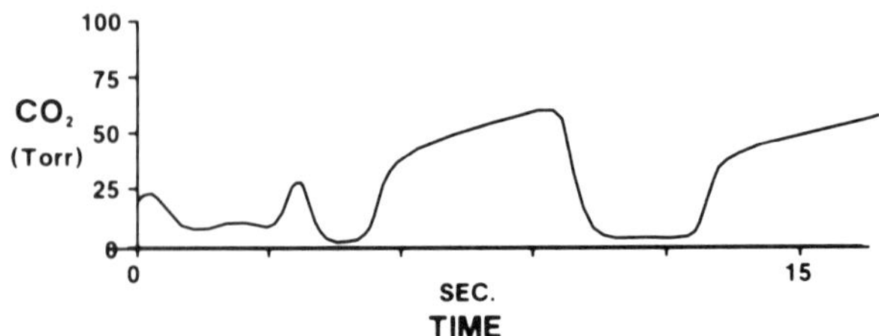

Figure 6-13. Mechanical obstruction. The flattened, ascending part of the capnogram reveals obstruction to expiration, either intrinsic or extrinsic. On inspiration, obstruction does not become apparent on the capnogram as fresh gas displaces the CO_2 at the sampling site.

and end-expired CO_2 values, we therefore interrupt high-frequency ventilation at regular intervals and interpose two large tidal volumes.

If the ascending or expiratory portion of the curve becomes flattened to a lazy slope (Fig. 6-13), expiratory obstruction must be considered. This can happen to a patient with obstructive lung disease, emphysema, or wheezing, or when the endotracheal tube is kinked, or when some other obstruction to expiratory flow impedes exhalation.

When patients are paralyzed during mechanical ventilation, the capnogram should show a monotonous, repetitive pattern. Once the diaphragm begins to move, one may begin to see a small dip in the latter third of the plateau of the capnogram, as shown in Figure 6-14. This often indicates air hunger, because it takes a considerable stimulus to move the diaphragm under general anesthesia in a patient who is partially paralyzed. These dips have sometimes been called "curare clefts," an unfortunate

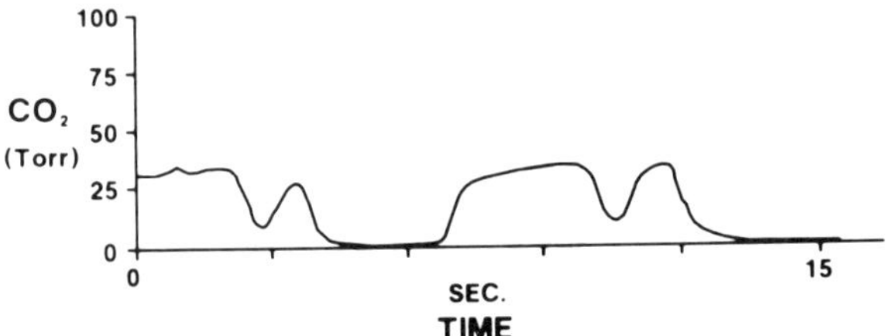

Figure 6-14. Capnogram showing spontaneous breaths superimposed on mechanical ventilation. This typical pattern demonstrates an inspiratory movement of gas before the mechanical ventilator initiates inspiration. Observe that the spontaneous inspiration is too shallow to remove all the CO_2 from the area of the sampling port. This often develops in patients who are underventilated and attempt to breathe on their own, but cannot do so successfully due to muscle weakness. This calls for more ventilation rather than more muscle relaxant drug.

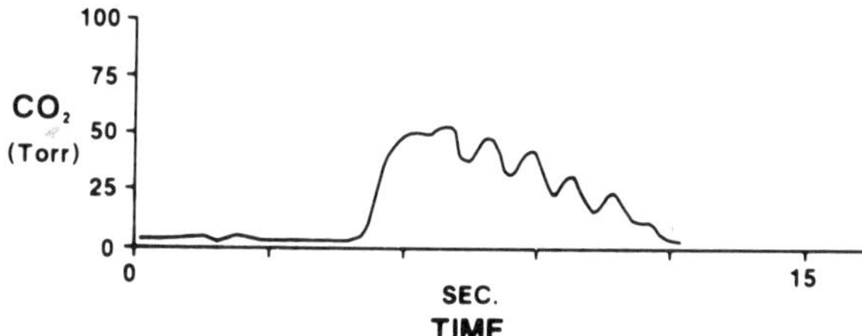

Figure 6-15. Capnogram with cardiogenic oscillations. Ventricular ejections generate changes in intrathoracic volume. These are reflected in the capnogram when small cardiogenic tidal volumes can move gas free of CO_2 under the CO_2 sampling port.

term that distracts from the recognition that such events should not occur under well-conducted anesthesia. The dips are usually accompanied by a weak tracheal tug, giving more evidence that strong signals are sent by the patient's respiratory center to remedy a state of hypoventilation. In patients not paralyzed, a dip can be viewed with equanimity; no tracheal tug will be seen; the patient is simply beginning to assume spontaneous control of his ventilation as dictated by his respiratory center.

Small, regular, toothlike oscillations in the descending portion of the curve (which is usually as steep as the ascending portion) usually represent cardiogenic oscillations, dramatic evidence of a pneumocardiogram (Fig. 6-15). With each systole the heart ejects enough blood to diminish the intrathoracic volume, giving rise to a little inspiratory flow of gas. The nature of these oscillations is quickly confirmed by counting and timing them against the electrocardiogram.

The shallow downward slope after the plateau (Fig. 6-16) may not represent the beginning of a slow inspiration, but may simply reflect that the end-expired CO_2 deposited in the vicinity of the sampling tube is being removed and that fresh gas from elsewhere in the breathing tubes is be-

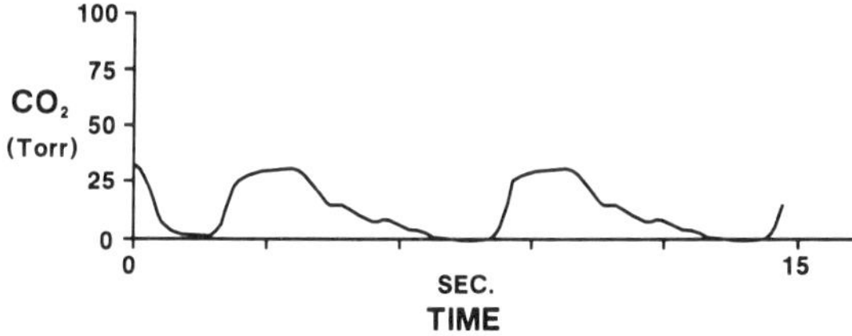

Figure 6-16. Long respiratory pause with aspiration of fresh gas into the sampling port. In patients with small tidal volumes or with rapid rates of sampling, fresh gas may be drawn into the sampling port before ventilation is initiated.

Table 6-5. MONITORING VENTILATION

	End-expired CO_2*	Inspired CO_2*
External		
Disconnect or stop ventilator—apneic patient	$\underline{\downarrow}$	NC†
Faulty unidirectional valve in circle system	$\uparrow$	$\underline{\uparrow}$
Exhausted CO_2 absorber	$\uparrow$	$\underline{\uparrow}$
Spontaneously breathing patients under drapes	$\uparrow$	$\underline{\uparrow}$
Increased dead space	$\uparrow$	$\underline{\uparrow}$
Internal		
Hyperthermia (ventilation constant)	$\uparrow$	NC
Hypothermia (ventilation constant)	$\downarrow$	NC
Pulmonary embolism (air or thrombus)	$\downarrow$	NC
Reduced cardiac output	$\downarrow$	NC
Hyperventilation	$\downarrow$	NC
Hypoventilation	$\uparrow$	NC

* Initial change for end-expired and inspired CO_2 is underscored.
† NC = no change

ginning to replace the CO_2. This is most commonly seen in children with small tidal volumes, with high flow rates of gases aspired to the analyzer, and with long expiratory pauses.

TRENDS

A normal CO_2 capnogram, recorded over time by a slow-speed recorder, looks rather monotonous. Table 6-5 gives differential diagnostic considerations should the capnogram demonstrate a downward or upward trend.

CAPNOGRAPHY UNDER DRAPES

Particularly elderly patients undergoing ophthalmologic operations are often heavily sedated because the procedure is carried out under local anesthesia; furthermore, their noses and mouths are covered with drapes. One can sample gas for capnography either by taping a collecting tube under the nose (Fig. 6-17) or by attaching it to nasal prongs. At the same time, air or oxygen should be insufflated under the drapes close to the mouth of the patient. Capnography under these circumstances is not accurate, but serves as a monitor of ventilation and helps to detect CO_2 in the inspired air.

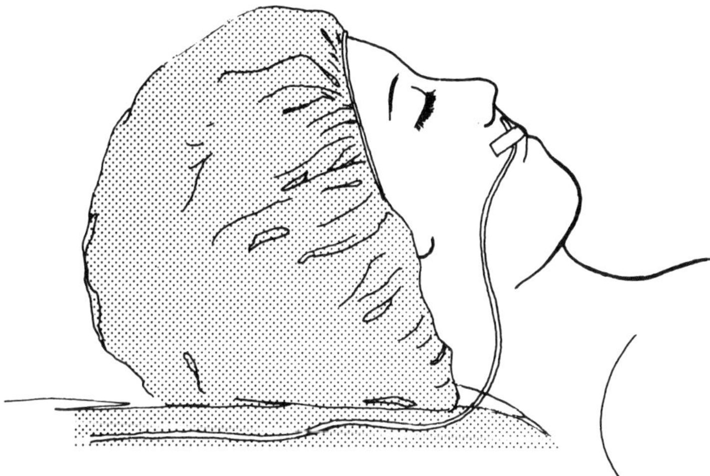

Figure 6-17. Under drapes, a patient under local anesthesia during eye surgery sometimes suffers respiratory insufficiency. Monitoring CO_2 of inspired and expired gas can help. When the atmosphere surrounding the patient's face becomes dead space, the CO_2 levels of inspired and expired air increase.

CAPNOGRAPHY ON AWAKE PATIENTS

Capnography on awake and sedated patients may also be done through a nasal airway. After a nasal airway of appropriate size is inserted into a naris using local anesthetic and lubricant, the sampling tube is inserted to 1 cm, from the pharyngeal opening of the airway. A satisfactory capnograph is usually obtained.[18]

Shunt and Dead Space

In clinical practice two findings often present puzzling paradoxes. One observation can be that oxygen tension in arterial blood is low (indicating hypoventilation) while CO_2 values are also low (indicating hyperventilation); the other that the gradient of CO_2 from alveolus to artery may be widening during anesthesia. These paradoxes are ascribed to shunts and dead space.

SHUNT Arterial blood gas shows a low Po_2 (*e.g.*, 60 torr) and also a low Pco_2 (*e.g.*, 30 torr); yet the patient breathes a gas mixture containing 40% oxygen. How can the oxygen be low when the patient not only gets enough oxygen in the inspired air but when his carbon dioxide level indicates adequate ventilation?

Such data are typical for a right to left shunt where some venous blood reaches the left atrium and ventricle without having undergone oxygenation. The following consideration makes clear why a discrepancy between arterial oxygen and CO_2 is so common under these circumstances.

Assume that the blood in the pulmonary artery is split, half going to well-ventilated alveoli, where it is exposed to oxygen and where it can become fully saturated, the other half flowing past unventilated alveoli and emerging in the pulmonary vein essentially as it entered the pulmonary artery. The mixture of oxygenated and unoxygenated blood will reflect the degree of the shunt. When we now hyperventilate the patient's lungs, the blood that flows past ventilated alveoli can absorb only a little additional oxygen, namely that which goes into solution; its hemoglobin is already fully saturated and it cannot carry more oxygen, regardless of the P_{O_2} to which we expose it. Hyperventilation in the face of a shunt will therefore accomplish little for oxygen.

For CO_2 the situation is different. With hyperventilation of the perfused lung, more and more CO_2 is blown off. The blood flowing from the ventilated portion of the lung will therefore have quite a low P_{CO_2} and this blood will mix with the blood coming from the lung that was perfused but not ventilated. Since the gradient for CO_2 from the venous to the arterial side is not large in the first place (46 torr on the venous side to 40 torr on the arterial side), it is understandable that blood emerging from the ventilated side with a P_{CO_2} of, say, 20 torr and mixing with the shunted blood (P_{CO_2} = 46 torr) can bring the P_{CO_2} down well below 40 torr in the face of significant hypoxemia.

The most striking example of a shunt is perhaps seen following the unintentional intubation of a main stem bronchus. Now one lung is well ventilated and perfused. Ventilation can be adjusted to assure good end-expired CO_2 values. But despite what appears to be adequate ventilation, the patient's arterial oxygen saturation begins to fall because hyperventilation of the ventilated lung cannot compensate for the large amount of blood shunted through the unventilated lung.

DEAD SPACE The other seeming paradox is the observation of a rising gradient between end-expired and arterial P_{CO_2}, a common observation during anesthesia. It is the hallmark of processes interfering with the perfusion of ventilated alveoli, where a ventilated alveolus no longer contributes CO_2 to the expired gas. The gas coming from the unperfused alveoli dilutes the CO_2 coming from the perfused alveoli; therefore the end-expired CO_2 will be lower than the arterial P_{CO_2}. Thus, a rising gradient between end-expired and arterial CO_2 signifies the development of alveolar dead space. The observations made for CO_2 also apply to oxygen.

Clinically, alveolar dead space arises with pulmonary embolism, for

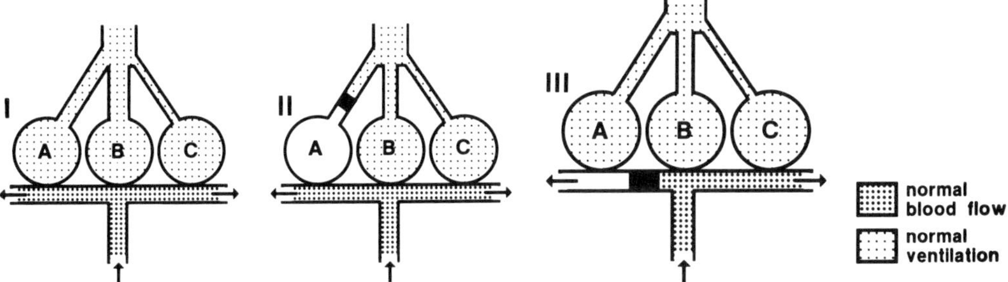

Figure 6-18. The diagram shows alveoli with a normal (*A*), a wide (*B*), and a narrow (*C*) airway. The rate of emptying will be influenced by the size of the airway. This explains the slope of the plateau of the capnogram. In *II*, one airway is blocked, which creates a right-to-left shunt. In *III*, one vessel is blocked, which leads to ventilation of an unperfused alveolus and increased dead space with a rising end-expired to arterial CO_2 gradient, with P_ACO_2 falling well below $PaCO_2$.

instance, air embolism. Perhaps more common is the observation during lengthy operations with patients in the lateral position, where a redistribution of pulmonary blood flow leads to an underperfusion of certain ventilated segments of the lungs.

Figure 6-18 summarizes the principles involved. It must be understood that the ventilation and perfusion abnormalities are never that clearcut. Usually, partial underventilation and underperfusion are mixed in changing patterns. Nevertheless, the diagram helps to explain the findings in the operating room and intensive care unit.

Infrared Analyzers

CO_2 in inspired and expired gas is monitored by two different methods: either with a mass spectrometer (see above) or with an infrared device. Infrared devices may themselves be subdivided into two categories: inline analyzers and sampling analyzers.

The in-line analyzer* has a sensing head mounted on the endotracheal tube as a breathe-through infrared cell and a transducer. Its quick response time and freedom from problems associated with long sampling catheters are advantageous; added dead space and weight and its cost are disadvantages.

The sampling analyzer withdraws, under suction, a continuous sample of inspired and expired gases. The gases are transported through a cap-

* Siemens-Elema, Elk Grove Village, Illinois; Hewlett-Packard, Waltham, Massachusetts

illary to an infrared analyzer. The advantages of these systems are that dead space is reduced, the attachment to the endotracheal tube is simple, the need for miniaturization is reduced, and the expense is small.

HOW INFRARED CO_2 ANALYZERS WORK

CO_2 absorbs infrared light at 2600 nm and 4300 nm wavelengths. The light is beamed through a calibrated, CO_2-filled chamber serving as a control and through the chamber with the gas that is to be analyzed. Infrared-sensitive photocells, with filters that select the wavelength to be detected, receive light from both chambers and calculate the concentrations of CO_2 in the sample gas by comparing it to the known concentration of CO_2 in the control.

Several difficulties had to be overcome in applying these principles. The first of these was the need for a correction factor for infrared absorption caused by nitrogen and nitrous oxide. This is referred to as pressure broadening, which occurs when a background gas, in this case nitrogen or nitrous oxide, accepts kinetic energy from CO_2 molecules. Most CO_2 monitors compensate for this either manually or automatically. A second problem is that water vapor can interfere with accurate CO_2 analysis. In sampling systems, water vapor can condense and block the sample capillary. It can also cause errors in breathe-through systems when the water condenses on the cell windows. Water vapor can also affect calibration. Clinically, however, this is insignificant. A third problem is that the absorption of infrared light by CO_2 is not linear. Manufacturers adjust for this in the design of instruments.

Other Gases

Nitrogen

Nitrogen is analyzed in the mass spectrometer. Instances of air embolism, discussed in Chapter 11, are diagnosed quickly by the unexpected appearance of nitrogen in expired gas. This occurs when air enters the venous system, passes through capillaries, and travels into alveoli. Because nitrogen is not typically administered to patients during anesthesia, the gas can serve as a leak detector. Since the mass spectrometer operates at subatmospheric pressure, any leak in the sampling system, including occasionally loose-fitting endotracheal tubing, results in entrainment of air, which is manifested as the appearance of nitrogen in the inspired *and* expired gases. This fact is helpful in distinguishing between air embolus and a sampling leak.

Nitrous Oxide

A mass spectrometer is usually needed for analysis of this frequently used gas, but infrared analyzers are also used. The mass spectrometer will show inspired and expired levels of the gas and thus allow the anesthesiologist to monitor the uptake of the drug. Since nitrous oxide is relatively insoluble in blood, uptake is fast and, after an hour, if the settings of the flow meters have not been changed, the inspired and expired values will begin to coincide.

Halogenated Anesthetic Agents

It is helpful to the anesthesiologist to monitor the concentration or partial pressure of inhaled and exhaled anesthetic vapors. Unexpected falls in blood pressure call for an analysis of depth of anesthesia, which is much facilitated when one can look at a gas analyzer to see how much drug the patient shows in the expired gas. Similarly, a patient slow to rally after anesthesia will cause less concern when the analyzer shows continued excretion of anesthetic vapors in the exhaled gas. The mass spectrometer, in particular, makes it possible to discover mistakes of filling a vaporizer with the wrong agent. Several case reports have been published recounting the problems encountered when agents have been mixed or a vaporizer had been filled incorrectly. If, for instance, the anesthesiologist thinks he is giving an agent with a low vapor pressure, but his vaporizer is filled with one of high vapor pressure, unpleasant clinical surprises are in store for him. Gas analyzers also permit the calibration of vaporizers. Some clinicians like to do this daily, making factory calibration necessary less often and thus saving money.

Anesthetic vapor analyzers also help us to use low-flow anesthesia more easily. Most vaporizers are nonlinear at flows at less than 1 liter per minute. With the analyzer it is possible to measure end-tidal anesthetic concentration, instead of being dependent on calculations incorporating many estimates to obtain vapor pressures.

Anesthetic gases can be analyzed by a number of methods. The "gold standard" is probably the mass spectrometer, already discussed. It is rapid, accurate, quite reliable, and capable of distinguishing different anesthetic vapors from one another. However, the mass spectrometer is expensive, serves multiple rooms, and has its limitations, as discussed. Other methods for analysis of anesthetic gases rely on the absorption of infrared and ultraviolet light. These methods resemble those described for CO_2. A difficulty with these analyzers is that they cannot positively identify a halogenated anesthetic agent; that is, the user must set the machine to the drug to be employed. Thus, infrared analyzers cannot protect against the mixing of drugs, or wrong filling of a vaporizer. They also tend to have slower response times than CO_2 analyzers or the mass spectrometer. Their advantage is that they are less expensive than the mass spectrometer, and can be dedicated to a single room.

For some years a silicone rubber device was available as a gas ana-

Table 6-6. EXPIRATORY INSPIRATORY ALARM PRESSURES OF VARIOUS GASES AND VAPORS

	Gas pressures (torr)						
	CO_2	O_2	N_2	N_2O	Halothane	Ethrane	Fluorane
Expiratory							
High	55	No	610	610	40	40	40
Low	No	100	No	No	No	No	No
Inspiratory							
High	No	No	610	610	40	40	40
Low	No	140	No	No	No	No	No

lyzer. The principle was based on the observation that these substances absorb anesthetic vapors and in the process change their physical characteristics, such as size under tension. These devices are quite nonspecific and difficult to calibrate.

Finally, a piezoelectric analyzer[19] has been produced that employs an oscillating quartz crystal covered by a film of material that absorbs anesthetic vapors. Again, the device is not specific, is sensitive to water vapor, and is difficult to calibrate.

Many companies are at work to develop new and less expensive systems that will have the advantages of the mass spectrometer without its drawback of high price. We look forward to these developments because monitoring anesthetic agents makes anesthesia safer for our patients.

ALARMS

Many analyzers offer alarms for O_2, CO_2, and anesthetic agents. Table 6-6 shows the alarm limits used in our hospital's mass spectrometer.

REFERENCES

1. Cooper JB, Newbower RS, Kitz RJ: An analysis of major errors and equipment failures in anesthesia management: Considerations for prevention and detection. Anesthesiology 60:34–42, 1984
2. Nunn JF, Ezi-Ashi TE: The accuracy of the respirometer and ventigrator. Br J Anaesth 34:422, 1962
3. Van Wagenen R, Westenskow DR, Benner R: Respiratory gas analysis by Raman scattering (abstr). Anesthesiology 63:A163, 1985
4. Gravenstein JS, Gravenstein N, van der Aa JJ, et al: Pitfalls with mass spectrometry in clinical anesthesia. Int J Clin Monit Comput 1:27–34, 1984
5. Baumberger JP, Goodfriend RB: Determination of arterial oxygen tension in man by equilibration through intact skin. Fed Proc 10:10, 1951

6. Huch A, Huch R, Arner B, et al: Continuous transcutaneous oxygen tension measured with a heated electrode. Scand J Clin Lab Invest 31:269, 1973
7. Barker SJ, Tremper KK: Transcutaneous oxygen tension: Physiological variable for monitoring oxygenation. J Clin Monit 1:130–134, 1985
8. Lofgren O: Transcutaneous oxygen measurement in adult intensive care. Acta Anaesthesiol Scand 23:534, 1979
9. Maekawa T, Okuda Y, McDowall DG: Effect of low concentrations of halothane on the oxygen electrode. Br J Anaesth 52:585, 1980
10. Yelderman M, New W: Evaluation of pulse oximetry (abstr). Anesthesiology 59:A349–A352, 1983
11. Fanconi S, Doherty P, Edmonds JF, et al: Pulse oximetry in pediatric intensive care: Comparisons with measured saturations and transcutaneous oxygen tension. J Pediatr 107:362–366, 1985
12. Sidi A, Rush WR, Paulus DA, et al: Effect of fluorescein, idocyanine green, and methylene blue on the measurement of oxygen saturation on pulse oximetry (abstr). Anesthesiology 65:A132, 1986
13. New W: Pulse oximetry. J Clin Monit 1:126–129, 1985
14. Strohl KP, House PM, Holic JF, et al: Comparison of three transmittance oximeters. Med Instrum 20:143–149, 1986
15. Barker SJ, Tremper KK, Gamel DM: A clinical comparison of transcutaneous PO_2 and pulse oximetry in the operating room. Anesth Analg 65:805–808, 1986
16. Gravenstein N, Lampotang S, Beneken JW: Bain circuit: Influences on capnography (abstr). Anesthesiology 61:A172, 1984
17. Beneken JEW, Gravenstein N, Gravenstein JS, et al: Capnography and the Bain circuit. I: A computer model. J Clin Monit 1:103–113, 1985
18. Norman EA, Zeig NJ, Ahmed I: Better designs for mass spectrometer monitoring of the awake patient. Anesthesiology 64:664, 1986
19. Cooper JB, Edmonson JH, Joseph DM, et al: Piezoelectric absorption anesthetic sensor. IEEE Trans Biomed Eng 28:459–466, 1981

CHAPTER 7

Temperature

Humans are homeostatic creatures. They generate heat by using endogenous chemical processes and lose heat to, or gain heat from, their surroundings via evaporation, radiation, conduction, and convection in order to stabilize body temperature. Premature babies are particularly sensitive to the temperature of their environment. Procedures requiring deep general anesthesia and subsequent muscle relaxation lead to impairment of temperature homeostasis in patients.

ENDOGENOUS TEMPERATURE DERANGEMENT

The patient who is genetically predisposed to hyperthermia during anesthesia is at particular risk. Known as *malignant hyperthermia,* this disease, reported first by Moschowitz[1] in 1916, has several symptoms. They include muscular rigidity after the administration of succinylcholine, tachycardia and other arrhythmias, hypertension, skin mottling, increasing P_aCO_2, myoglobinuria, renal failure, electrolyte abnormalities, defective coagulation, and neurologic disorders. Signs, symptoms, and the suggested management of this acute crisis are provided below.[2,3] Often the rise in temperature is actually a late manifestation of the disease. When temperature rises above 42°C, the mortality rate is 80% to 90%.

Malignant Hyperthermia

DEFINITION

Malignant hyperthermia (MH) is a fulminant hypermetabolic crisis triggered by anesthetic agents.

INCIDENCE

The incidence of the disease is as follows: 1 per 15,000 to 1 per 150,000 in North America depending on race; 1 per 15,000 children; men more than women; familial genetic transmission; 50% of offspring affected; mortality rate of 50% to 60%.

CHOICE OF ANESTHETIC FOR ELECTIVE ANESTHESIA IN SUSCEPTIBLE INDIVIDUALS

The following recommended precautions to prevent MH in susceptible patients are based on information compiled by Britt and the Malignant Hyperthermia Association of the United States (MHAUS):[2,4]

1. Institute dantrolene prophylaxis. *per os* over 3 days prior to anesthesia with 1 to 1.5 mg/kg four times per day, 2 to 4 mg/kg IV over 1 to 4 hours prior to anesthesia.
2. Clean the anesthesia machine. Flush the system with 3 liters/min O_2 for 6 hours. Install fresh soda lime.
3. Administer regional, spinal, or epidural anesthesia, if possible, with chloroprocaine, procaine, or tetracaine. Lidocaine and other aminos are now considered safe for regional anesthesia.
4. Premedicate the patient with a narcotic, a barbiturate, or a benzodiazepine drug, or some combination thereof.
5. Continue with a barbiturate, a narcotic, a benzodiazepine, or droperidol drug during induction.
6. For maintenance, N_2O–O_2, a narcotic, or droperidol is suggested with a nondepolarizing muscle relaxant as needed. Atracurium, vecuronium, and pancuronium have all been safely used in MH patients.
7. The question of whether to reverse the nondepolarized muscle block is controversial. Most clinicians, however, do reverse the muscle block.
8. In the absence of muscle rigidity and hyperthermia, dantrolene

may be administered, for 6 hours to 12 hours afterward, as indicated by history and clinical findings.

The following should *not* be administered to MH-susceptible patients:

1. *Inhalation Anesthetics:* Enflurane (Ethrane), halothane (Fluothane), isoflurane (Forane), cyclopropane, methoxyflurane (Penthrane), diethyl ether
2. *Depolarizing Muscle Relaxants:* Succinylcholine and decamethonium
3. *Others:* Phenothiazines, calcium preparations

The following are controversial drugs for MH-susceptible patients:*

1. Anticholinesterases (*e.g.,* neostigmine, pyridostigmine, edrophonium)
2. Vasopressors (*e.g.,* epinephrine, ephedrine, dopamine)
3. Anticholinergics (*e.g.,* atropine, scopolamine)
4. Digitalis preparations
5. *d*-Tubocurare

Management of Malignant Hyperthermia Crisis

CLINICAL FINDINGS

Clinical findings include the following: variable course; tachycardia and tachypnea; fever usually *not* the presenting sign.

EARLY Sometimes muscle rigidity following succinylcholine: tachycardia; also tachypnea, unstable blood pressure, arrhythmias, cyanosis, profuse sweating, rapid increase in temperature.

LATE Skeletal muscle swelling; left heart failure; disseminated intravascular coagulopathy; acute renal failure.

LABORATORY Respiratory and metabolic acidosis; increased serum levels of potassium, magnesium, myoglobin, and creatinine phosphokinase; hypoxemia; hypercapnia (P_aCO_2 to 200 torr), *p*H 7.20 to 6.80; myoglobinuria; test for levels of creatine phosphokinase (CPK), lactate dehydrogenase (LDH), serum aspartate aminotransferase (SGOT), alkaline phosphatase, bilirubin, calcium, magnesium, blood urea nitrogen (BUN),

* Some experts believe these drugs are unsafe or confuse the clinical picture of the MH reaction.

creatinine, triiodothyronine (T_3), prothrombin time (PT), partial thromboplastin time (PTT), platelet count, lactic acid.

MANDATORY MONITORING

Electrocardiogram, temperature, arterial blood capnography, potassium, sodium, central venous pressure or pulmonary artery catheter depending on patient's condition; arterial catheter for blood pressure and blood sampling; urinary output (Foley catheter).

SUPPLIES

Have the following immediately available: sodium bicarbonate (12 × 50 mEq amps); dantrolene sodium (20–30 vials); iced IV saline (12 × 1000 ml bottles); furosemide (10 × 20 mg amps); mannitol (4 × 12.5 g amps); procainamide (1000 mg); regular perfusion apparatus in hospitals with experience in its use.

TREATMENT

The following procedures are recommended by MHAUS for the treatment of an MH crisis:[4]

1. Discontinue all inhalation anesthetics and hyperventilate with 100% oxygen.
2. End surgery as quickly as possible and, if needed, switch to safe anesthetics.
3. Initially, administer dantrolene sodium, 1 to 10 mg/kg, mixed with sterile distilled water IV at a rate of 1 mg/kg/min. Continue dantrolene until symptoms of hypermetabolism subside.
4. Administer bicarbonate 1 mEq to 2 mEq/kg IV unless arterial blood gas analysis indicates otherwise.
5. Combat fever with active cooling.
6. Change anesthetic tubing and, if possible, soda lime.
7. If arrhythmias persist after treatment of acidosis and hyperkalemia, give repeated doses of procainamide.
8. Titrate dantrolene as necessary to heart rate, muscle rigidity, and temperature. Although the average successful dose of dantrolene is about 2.5 mg/kg, much higher doses may be needed (10 mg/kg over each 4-hour span and more). Fortunately dantrolene does not produce significant myocardial depression at these doses unless the patient simultaneously receives calcium channel blockers.
9. Determine and monitor closely urine output, serum potassium, calcium, arterial blood gases, and clotting status. Hyperkalemia is common in the acute phase of MH and should be treated with intravenous glucose and insulin.

10. Watch the patient closely for at least 24 hours as MH can recrudesce.
11. Follow the levels of CPK, calcium, and potassium until such time as they return to normal.
12. Monitor the electrocardiogram (ECG) throughout treatment.
13. Monitor body temperature closely since vigorous treatment of MH may lead to hypothermia. Temperature instability may persist for several days after the acute episode. Core body temperatures of 42–43°C are compatible with survival and normal brain function if treated promptly.
14. Ensure urine output of greater than 1 ml/kg/hr. Consider central venous pressure (CVP) monitoring to guard against hypovolemia or cardiac failure.
15. When the patient's condition has stabilized, convert from intravenous to oral dantrolene. Optimal doses and duration of treatment with dantrolene are not known. Many patients have received a total dose of 4 mg/kg/day in divided doses for 48 hours postoperatively.

The above recommendations may not apply to every case, however, and should be altered if required.

EXOGENOUS TEMPERATURE DERANGEMENT

Before operating rooms were cooled, patients often developed fever once placed under drapes. Air-conditioned operating rooms have reduced, but not eliminated, this problem.

Two forms of hypothermia are of interest. The first is intentional, for example, during neurosurgical or cardiac procedures. During intentional hypothermia, cooling can lead to ventricular fibrillation. During the rewarming process at the end of cardiopulmonary bypass, the patient's heart may initially be refractory to a spontaneous rhythm until sufficient rewarming has taken place.

Hypothermia can also occur inadvertently. There are several avenues by which the patient dissipates heat. They include low environmental temperatures, low humidity, inspiration of cold gas, vasodilatation, decreased muscle activity, infusion of cold fluids, and the influence of anesthetic and paralyzing agents on thermoregulation.[5] Evaporation, especially when the patient is soaked with antiseptic solution, can cause the patient's temperature to fall.

Morris found, during intra-abdominal operations, that a temperature of 21°C in the operating theater was critical.[6] If exposed to temperatures below 21°C for 2 hours of anesthesia and operation, the patient's esophageal temperature dropped below 36°C regardless of his age.[7]

HEAT-LOSS REDUCTION

Heat loss can be conserved by several methods, intraoperatively as well as pre- and postoperatively. The first is by controlling the temperature of the operating room. When it is below 21°C, all patients will become hypothermic. Between 21°C and 24°C, about 70% of the patients will remain normothermic. If the temperature of the operating room is maintained between 24°C and 26°C, patients remain normothermic. Young children and elderly patients are particularly susceptible to inadvertent hypothermia because they have less ability to produce heat. Infants, of course, have an increased ratio of body surface area to mass, further contributing to heat loss. Since most operating rooms are kept cool and because the greatest heat loss occurs during the first hour of anesthesia, few patients will escape an intraoperative temperature drop. Warming blankets are helpful in maintaining temperatures only in small patients of less than 1 m^2 body surface area.

Heating and humidifying inspired gases to 38 ± 1°C and 100% relative humidity safely assists in supporting body temperature. There are several heated humidifiers currently on the market. The temperature of the gas flowing to the patient must not exceed 43°C, in order to prevent airway burns.

Another method of maintaining body temperature is to warm any fluid being administered to the patient. Thermostatically controlled warmers for intravenous fluids are available. Warmers currently manufactured (Fenwal, American Hospital Supply, and others) can increase the temperature of administered fluid to body temperature nearly independent of the rate at which the fluid is infused.

Anesthetic agents contribute to heat loss in two ways.[8] First, the agents cause subcutaneous vasodilatation. Increased amounts of blood circulate to the skin, which is already cooler than the aorta or cerebellum. This cutaneous blood cools, returns to the heart, and, in turn, cools vessel-rich organs. The cycle continues and more heat is lost. A second mechanism affects the hypothalamic, thermoregulatory center. Anesthetic agents seem to reset or turn off its thermostat.[9] Interestingly, in many patients, ketamine increases temperature.

Figure 7-1 explains why heat loss is greatest early during anesthesia. If all mechanisms by which the body maintains its temperature cease at once, and if the room were much colder than the body, the temperature gradient would be steep at first, and small after much heat loss. Thus, the initial heat loss will be relatively pronounced. The implication is that, if normothermia is important, it must be maintained even during relatively short procedures.

Hypothermia has several physiological consequences. At 30°C metabolic rate may fall to 50% of normal. Oxygen uptake and carbon dioxide production decrease. Blood pressure may rise at first, then fall. Ventric-

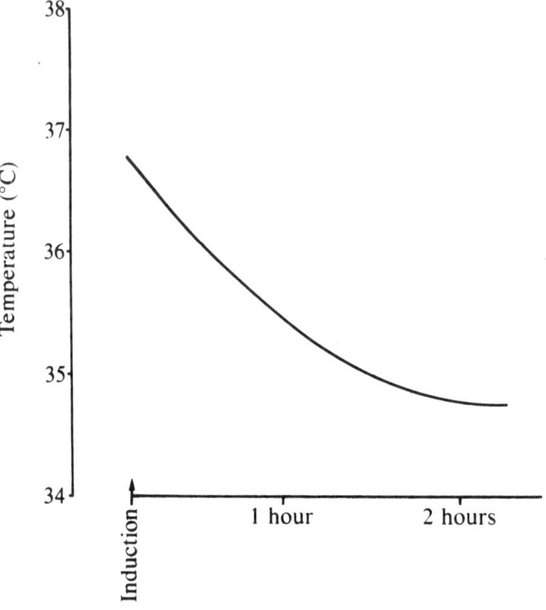

Figure 7-1. Temperature change during anesthesia. Observe the typical rapid fall of temperature early during anesthesia.

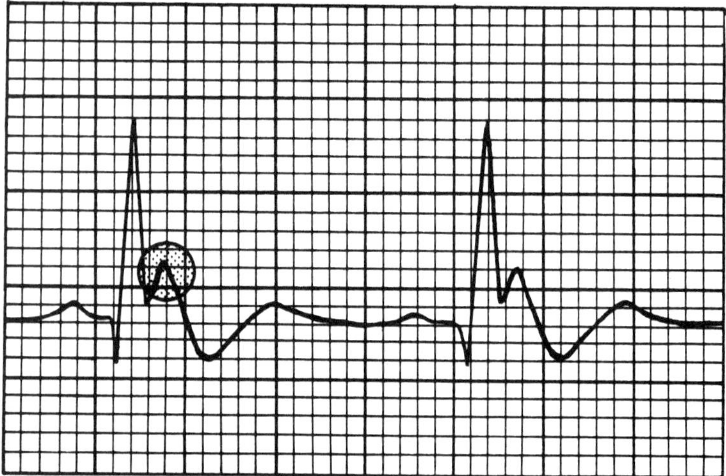

Figure 7-2. Electrocardiogram in hypothermia. A J-wave (*shaded*) is sometimes seen during hypothermia below 30°C.

ular arrhythmias become frequent below 28°C. If fibrillation does not supervene, hypotension occurs at approximately 25°C. A decreased sinus rate, T-wave inversions, QT interval prolongation, as well as the pathognomonic J-wave may develop (Fig. 7-2). Depending upon the drugs used, spontaneous ventilation may be maintained in moderate hypothermia. Although hypothermia does affect the oxyhemoglobin dissociation curve, the resultant shift to the left is not clinically significant. Acid–base balance is difficult to assess. Urine flow will increase with decreasing temperature, decreasing only with profound hypothermia. Alterations in blood flow are manifest in the nervous system, where the cerebral blood flow decreases 6% to 7% per 1°C drop.

Postoperative shivering may substantially increase oxygen consumption. The average maximum oxygen consumption increase in Roe's study of 24 unselected adult patients undergoing elective operations was 80% above the resting preoperative value, while average rectal temperature had dropped 1.1°C.[10] A fall of between 0.3°C and 1.2°C increased average oxygen consumption 92% postoperatively.

TEMPERATURE-MONITORING EQUIPMENT

Several different types of equipment may be used to measure the patient's temperature intraoperatively. These include probes, tapes, and surface electrodes. Each type has its advantage in specific clinical settings.

Temperature Probes

Temperature probes make use of either a thermocouple or a thermistor. A thermistor is a well-aged semiconductor that is a thermally sensitive resistor. A thermocouple consists of two different types of metal joined at two junctions that are maintained at different temperatures. An electromotive force is generated which, in turn, drives a measurable current. The current is proportional to the difference between the temperature of the two junctions.[11] Measurement of either resistance or current, then, indicates the temperature that is displayed.

Location of Temperature Probe

Where the temperature probe should be placed has been investigated in numerous studies. Location of the probe is important, but, no matter where it is placed (*e.g.*, nasopharynx, skin, rectum), remember that the temperature displayed represents the value at a particular point and does not necessarily reflect temperature elsewhere.

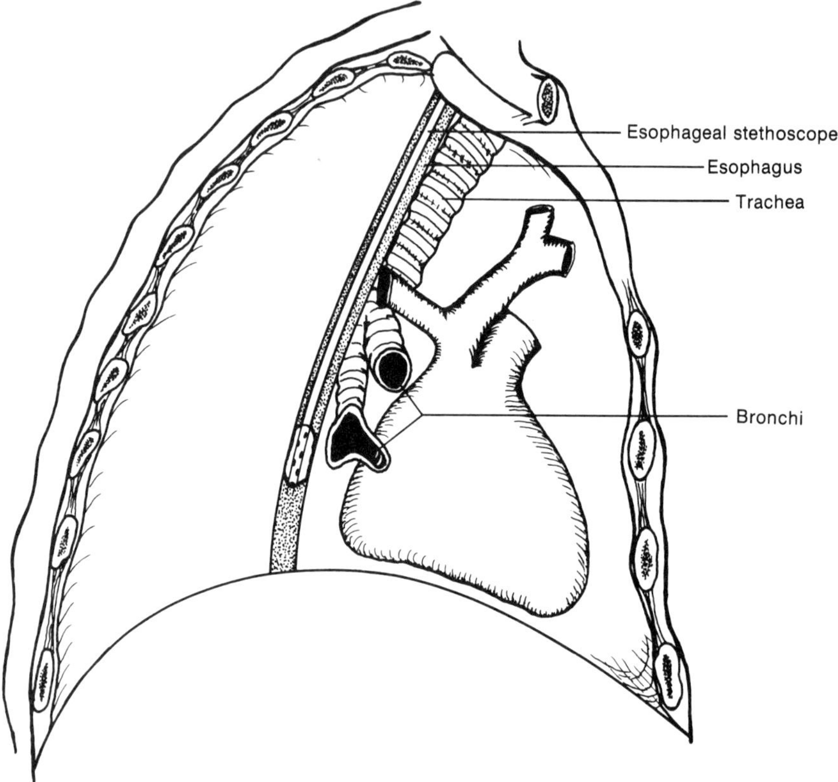

Figure 7-3. Location of esophageal temperature probe. The best place is the lower third of the esophagus behind the heart. At this spot, heart sounds are loudest. An esophageal stethoscope armed with a temperature probe makes correct placement of the temperature probe easy.

Esophagus

Whitby and Dunkin examined cerebral, esophageal, and nasopharyngeal temperatures and confirmed that temperatures measured in the lower esophagus approximate cerebral temperature.[12] This is no longer true once the thorax is open or if cold fluids have been rapidly infused.

The ideal location for the esophageal temperature probe is in the lower one-third to one-fourth of the esophagus. In the adult, 45 cm from the nostril gives a good approximation of cerebral temperature;[13] if the mid- or upper esophagus is used, the temperature readings may be affected by cool air in the trachea. Placing a temperature probe-equipped esophageal stethoscope at the point where heart sounds are most prominent gives good results and works well in patients of all ages (Fig. 7-3).

Nasopharynx

Ideally, the probe should be adjacent to the nasopharyngeal mucosa, so that the probe accurately measures the temperature there, which is greatly influenced by the carotid blood passing nearby. Except for an occasional case of epistaxis, the method is quite safe. In the pregnant patient, children with large adenoids, and patients with clotting disorders, the incidence of epistaxis is high. Iatrogenic epistaxis in these and the hypertensive patient may be difficult to halt and may lead to significant blood loss.

It is our experience that the probe is frequently passed into the oral cavity, where it rests in close proximity to the endotracheal tube, which may cool the probe.[14] The proper location is usually reached when the probe meets resistance to further passage and it must bend to enter the nasopharynx.

Rectum

Rectal probes have been used for many years, although not well tolerated by awake patients and often objectionable to others. The rectum does not reflect the core temperature well and feces slow the response time. The probe may be dislodged during a procedure and replacement may be difficult. When we wish to monitor core temperature, we think of the brain or heart. There is no evidence that the rectum would reflect the temperature of either.

Tympanic Membrane

Probes can be placed adjacent to the tympanic membrane.[15] Benzinger advocates tympanic thermometry because of the precise location of the probe, the cleanliness, and the minimal inconvenience, embarrassment, or discomfort to the patient.[16] Because of the danger of perforating the tympanic membrane, there is a tendency to place the probe not quite far enough into the external canal. Therefore, at times, the temperature of the pinna, rather than a more central temperature, is recorded.

The abundant arteriolar blood supply to the tympanic membrane derives from the posterior auricular and internal maxillary arteries, both of which are direct branches of the external carotid, which correlate well with cerebral blood temperature.

Skin

The temperature of the axilla is usually 0.5°C less than the oral temperature, and 1°C lower than the rectal temperature. It will, as does skin temperature measured elsewhere, reflect changes of core temperature, but still be cooler than the core and warmer than exposed skin by an unpredictable amount. Abduct the arm before positioning the sensor, then return it to the adducted position. We use axillary temperature only in awake patients under regional anesthesia when we cannot place probes conveniently or safely in an orifice.

Skin temperature can also be monitored with liquid crystal thermometry. Milar strips impregnated with microencapsulated cholesteric liquid crystals are placed on the skin. The molecular arrangement of the liquid crystals changes as skin temperature varies. When placed on a black background, the crystals scatter light and become visible. The temperature of the forehead skin and the esophagus have reasonably good linear agreement. Because the skin is normally several degrees cooler than the esophagus, an offset is to be expected. Rapidity and linearity of response is also comparable to that achieved with thermistor probes placed in the esophagus. There are several advantages to using liquid crystal thermometry.[17] It is inexpensive, convenient, easily applied, readily accessible to the anesthesiologist, noninvasive and nonirritating to the patient, self-contained and devoid of electronic circuitry, thus eliminating electrocution or burn hazards, and disposable, thereby eliminating cross contamination. A disadvantage is that the monitor cannot be connected to a recording system. Also, the skin may reflect core temperature more faithfully during anesthesia, when the skin tends to be well perfused. In awake patients, or whenever blood flow to the skin is reduced, significant discrepancies between skin and core temperature may develop.[18]

During passive or active cooling or heating, one part of the body may be markedly warmer than another. It is then helpful to monitor two sites—for instance, esophagus and blood in the heart-lung machine, or skin and esophagus. In addition to the core temperature, the difference between core and a second site can be watched. The rate at which this "Δ temperature" changes provides indirect information on blood flow (slow change of Δt = poor blood flow) and is helpful in guarding against overshooting during warming or cooling.

Correlation of Temperatures Measured at Different Sites

Many studies have been published describing thermometry of the esophagus, rectum, tympanic membrane, and skin, and correlating one with the other.[12,13,15,19–23] Some of these reports present conflicting results, which simply shows that the temperature of tissues is variable and is influenced by blood flow, which in turn is governed by physiologic and pharmacologic factors. Thus, the temperature of the great toe increases with sleep, ear lobes turn red and warm with embarrassment, hands and feet turn cold with fright, and during anesthesia the skin is better perfused than during preoperative anxiety, a fact well known to an anesthesiologist who needs to puncture a vein. Hormonal influences, of course, can affect temperature, as for instance with ovulation or thyroid dysfunction. The fact that disease processes such as endotoxins can raise core temperature before skin temperature is also well appreciated. Clinical thermometry must take these factors into account, and no one should be surprised to find differences between temperature probes placed at this or that site. Nevertheless, comparing core and skin temperatures may at times give helpful trends, when for instance the core temperature is well maintained whereas skin temperatures fall, indicating cutaneous vasoconstriction (and a cool environment!).

Equipment Checking

Calibration of thermometric equipment is frequently difficult. With electrical equipment one first checks for continuity of electrical circuitry, with a switch that activates a signal indicating either function or malfunction of the apparatus. Another way to check is to place an item of known temperature in contact with the thermometer and check for accuracy. Do this with a calibrated mercury thermometer and a solution that is in the desired temperature range. If the monitor is not accurate, usually an internal problem exists requiring trained personnel to solve it.

Be certain to use temperature probes that are electronically compatible with the monitor used. Jacks that fit the monitor receptacle, but have internal thermistor electronics incompatible with the monitor, will give false readings. To avoid the problem, check the manufacturer's recommendation for a suitable probe, usually identified by a number.

Aside from local, mechanical tissue trauma causing epistaxis or perforation by probe placement, other less obvious health hazards may arise. Probes are potential current conductors and can cause electrical burns. For this reason, the monitor should be electrically isolated to preclude current passage. If a multipurpose physiologic monitor is used, the temperature-monitoring portion of it should be electrically isolated. Using a battery-operated device is no guarantee of electrical safety, since the chassis may be grounded through a metal support. At least one case has been reported in which the use of an electrosurgical machine led to severe burns through a skin temperature probe.[24] Placing the unit on a piece of nonconductive material provides insulation.

REFERENCES

1. Moschowitz AV: Post-operative heatstroke. Surg Gynecol Obstet 23:443, 1916
2. Britt BA: Malignant hyperthermia. Can Anaesth Soc J 32:666–677, 1985
3. Ryan JF: Treatment of acute hyperthermia crisis. In Britt BA (ed): Malignant

Hyperthermia. International Anesthesiology Clinics, Spring 1978, pp 153–168, Little, Brown & Co, 1978

4. Medic Alert Foundation International, PO Box 3231, Darlen, Connecticut 06820
5. Holdcroft A, Hall GM: Heat loss during anaesthesia. Br J Anaesth 50:157, 1978
6. Morris RH: Influence of ambient temperature on patient temperature during intraabdominal surgery. Ann Surg 173:230, 1971
7. Goldberg MJ, Roe CF: Temperature changes during anesthesia and operations. Arch Surg 93:365, 1966
8. Hare HA: Experiments to determine the influence of etherization on the normal bodily temperature with reference to the use of external heat. The Therapeutic Gazette 12:317, 1888
9. Hammel HT, Hardy JD, Fusco MM: Thermoregulatory responses to hypothalamic cooling in unanesthetized dogs. Am J Physiol 198:481, 1960
10. Roe CF: Temperature regulation and energy metabolism in surgical patients. Prog Surg 12:96, 1973
11. Hill DW: Electronic Measurement Techniques in Anaesthesia and Surgery, pp 366, 369. New York, Butterworth, 1970
12. Whitby JD, Dunkin LJ: Temperature differences in the oesophagus. Br J Anaesth 40:991, 1968
13. Webb GE: Comparison of esophageal and tympanic temperature monitoring during cardiopulmonary bypass. Anesth Analg 52:729, 1973
14. Hendrickx HHL, Trahey GE, Argentieri MP: Paradoxical inhibition of decreases in body temperature by use of heated and humidified gases. Anesth Analg 61:393–394, 1982
15. Dickey WT, Ahlgren EW, Stephen CR: Body temperature monitoring via the tympanic membrane. Surgery 67:981, 1970
16. Benzinger M, Benzinger TH: Tympanic clinical temperature. In Temperature, Its Measurement and Control in Science and Industry, Vol 4, pp 2089–2102. Pittsburgh, Instrument Society of America, 1972
17. Lees DE, Schuette W, Bull JM et al: An evaluation of liquid-crystal thermometry as a screening device for intraoperative hyperthermia. Anesth Analg 57:669, 1978
18. Vaughan MS, Cork CR, Vaughan RW: Inaccuracy of liquid crystal thermometry to identify core temperature trends in postoperative adults. Anesth Analg 61:284, 1982
19. Wilson RD, Knapp C, Traber DL et al: Tympanic thermography: A clinical and research evaluation of a new technic. South Med J 64:1452, 1971
20. Lacoumenta S, Hall GM: Liquid crystal thermometry during anaesthesia. Anaesthesia 39:54, 1984
21. Holdcroft A, Hall GM: Heat loss during anaesthesia. Br J Anaesth 50:157, 1978
22. Cabanac M, Caputa M: Open loop increase in trunk temperature produced by face cooling in working humans. J Physiol (Lond) 289:163–174, 1979
23. Cork RC, Vaughan RW, Humphrey LS: Precision and accuracy of intraoperative temperature monitoring. Anesth Analg 62:211–214, 1983
24. Schneider AJL, Apple HP, Braun RT: Electrosurgical burns at skin temperature probes. Anesthesiology 47:72, 1977

CHAPTER 8

Neuromuscular Function

MUSCLE RELAXATION

The surgeon's work can be facilitated by decreasing central and reflex stimulation of muscles (with general anesthesia), by blocking nerves (with regional anesthesia), and by blocking neuromuscular transmission (with special neuromuscular blocking drugs). In today's anesthesia practice, the use of neuromuscular blocking drugs—often called *relaxants*—is widespread, yet various other means that aid the surgeon are still practiced and should not be forgotten. Relaxants are also used in the intensive care setting. It is, therefore, necessary to review ways of monitoring the adequacy of relaxation, regardless of the means by which it was achieved.

Spontaneous Ventilation

Today, intra-abdominal operations are performed only rarely in patients breathing spontaneously. Yet, it is useful to discuss how such patients used to be monitored by watching the patterns of spontaneous ventilation, as these patterns provide clues that are also important in comatose or obtunded patients breathing spontaneously.

If, during inspiration, the abdominal content is pushed down with a jerking rather than a smooth motion, by abrupt and brief diaphragmatic contractions, and if these contractions are also transmitted to the mediastinum and the trachea, and if they cause the larynx to move down with every breath (a tracheal tug), a discrepancy exists between the force of the contraction of respiratory muscles and the amount of air being moved. This discrepancy may be caused by a partial paralysis of respiratory muscles, depression of the respiratory center, very poor compliance of the lungs, or obstruction of the airways. It is common in patients in the intensive care unit who show respiratory distress which is not yet developed to the point where mechanical ventilation has been instituted, and in postoperative patients who suffer the lingering effects of inadequate reversal of relaxants and anesthetic depression. In the early phases of this respiratory pattern, arterial blood gases may still show acceptable values for P_{O_2} and P_{CO_2}, but eventually fatigue, and subsequently respiratory decompensation, may prevail. This particular pattern of breathing, when allowed to develop fully, finally leads to the characteristic picture of agonal breathing and cardiac arrest. A typical story is that of the recovery room patient who was responsive upon arrival from the operating room. Early signs of respiratory insufficiency were ignored and, an hour later, the patient was found apneic.

If, during expiration, the abdominal wall tightens and the abdomen rises (or, if the abdomen is open, the abdominal contents are pushed out), the patient is probably in a light coma or recovering from general anesthesia. In the absence of an endotracheal tube, such patients usually phonate as they increase their intra-abdominal pressure during expiration. For intubated patients with normal lungs, spontaneous ventilation is likely to be adequate. In either case, the regurgitation of gastric contents is a threat. Here the force of muscle power is adequate, but a CNS affected by trauma, disease, or drugs generates unusual breathing patterns.

Mechanical Ventilation

During surgical procedures under general anesthesia and employing mechanical ventilation, the symptoms to be monitored will depend on the amounts of neuromuscular blocking drugs and anesthetic agents in use. If the patient is not utterly flaccid from such drugs, a surgeon who lifts the abdominal wall up smartly will find resistance. Spinal reflexes will cause the muscles to resist. Gentle and firm traction rather than sudden, jerky stress testing by the surgeon will alleviate this problem. During a difficult operation where little wants to go right, the stressed surgeon may call for more relaxation; however, inspection and neuromuscular testing (see below) may not reveal lack of relaxation. Just as the degree of neuromuscular blockage in the adductor pollicis muscle (predominately slow fibers) may not tell the whole story of neuromuscular relaxation of the abdominal muscles (mixed slow and fast fibers), one may not conclude that the hand can be relaxed while the muscles of the abdomen are too tight for the surgeon to do his work.

Extensive clinical experience has amply demonstrated the utility of neuromuscular monitoring in providing the surgeon with optimal operating conditions. Once the neuromuscular apparatus of the hand is completely blocked, or nearly so, very little muscular resistance can be offered by the patient in abdominal or other muscles, even though they may be differently constituted than those of the hand. In some muscular patients, the muscle mass rather than the muscle tone may make surgical exposure difficult. Giving more neuromuscular blockers to a patient whose hand is already blocked means losing the best means of measuring the degree of relaxation. Anesthesiologists who allow themselves to be pushed into giving more neuromuscular blocking drugs than can be monitored are unlikely to improve the operative conditions, but will face considerable difficulties when the time comes to judge the dosages of drugs to be given for reversal of the neuromuscular block. Rather than give more drugs when there is no evidence that they will be beneficial, the clinician should try other maneuvers to help the surgeon, such as flexing the table or deepening anesthesia.

During assisted or controlled ventilation by hand, you may notice that the compliance of the anesthesia bag decreases. This can be caused by an increased tone of intercostal and abdominal muscles (light anesthesia, inadequate relaxation), a surgeon leaning on the chest, airway obstruction, or bronchospasm. Frequently, a change in compliance is noticed later than desirable if the patient's lungs are ventilated by machine. With diminishing relaxation, a fixed pressure-variable volume ventilator will put less volume into the patient's lungs. A fixed volume-variable pressure machine, however, will develop more pressure. Watch ventilator, pressure gauges and, most importantly, the patient's chest. When you observe changes, check for obstruction, pressure on the chest, or loss of muscle relaxation, and treat accordingly.

In pediatric anesthesia, the anesthetized infant's hand is often placed next to his head. This allows us to test the tone in the fingers. Utter flaccidity is usually a sign of generalized muscle relaxation.

If during the operation a muscle relaxant (*e.g.*, pancuronium) was used, toward the end an antagonist to the muscle relaxant (*e.g.*, neostigmine with atropine) is usually employed. Assume that the patient had no problems with his ventilation before anesthesia. Now the question arises whether he has regained the strength to breathe without help. If he is awake enough to follow instructions, ask him to lift his head off the pillow for 5 seconds. If he can do that, we assume he has enough control over his muscles to breathe adequately without assistance. If he is not awake enough, or for other reasons he is incapable of understanding or responding to this command, we can assess his muscle power by stimulating a motor nerve (usually the ulnar nerve) and gauging his response. Finally, we can cause his airway to be obstructed and measure how much negative pressure (inspiratory force) he will generate—in desperation—to inhale. If it is 20 torr or more, muscle power is judged to be adequate to sustain spontaneous, unassisted ventilation.[1] Others assess the amount of positive pressure generated and compare the value before the relaxant was given to that observed afterwards. In either case, the airway must be obstructed. This is usually done by removing the breathing bag and occluding the hole, or by attaching a pressure gauge to the endotracheal tube or the face mask and occluding the airway. These tests should only be performed in patients who have a normal or high arterial P_{O_2}, who have their lungs filled with oxygen, and who can tolerate quite a bit of straining and an elevation of arterial P_{CO_2}.

In conscious patients one can test vital capacity, or maximal gas flow rates. Often the patients are not able to perform these tests because of after-effects from anesthesia or incisional pain, bandages, or casts.

No single test should be relied on. A patient may well be able to lift his head off the pillow for 10 seconds and then suffocate from obstruction or oversedation.

Assessment with Instruments

When instruments are brought into play to assess the degree of relaxation, the following facts of neuromuscular activity must be understood: Muscle relaxants act primarily (but not exclusively) on the junction of motor nerve with muscle fiber. Since muscle can be stimulated electrically even in the presence of a relaxant, take care to stimulate the nerve rather than the muscle in order to test the neuromuscular junction. The electrodes should, therefore, be placed over a nerve. While any motor nerve will do, the ulnar is usually used, since the patient's hand can be monitored in most anesthetic procedures. The course of the ulnar nerve is traced in Figure 8-1. The ulnar nerve supplies motor fibers to the flexor carpi ulnaris and the medial half of the flexor digitorum profundus, the palmaris brevis, the flexor brevis digiti quinti, abductor digiti quinti, opponens digiti quinti, dorsal and volar musculus interosseus, and the third and fourth musculi lumbricales. Finally, it innervates the oblique and transverse heads of the adductor pollicis brevis and the deep part of the flexor pollicis brevis.

The closer to the wrist the electrode is placed, the more circumscribed the effect of stimulation of the ulnar nerve. Electrodes close to the wrist

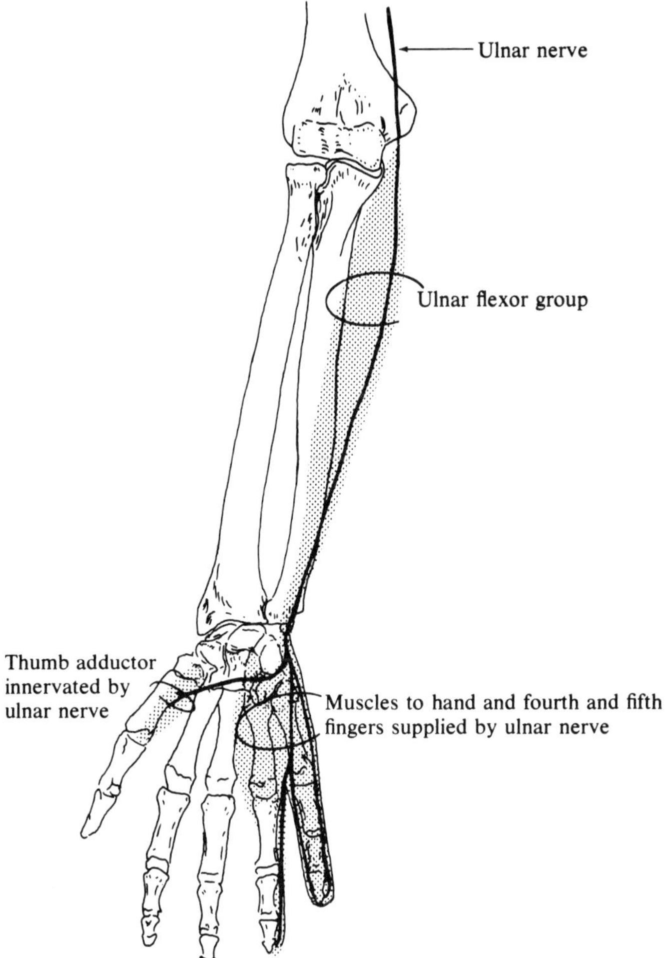

Figure 8-1. Semi-diagrammatic picture of muscles supplied by the ulnar nerve. The ulnar nerve supplies, in the forearm, a group of muscles causing flexion of the wrist and fingers. It is not desirable to stimulate these. Therefore, do not place the negative electrode over the ulnar nerve at the elbow. The ulnar nerve also supplies muscles of the hand, fourth and fifth fingers, and thumb. Stimulating the ulnar nerve at the wrist causes these muscles to contract. The names of these muscles are listed in the text.

will spare the flexor carpi ulnaris and one will primarily see thumb and finger effects. Electrodes over the ulnar nerve close to the olecranon will allow stimulation of the wrist flexors and the entire hand will be flexed toward the ulna. When one uses one of the recording devices attached to thumb or fingers, or placed into the palm (see below), the electrode should be close to the wrist to limit motion of the hand to thumb and fingers.

EQUIPMENT USED TO TEST MUSCLE RELAXATION

Currents Used

Use a current designed to stimulate nerve rather than muscle. Physiologists have described a *strength–duration curve*, as shown in Figure 8-2. A stimulus can be quite strong but fail to cause a neuromuscular response because it is too brief. Conversely, stimulation for a long time will not evoke a response if the stimulus is too weak. The threshold for muscle fiber stimulation may be 20 times higher than that necessary for nerve stimulation.

Since nerves are complex bundles made up of many fibers, it is important to use a stimulus intensity sufficient to depolarize all components of the nerve. For this reason, the so-called *supramaximal* stimulus is used, or a stimulus that is 10% to 20% greater than needed to produce a maximal motor response. In clinical practice, assessment of what constitutes a supramaximal stimulus is based upon an inexact estimate. Ideally, we apply a stimulus to the anesthetized patient (because it hurts) before the neuromuscular blocking drug is given and establish the amperage at which a maximal response is elicited. Then, the current is increased by 10% of the scale and it is assumed that this constitutes a supramaximal stimulus.

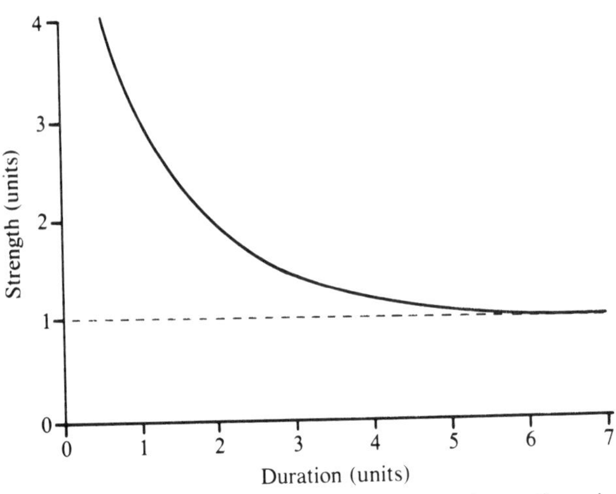

Figure 8-2. The strength–duration curve shows the minimal strength and duration of a current to stimulate a nerve or muscle. The broken horizontal line is the *rheobase* or the minimal strength of current to produce a response, regardless of stimulus duration.

A single stimulus of 0.2 msec and adequate amperage will cause a muscle twitch. Single twitch responses can be elicited at a rate of about 0.1 Hz (1 every 10 seconds). Rapidly repeated (30–100 Hz) individual stimuli cause a tetanus. Prolonged tetanic stimulation produces fatigue of the neuromuscular unit. Consequently, tetanic stimulations are kept brief, usually at about 5 seconds. Rest periods of about 2 minutes are needed between tetanic stimulations when the tetanus is maintained for 10 seconds.

Nerve stimulators allow adjustment of the voltage or amperage output of the instrument. The amount of current reaching the nerve will be affected by the resistance offered by the tissue overlying the nerve, by the conduction between electrode and tissue, and by the nature of the electrode. The instruments on the market, unfortunately, are not uniform in the voltage waveform they generate nor in the maximal current they can deliver into a constant resistance load.[2] It is, therefore, desirable to have a stimulator that will display the milliamperage output of the device. The current delivered through a stick-on skin electrode and just sufficient to trigger a muscle contraction lies between 5 and 25 mA, and that for supramaximal stimulation between 30 and 60 mA. Patients with smaller wrists tend to require less current.[3] Indeed, in very obese patients skin electrodes may not permit the delivery of supramaximal currents and needle electrodes may become necessary, even though we like to avoid needle electrodes because of the danger of infection and injury. With well-placed needle electrodes the current requirements are lower, usually under 10 mA.

Recently, monitors have appeared on the market that use the same strategy of stimulating nerves, but they record an electromyographic, rather than a mechanical, response. The action potentials of the muscle are sensed with the help of stick-on electrodes and are displayed on a digital read-out or are recorded on paper. This system offers attractive features because it relies on a microprocessor to handle the electromyographic signal. Incorporating a microprocessor opens many options, such as automatic adjustment of levels of stimulation, calibration of the response, and versatile displays, alarms, and the generation of permanent records.

Electrode Placement

Either needle electrodes (short, 25-gauge, steel needles with a metal, not plastic, hub) or skin electrodes (small, sticky pads with an electrolyte jelly in the center) are placed close to a nerve. We prefer to avoid needle electrodes; so do patients!

Battery-powered nerve stimulators ("twitch monitors") on the market generate a direct current: one electrode being negative, the other

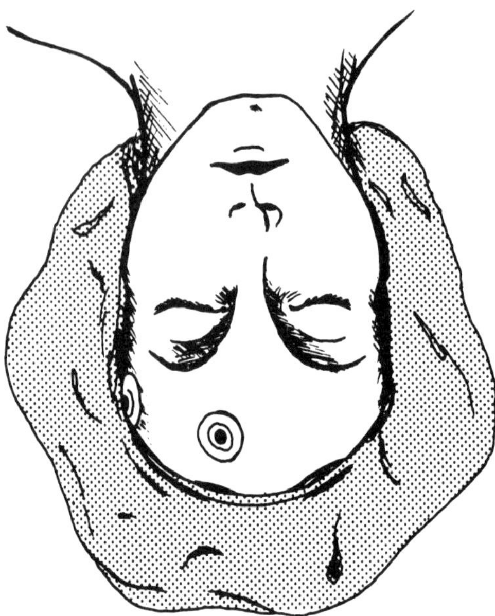

Figure 8-3. Electrodes can be placed on the forehead and contraction of the frontalis muscle can be observed. Place the negative electrode over the lateral forehead where you suspect the temporal branch of the facial nerve lies. The positive electrode can be placed where convenient. (This figure is not upside-down. The anesthetist usually views the patient from this vantage point.)

positive. Some monitors are so marked. If the electrodes are placed close together over the distal ulnar nerve, it makes little difference where the positive or negative electrode is located. However, when only one electrode lies over a nerve while the other does not (*e.g.,* one at the wrist over the ulnar nerve, the other over muscle without a major nerve, *i.e.,* on the hypothenar eminence), electrode polarity becomes important: the negative electrode should lie over the nerve to be stimulated. Less amperage is required to depolarize the nerve lying under a negative than under a positive electrode.

Electrodes can also be placed on the forehead (Fig. 8-3); however, facial stimulation may underestimate the intensity of the neuromuscular block.[4] One can also apply the electrodes to the medial aspect of the ankle over the posterior tibial nerve and observe the flexion of the big toe.*

Skin offers greater electrical resistance, so more current is required for skin than for needle electrodes. Sticky skin electrodes and intense cutaneous stimulation may leave the skin red and irritated. Needle elec-

* L. P. Frank, personal communication

trodes, of course, make holes which can become infected. The needles should be placed subcutaneously. Inserting them deeper, close to a muscle, may produce muscle excitation. If by chance the nerve stimulator is electrically grounded while the indifferent electrode of the electrocautery unit has a defective ground wire, the needle electrodes of the nerve stimulator can become the ground. A third degree burn can result.

CLINICAL FINDINGS ON NERVE STIMULATION

A number of different strategies of stimulating the nerve have been studied. At this time, two methods are most widely used: single twitch (usually one every 10 seconds) and tetanic stimulation (usually between 30 and 100 stimuli per second). With depolarizing drugs, these responses and the tetanic contractions are uniformly depressed. With nondepolarizing drugs, or after prolonged use of a depolarizing drug and the development of a so-called desensitization, or dual block, the picture is different. The response to the individual twitch is decreased, the tetanus is not sustained, and post-tetanic facilitation is seen.

The train-of-four stimulation is the second type commonly employed.[5] Four supramaximal stimuli of equal intensity and duration are given at a rate of 2 Hz (four stimuli in 2 seconds). The train-of-four should not be repeated more often than every 10 seconds. One advantage recommends the train-of-four over the twitch and tetanus: with single twitch stimuli, one cannot tell whether a twitch is of reduced or normal amplitude since they all look alike, whether normal or depressed. Indeed, a single twitch response may have returned to control values while the train-of-four still shows neuromuscular depression.[6] With the train-of-four, the first twitch serves as a yardstick against which the three subsequent twitches are measured. With nondepolarizing blocks this is helpful. In depolarizing blocks, however, the train-of-four shows uniform depression and loses its distinctive advantage over twitch and tetanus.

Savarese and Ali[7] suggest that the ratio of the fourth response to the first response be expressed in percent. If the first response is A and the fourth is B, then B/A × 100 equals the percentage of neuromuscular block. Clinical experience suggests that a response to the fourth stimulus, which is 75% that of the first stimulus (in other words, it is 25% smaller than the first response), provides adequate muscle power for most patients to maintain spontaneous ventilation. Lee uses a slightly different approach.[8] He states that the patient will have a block of about 75% when the last twitch can no longer be seen, 80% when the third twitch is gone, 90% when only the first twitch is left, and 100% when a train-of-four stimulation elicits no response at all. Adequate muscle relaxation for intra-abdominal procedures can be expected with a 75% to 90% block. Remember that these tests are only diagnostic aids. They are helpful, but only in conjunction with an assessment of the patient, his state of consciousness, and his ventilation.

Electrolyte imbalances, hypothermia, and burns may alter the sensitivity of the patient to neuromuscular blocking drugs, but the responses to neuromuscular monitoring will not mislead the clinician in these instances. The situation is different in a patient with upper motor neuron lesions, in whom a nondepolarizing neuromuscular blocking drug may produce good relaxation, but testing the muscles in an affected (paretic) limb with a stimulator may falsely show resistance to the neuromuscular blocking drug.[9] This phenomenon is more pronounced in paretic limbs afflicted for more than 3 weeks than in those of more recent onset.[10]

Measuring the Response

In clinical practice the muscular response to nerve stimulation is usually gauged by inspection. Particularly with the train-of-four, where the four contractions can be compared to each other, visual assessment may be sufficient. However, it is not exact. A number of devices have been described to allow quantification of the contractions.[11–13] Strain gauges can be hooked to the thumb (Fig. 8-4), placed under the thumb, or put into the palm of the hand. The hand must be restrained with a splint to make these devices work well and for output to be of reproducible quality. The output of the strain gauge must be amplified and displayed or recorded on paper. Because the resting tension on the muscle to be tested can

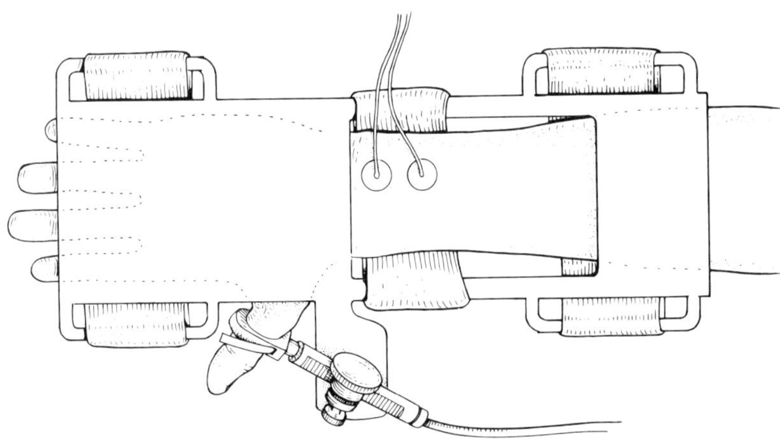

Figure 8-4. One of several commercially available monitors to test neuromuscular function under anesthesia. The hand is immobilized on a board and the thumb hooked to a strain gauge that records the strength of thumb adduction. (Medar Corporation, Scarsdale, New York)

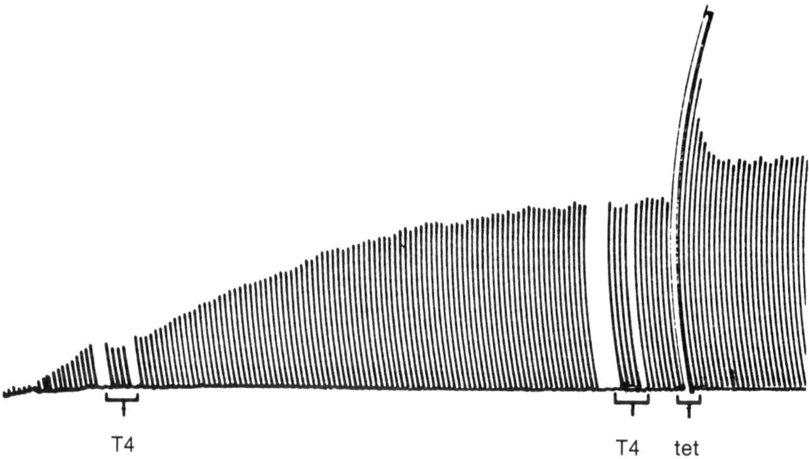

Figure 8-5. The output from a strain gauge measuring the contractions of the thumb adductor was recorded on slowly moving paper. With each supramaximal stimulus (of the ulnar nerve) spaced 5 seconds apart, a contraction occurred. For the train-of-four (*T4*) the paper speed was increased so that the four individual contractions could be identified. A tetanic stimulation (*tet*) produced a well-sustained tetanus and post-tetanic facilitation. The tracing shows recovery from a single dose of 120 mg succinylcholine. (Courtesy of E. S. Munson, MD)

affect the response, Donlon and co-workers recommend that the resting tension be checked and maintained at about 200 g to 300 g.[14] Some commercial systems make it convenient to record the responses to nerve stimulation during routine clinical anesthesia.

When the output of a strain gauge is amplified and then recorded on slowly moving paper, typical tracings result. Figures 8-5 through 8-7 show the characteristic patterns obtained in patients in whom the twitch, train-of-four, and tetanic response to stimulation of the ulnar nerve were recorded with a pistol-grip strain gauge.

Figure 8-5 shows a recovery pattern. The patient, who had been given 120 mg succinylcholine without precurarization, became flaccid and then gradually began to respond to single twitch, train-of-four, and tetanic stimulation. Observe that in this almost pure depolarizing block the two train-of-four tests are approximately as much depressed as the single-twitch responses preceding and following the train-of-four. The tetanic response shows a well-sustained plateau of contraction, which would indicate cither complete recovery or at least absence of a desensitization or dual block. However, following the tetanus we observe post-tetanic facilitation, which reveals that the neuromuscular junction had not yet returned to normal or is affected by a general anesthetic.

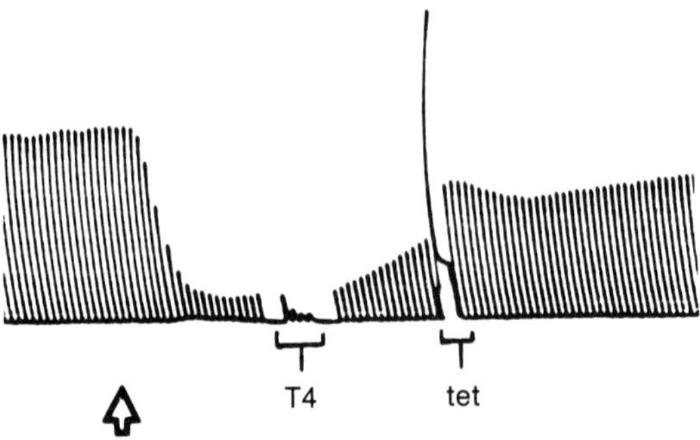

Figure 8-6. Data from the patient described in Figure 8-5. Twenty milligrams of succinylcholine was given (*arrow*). The pattern of a densensitization or dual block is observed. The train-of-four (*T4*) shows a block of about 90%. Tetanic stimulation (*tet*) is not sustained but fades, and post-tetanic facilitation is evident. (Courtesy of E. S. Munson, MD)

After 1 hour and a total dose of 240 mg succinylcholine, the patient was given an additional 20 mg succinylcholine (Fig. 8-6). Observe how the twitch responses diminish as the succinylcholine takes effect. The train-of-four now clearly demonstrates a desensitization or dual block; the first of the train-of-four responses is significantly larger than the three subsequent responses, which are barely discernable. The tetanus shows a poorly sustained tetanic contracture; that is, instead of a plateau we see a "fade" and then mild post-tetanic facilitation.

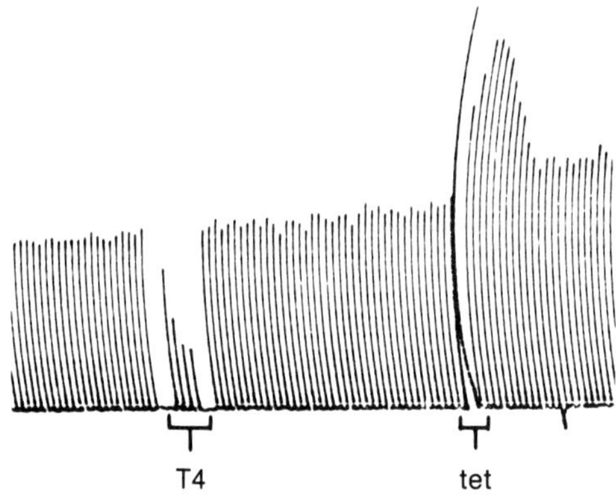

Figure 8-7. Recording set-up as described in Figure 8-5. The pattern of a 50% block after *d*-tubocurarine is seen. The train-of-four (*T4*) shows the fourth twitch to be about half as large as the first twitch. The tetanus (*tet*) is not sustained but fades and is followed by marked facilitation. (Courtesy of E. S. Munson, MD)

The pure effects of a nondepolarizing drug, in this instance *d*-tubocurarine, are presented in Fig. 8-7. The patient had previously received 15 mg of *d*-tubocurarine, resulting in partial neuromuscular blockade. The twitch responses were present and, without a previous twitch response available for comparison, the responses by themselves would not enable us to diagnose the degree of neuromuscular depression. Here a train-of-four response is helpful. The fourth response is about half as high as the first; that is, we can assume a neuromuscular blockade of approximately 50% secondary to a nondepolarizing muscle relaxant. The tetanus is not sustained but shows distinct fade. Post-tetanic facilitation is clearly seen.

When a train-of-four response cannot be elicited (100% block) after giving a large dose of a nondepolarizing neuromuscular blocking drug, it may still be possible to elicit a measurable response to single stimulations at 1 Hz. This is accomplished by exploiting the fact that tetanic stimulation is followed by facilitation. Howardy-Hansen and co-workers[15] have shown this for pancuronium. The more numerous the facilitated single twitches that could be elicited 3 seconds after a 50-Hz tetanus, the sooner the return of a nonfacilitated train-of-four could be expected. On the average, when two, five, or eight such twitches at 1 Hz could be elicited 3 seconds after a 50-Hz tetanus, it took close to 40, 20, or 10 minutes, respectively, before the nonfacilitated train-of-four returned. This is a useful observation (regardless of the drug employed) in cases where an operation ends sooner than expected and no muscle contraction to unfacilitated stimulation can be triggered or observed.

CLINICAL COMMENTS

We urge careful clinical observation of patient and the operative field during the operation and recommend the use of a nerve stimulator when muscle relaxants are used.

Succinylcholine is hydrolyzed by plasma pseudocholinesterase. This enzyme may be inhibited by drugs or poisons; furthermore, it may not be present in normal amounts—as in severe liver disease—or it may occur in an ineffective, atypical form, secondary to genetic influences. About 1 in 2500 to 3000 patients have a homozygous atypical pattern. In such a patient, after a customary dose of succinylcholine (40–100 mg IV for the average adult), paralysis may last for hours rather than a few minutes. If spontaneous ventilation fails to return shortly after intubation, it is difficult to determine whether the patient is apneic because of hypocarbia from hyperventilation, or if paralysis is due to extended action of succinylcholine. Continuous respiratory gas or an arterial blood gas analysis (see Chap. 6) will tell the level of alveolar-arterial P_{CO_2} and a nerve stimulator will answer the question about paralysis quickly. If succinylcholine is the only relaxant to be used, if it is used only during intubation, and if we know from the record of previous anesthetics that the patient hydrolyzes succinylcholine normally, a nerve stimulator is not needed.

No definitive studies exist that would allow us to state that respiratory insufficiency cannot threaten a patient who shows no fade on twitch, only 25% depression on the train-of-four test, who can lift his head off the pillow for 5 seconds, or who can generate 20 torr inspiratory force against a closed airway. A patient may be able to muster his reserves for a short effort but be too debilitated or depressed to sustain the power required to overcome respiratory obstruction. The combined effects of relaxants and opioids (and other CNS depressants) may set the stage for respiratory failure where either alone would not have jeopardized the patient.[16]

REFERENCES

1. Bendixen HH, Surtees AD, Oyama T et al: Postoperative disturbances in ventilation following the use of muscle relaxants in anesthesia. Anesthesiology 20:121, 1959
2. Mylrea KC, Hameroff SR, Calkins JM, et al: Evaluation of peripheral stimulators and relationship to possible errors in assessing neuromuscular blockade. Anesthesiology 60:464–466, 1984
3. Kopman AF, Lawson D: Milliamperage requirement for supramaximal stimulation of the ulnar nerve with surface electrodes. Anesthesiology 61:83–85, 1984
4. Stiffel P, Haweroff SR, Blitt CD: Electrode type and placement during train-of-four affects assessment of neuromuscular blockade. Anesth Analg 59:560, 1980
5. Grob D, Johns RJ, Harvey AM: Studies in neuromuscular function. Bull Johns Hopkins Hosp 99:195, 1956
6. Ali HH, Savarese JJ, Lebowitz PW et al: Twitch, tetanus and train-of-four as indices of recovery from non-depolarizing neuromuscular blockade. Anesthesiology 54:294, 1981
7. Savarese JJ, Ali HH: Monitoring in the operating room: The neuromuscular function. In Gravenstein JS, Newbower RS, Ream AK, et al (eds): Monitoring Surgical Patients in the Operating Room, pp 31–50. Springfield, IL, Charles C Thomas, 1979
8. Lee CM: Train of four quantitation of competitive neuromuscular blockade. Anesth Analg 54:649, 1975
9. Graham DH: Monitoring neuromuscular block may be unreliable in patients with upper-motor-neuron lesions. Anesthesiology 53:74–75, 1980
10. Iwasaki H, Namiki A, Omote K, et al: Response differences of paretic and healthy extremities to pancuronium and neostigmine in hemiplegic patients. Anesth Analg 64:864–866, 1985
11. Ali HH: A new device for monitoring force of thumb adduction. Br J Anaesth 42:83, 1970
12. Walts LF: The "boomerang"—A method of recording adductor tension. Can Anaesth Soc J 20:706, 1973

13. Walts LF, Lebowitz M, Dillon JB: A means of recording force of thumb adduction. Anesthesiology 29:1054, 1968
14. Donlon JV, Savarese JJ, Ali HH: Cumulative dose–response curves for gallamine: Effect of resting thumb tension and mode of stimulation. Anesth Analg 58:377, 1979
15. Howardy-Hansen P, Viby-Mogensen J, Gottschau A, et al: Tactile evaluation of the post-tetanic count (PTC). Anesthesiology 60:372–374, 1984
16. Bellville JW, Cohen EN, Hamilton J: The interaction of morphine and *d*-tubocurarine on respiration and grip strength in man. Clin Pharmacol Ther 5:35, 1964.

CHAPTER 9

Intracranial Pressure Measurement

INTRODUCTION AND TERMINOLOGY

When intracranial pressure (ICP) rises too high, the cerebral vascular bed becomes inadequately perfused, and the brain suffers ischemia. Signs and symptoms of increased ICP include headache, lethargy, nausea, vomiting, oculomotor, or abducens paresis, and papilledema. These signs and symptoms lack specificity and precision as indicators of ICP, as do the results of the CT scan, and during general anesthesia most of these symptoms are obscured. Although controversy exists over whether or not measurement of ICP alters morbidity and mortality,[1–3] particularly in adults, many clinicians monitor ICP. The pioneering effort of Guillaume and Janny in the measurement of ICP paved the way for the development of routine techniques for clinical practice.[4] Before we discuss these methods, a review of the dynamics of ICP, cerebral blood flow (CBF), and cerebral perfusion pressure (CPP) will prove useful.

PHYSIOLOGY OF INTRACRANIAL PRESSURE

Brain, cerebral spinal fluid (CSF), and blood are encased by a rigid container, the skull, with a small outlet, the foramen magnum. The CSF produced by the choroid plexus surrounds the brain and spinal cord, and occupies the ventricles. Some CSF flows through the foramen magnum into the spinal subarachnoid space. In health, CSF is produced and absorbed at a rate of 0.4 ml/min and normally occupies about 10% of the intracranial volume. When brain edema, tumor, hemorrhage, or an aberration in CSF mechanics increases the intracranial volume, the CSF absorption can be accelerated, and some CSF can be displaced into the spinal subarachnoid space. At very high ICP, CSF production can be throttled. When the "pressure relief valve," the foramen magnum, becomes occluded, only compensation by the production and absorption of CSF remains. This compensatory mechanism is easily overwhelmed, leading to drastic elevations in ICP and sudden calamities. In a healthy person, ICP remains less than 15 torr in spite of the dynamic change of the fluids—blood and CSF—that influence that pressure. As shown in Figure 9-1, intracranial volume can increase a little before compliance changes dramatically, and thereafter, with each additional milliliter of intracranial volume, the ICP increases markedly.

Blood flow through the brain is carefully regulated, not only to ensure a continuous supply of nutrients, but also to guarantee a reasonably constant volume of blood in the brain. The control of CBF over a range of CPP is called *autoregulation*. CPP is defined as the difference between the mean intracranial arterial pressure and the mean ICP (Fig. 9-2). Blood flow is autoregulated by the dilatation or constriction of blood vessels.

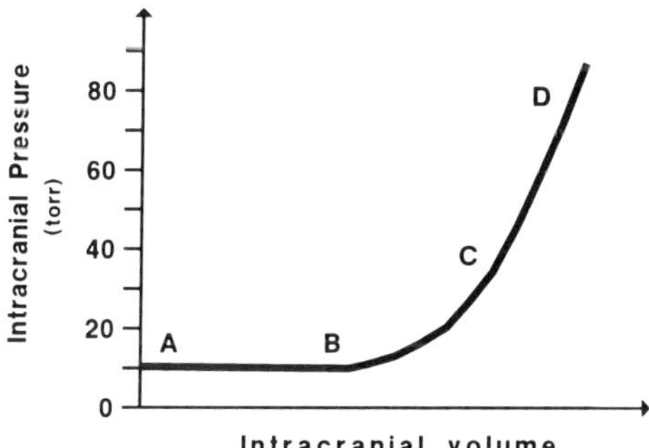

Figure 9-1. Intracranial volume–pressure relationships. When the intracranial volume is increased in a healthy person, significant compensatory mechanisms serve to maintain nearly normal pressure (*A–B*); however, once these mechanisms are exhausted, even small increments of volume lead to drastic changes in pressure (*C–D*).

Once CPP has fallen to less than 50 torr, the arterioles, capillaries, and veins have dilated maximally. Any further fall of CPP leads to cerebral ischemia. At a CPP greater than 150 torr, vasoconstriction is maximal, and any further increase in CPP causes cerebral edema as the intravascular pressure exceeds the extravascular pressure. Between mean perfusion pressures of 50 torr and 150 torr, autoregulation keeps CBF constant.

Arterial hypertension resets the autoregulation of CBF.[5] It is important to recognize this because at 50 torr or 60 torr mean arterial pressure measured at the level of the head, CPP may already be inadequate in a patient with essential hypertension, whereas similar values are acceptable in a healthy, normotensive patient. Strandgaard and colleagues, for example, reported that for hypertensive patients whose mean awake arterial pressure varied from 125 torr to 180 torr the lower levels of autoregulation were 90 torr to 125 torr.[5]

Intracranial pressure is affected not only by the balance of CSF production and absorption, and blood and brain volume, but also by venous pressure. Coughing, for instance, can increase ICP acutely by increasing venous pressure. By the same token, intraoperative positions such as a sharp turning or severe flexing of the neck or a face-down position may cause venous obstruction and thus inhibit cerebral venous drainage and increase ICP.

The physiologic gases, oxygen and CO_2, also have powerful effects on vascular tone in the brain. Figure 9-2 shows how cerebral flow varies

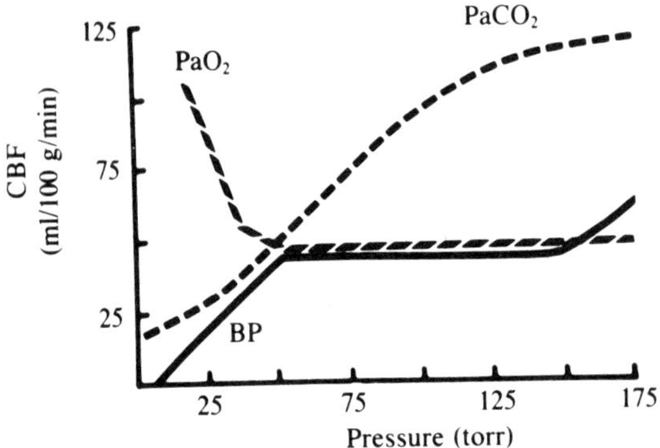

Figure 9-2. CBF versus CPP. CBF remains constant over a range of blood pressures. CBF is affected with severe hypoxemia. CBF varies nearly linearly as P_aCO_2 changes over a relatively large range. (Shapiro HM: Physiologic and pharmacologic regulation of cerebral blood flow. In Hershey SG [ed]: Refresher Courses in Anesthesiology, Vol 5, p 167. Copyright © 1977 by the American Society of Anesthesiologists, Inc.)

Table 9-1. LEVELS OF NORMAL AND ELEVATED ICP

Intracranial Pressure (torr)	Interpretation
5–15	Normal
15–20	Minimal elevation
20–40	Moderate elevation
>40	Severe elevation

directly with P_aCO_2. At a P_aCO_2 of 20 torr, CBF is half the normal amount; at a P_aCO_2 of 80 torr, CBF is doubled. Oxygen level also alters CBF. At severely hypoxic levels CBF increases rapidly. These hypoxemic effects add to the hypercarbic effects, and a combination of hypoxemia and hypercarbia can dramatically increase ICP.

ABNORMAL INTRACRANIAL PRESSURES

Relatively high ICP is tolerated when these pressures have developed very slowly; conversely, rapid elevations of ICP—for instance, after trauma—are poorly tolerated, even though the absolute change may be far less than that observed in a patient with hydrocephalus or pseudotumor cerebri. Table 9-1 shows normal and elevated ICP values. The danger of insufficient CPP arises when normal ICP is suddenly elevated to more than 20 torr.

Increased ICP is particularly malignant in patients with severe head injury. Severe trauma initiates a vicious cycle of tissue damage leading to cerebral edema, elevated ICP, decreased CPP, tissue ischemia, and decreased CBF, which all result in further tissue damage. General anesthesia brings additional concerns.

EFFECTS OF ANESTHETIC DRUGS ON INTRACRANIAL PRESSURE

Table 9-2 shows the alterations in CBF and ICP with various anesthetic agents and muscle relaxants. Volatile agents alter the plateau position of the CPP–CBF curve, resulting in increased CBF at the same CPP (see Fig. 9-2).[6] Halogenated anesthetic vapors generally increase CBF and ICP. In the normal patient CSF is displaced, minimizing the anesthetic effect on ICP. A patient with normal $PaCO_2$, a space-occupying lesion, and chronically elevated ICP may suffer a substantial and dangerous increase in ICP under anesthesia.

Table 9-2. EFFECT OF ANESTHETIC AGENTS ON ICP AND CBF

Agent	CBF and ICP
Induction	
Althesin	↓
Ketamine	↑
Thiopental	↓
Muscle relaxants	
Atracurium	0?
d-Tubocurarine	↑
Pancuronium	0 or ↓
Succinylcholine	?
Vecuronium	0
Inhalational agents	
Enflurane	↑
Halothane	↑
Isoflurane	↑
Nitrous oxide	↑
Intravenous	
Narcotics	↓

(Modified from Samuels SI: Anesthesia for supratentorial tumor. In Cottrell JE, Turndorf H [eds]: Anesthesia and Neurosurgery, 2nd ed, p. 119. St Louis, CV Mosby, 1986)

INDICATIONS FOR INTRACRANIAL PRESSURE MEASUREMENT

Turner and McDowall have prepared a list of causes of increased ICP; the conditions that place patients at risk are shown in Table 9-3.[7] They, as well as Sullivan and Becker, institute ICP monitoring preoperatively in patients with severe closed head injuries and in patients with high ICP, such as occurs with intracranial tumors, hydrocephalus, ruptured intracranial aneurysms, and Reye's syndrome.[8] Neurosurgical patients who require artificial ventilation are often sedated and are sometimes paralyzed, making clinical evaluation difficult. The ICPs of these patients must be frequently monitored. By initiating ICP monitoring preoperatively the anesthesiologist can provide safer management. Once the dura is opened, ICP measurement loses its value. However, once the dura and skull are closed, ICP may again require monitoring.

The causes of increased postoperative ICP include hypercarbia, cerebral edema, and intracranial bleeding. Cerebral edema almost always accompanies major neurosurgical operations where retractors have compressed brain tissue. ICP monitoring does not alert the anesthesiologist to edema formation, but indicates what effect it has on ICP. The edema

Table 9-3. CAUSES OF INCREASED ICP

Disease	
Hydrocephalus	
Cerebral tumor	
Intracranial hematoma	
Cerebral edema	
Benign intracranial hypertension	
Iatrogenic	
Severe hypoxia Hypercarbia Halogenated anesthetics	Cause increased cerebral blood flow and cerebral blood volume
Coughing and straining Physiotherapy Head-down tilt Poorly adjusted pressure ventilation Compression of jugular vein	Impair cerebral venous drainage and increase cerebral blood volume

may result from retraction or vascular insufficiency, particularly following intense vasoconstriction, for example, after the clipping of an aneurysm.

METHODS OF MEASURING INTRACRANIAL PRESSURE

Several methods and devices have been developed to measure ICP. Three of these are shown in Figure 9-3.

Intraventricular Catheter

Intraventricular catheters, now widely employed, were used by the first investigators in the field. Initially, catheters were placed in the lumbar CSF space. It was not until 1938 that the consequences of brain-stem herniation were outlined by Moore and Stern, who stated that herniation causes a change ". . . in the pressure relationship between the supra- and infratentorial spaces [which] leads to disturbance of circulation in the basilar artery."[9] From this and subsequent articles it became apparent that ICP has to be measured supratentorially.[10]

Today neurosurgeons insert a catheter into a lateral ventricle through a burr hole or a twist drill hole in the skull at the coronal suture in line with the pupil and direct the catheter medially toward the medial canthus of the ipsilateral eye or the ridge of the nose if the ventricle is small.[11] The catheter is connected to an external electronic pressure transducer (not a manometer). We can mount the transducer on the patient's head, zero it to the head level, or zero it to the heart level. Whichever method is used, it is important to zero to a known and constant reference point.

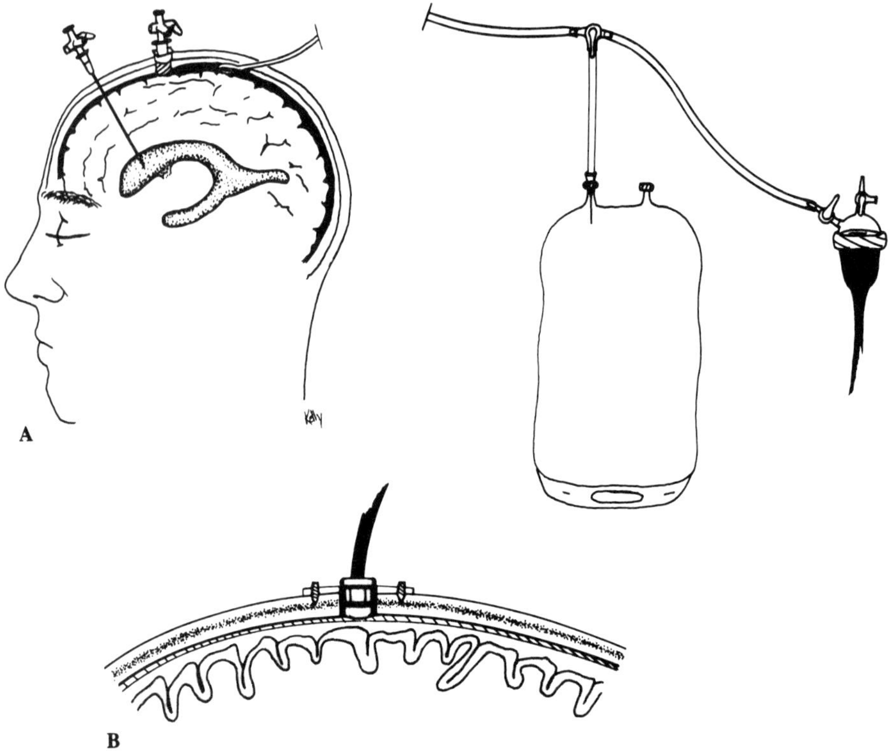

Figure 9-3. (*A*) Subdural monitoring sensors. Three different types of devices are shown. The intraventricular catheter is placed in a lateral ventricle. The hollow bolt (here subdural) is threaded into the skull. The ICP monitoring cup catheter is also shown in a subdural location. The plastic bag serves as a reservoir for CSF drainage. The transducer is placed at the level of the head. (*B*) Extradural monitoring sensors. A transducer-faced bolt is threaded into the skull and placed in an extradural location. The hollow bolt and cup catheter may also be placed in the extradural space. (*A*, adapted from Miller JD: Intracranial pressure monitoring. Br J Hosp Med 19:497, 1978)

We use the external auditory meatus, but other landmarks on the head are satisfactory.

By using a ventriculostomy, not only can we measure pressure, but we can also withdraw CSF both to reduce ICP and to retain the CSF for laboratory studies. The technique entails several risks to the patient. CSF may drain inadvertently and cause upward herniation if a lesion of the posterior fossa exists. Probing through tissue while attempting to locate a ventricle may cause bleeding and neurologic damage. In the presence of brain edema the ventricles may be compressed to a very small size, and with a shift at the midline structure the ventricles may be displaced: either event makes ventricular cannulation difficult.

Infection is of great concern when using a ventriculostomy catheter. Rates of infection are variously quoted from 0% with the percutaneous tunnel ventriculostomy[12] to 10%.[13] Brief monitoring duration may reduce the incidence.[14] Levin and co-workers recorded a 33% rate of infection after 5 days of monitoring, while essentially all of the patients were infected after 10 days.[13] After prolonged ventricular ICP monitoring the catheter may become obstructed. Although flushing may reestablish patency, it may also set the stage for infection. To minimize the danger of infection, meticulous attention to sterile technique is mandatory. Figure 9-3*A* shows a "closed" setup for monitoring pressure (sterile dome and tubing) and a collection bag (sterile bag and tubing). Whenever this system is opened, a syringe attached, or a transducer exchanged, bacteria may gain access (see also Chap. 4).

Subdural and Extradural Bolts

Two types of bolts have been used in an attempt to reduce the risks of using intraventricular catheters on patients. One is a hollow bolt connected by pressure tubing to a transducer; the other is a bolt that has an electronic transducer mounted on its face (see Fig. 9-3*B*). Both are screwed into a previously tapped burr hole either for extradural or for subdural monitoring after a small dural incision establishes communication with the arachnoid and CSF. If the subdurally placed bolt is hollow, brain material tends to occlude it. Subdural monitoring also carries a greater risk of infection, perhaps as great as the intraventricular approach. The extradural bolt eliminates this problem by omitting the dural incision. Extradural pressure readings are usually higher (by 2 torr to 3 torr, but at times by up to 30 torr) than CSF measurements.[15] If the transducer-tipped bolt is implanted at an angle to the dura or with excessive indentation, the pressure recorded exceeds the actual pressure. Local edema during insertion and different reference points account for some of the difference, but all differences cannot be attributed to methodologies. During hypercarbia the subarachnoid space may be obliterated, in which case the bolt no longer measures CSF pressure but rather brain pressure. Since hypercarbia increases CBF and results in brain swelling, brain pressure will be higher than CSF pressure.

In spite of these problems, Turner and colleagues showed that the agreement between the measurements of extradural and CSF pressures is good and found no patient in whom "raised intraventricular pressure is associated with normal extradural pressure."[16]

The bolts are simple to insert and may be placed almost anywhere in the skull. The operative site is avoided, and the incidence of infection is usually low, particularly with the extradural site. Unfortunately CSF cannot be withdrawn through this system.

Whether using an intraventricular catheter, hollow bolt, or other fluid-coupled system (relying on a fluid to transmit ICP signals to a transducer), be certain to check for leaks in the external pressure measuring system. As contrasted to measuring intravascular pressure where blood "backing up" towards, and into, the transducer assembly signals a leak, clear CSF gives no such signal. Shields and co-workers suggest isolating the external from the internal fluid pathways and applying an initial pressure of 50 torr.[17] If the pressure falls, a leak is present. Tissue occluding the bolt orifice results in falsely low ICP readings. Flushing the internal fluid path with 0.1 ml of saline may give a brief overpressure indication. Careful observation of the waveform will reveal the initial overpressure followed by a pulsatile waveform that indicates the true ICP value. Often, ICP again diminishes slowly, which indicates another occlusion of the bolt orifice with tissue.

Subdural and Epidural Catheters

Subdural and epidural catheters offer an alternative to bolts and intraventricular catheters. The Cordis Intracranial Pressure-Monitoring Cup Catheter,* developed by Wilkinson, is intended for continuous ICP monitoring.[18] It is inserted either through a burr hole or after a craniotomy. The catheter is placed in the subdural space with the cup (open side) facing the arachnoid membrane. The catheter is flushed every 2 hours to maintain the patency of the lumen (see Fig. 9-3A).

Goitein and Amit suggest an even simpler catheter method for ICP measurement in small children.[19] The open frontal fontanel in newborns and young children allows the percutaneous placement of a 22-gauge intravenous catheter. Following sterile preparation of the anterior fontanel and surrounding area, the lateral angle of the fontanel is palpated, and a 22-gauge intravenous catheter introduced laterally through the skin at a 30° angle. When the "pop" of pierced skin is perceived, the stylet is withdrawn and the catheter advanced. If CSF is to be visualized, the catheter is connected to the monitoring system, as shown in Figure 9-4. If not, 0.2 ml to 0.3 ml of sterile saline without preservatives is used as a flush solution and, again, the monitoring system is activated. For adults, Villanueva suggests placement of a silastic catheter through a 4.8-mm ($\frac{3}{16}$-inch) hole at 45° to 60° in the right frontal area of the skull, and a 2.4-mm ($\frac{3}{32}$-inch) hole in the dural.[20] He cites good agreement between intraventricular catheters and subdural bolt methods.

* Cordis International, Miami, Florida.

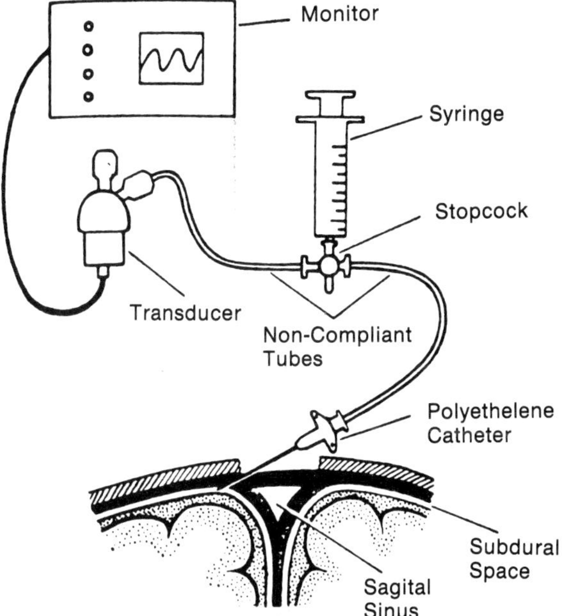

Figure 9-4. A schematic diagram of the monitoring system for measurement of intracranial pressure in small children. (Goitein KG, Amit Y: Percutaneous placement of subdural catheter for measurement of intracranial pressure in small children. Crit Care Med 10:46–48, 1982, © by Williams & Wilkins.)

Fiberoptic Intracranial Pressure Monitor

Paulus, in cooperation with Numoto and colleagues, developed a pressure-sensitive switch that was later modified to include fiberoptics.[21] The device consists of a small chamber with a pressure-sensitive membrane (Fig. 9-5). Changes in external pressure on the device cause movement of the membrane. By means of a servomechanism the membrane is returned to its original position by altering the pressure in the chamber. The pressure reflects ICP. Placed in the extradural (or subdural) space, the instrument permits ICP measurements but does not allow for CSF withdrawal. The resultant infection rates are exceedingly low.

Noninvasive Measurement of Intracranial Pressure

For years clinicians have palpated the anterior fontanel of the neonate to judge ICP. The method, though time-honored, does not allow quantitation, and a slowly increasing ICP will not be detected. Davidoff and Chanlin adopted the Schiøtz tonometer to measure extradural pressure.[22]

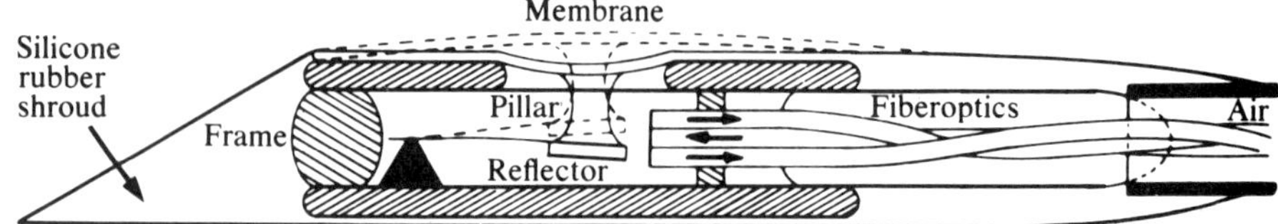

Figure 9-5. Fiberoptic intracranial pressure monitor. Shown is a cross section of the intracranial portion of a pressure sensor. Changes in intracranial pressure cause the membrane, and with it the reflector, to move. Light transmitted to the reflector by the afferent fiberoptic bundle is reflected to two efferent bundles. Displacement of the reflection off center causes unequal levels of light in the two efferent bundles. This inequality activates an air bellows to inflate (or deflate) the chamber, which returns the reflector to center. A transducer mounted in the bellows measures the air pressure in the sensor, which represents intracranial pressure. (Levin AB: The use of a fiberoptic intracranial pressure monitor in clinical practice. Neurosurgery 1:267, 1977)

Later, Numoto's implantable switch was modified by Epstein and colleagues to measure ICP noninvasively.[23] The Ladd ICP monitor* is placed over the anterior fontanel and held in place with a pad, tape, or electrocardiograph skin electrode.[24] To avoid "preloading" the sensor, no pressure should be applied to the sensor by the tape or frame. Correlation between this method and measurements by means of ventriculostomy or lumbar puncture is excellent.

INTERPRETATION OF INTRACRANIAL PRESSURE WAVEFORMS

Key and Retzius in 1875 were the first to record graphically the cerebrospinal pressure in animals.[25] The later findings of Lundberg formed the basis of subsequent work in ICP monitoring.[26] He analyzed the ventricular pressure curves in neurosurgical patients and was able to distinguish three types of spontaneous fluctuations, which he identified as A-, B-, and C-waves with the following characteristics:

- *A-waves* (Fig. 9-6*A*): a pattern of sustained pressures recurring at intervals of varying length (usual range: height of 50 torr to 100 torr, duration of 5 minutes to 20 minutes)
- *B-waves* (Fig. 9-6*B*): smaller, sharper waves usually occurring as rhythmic oscillation with a dominating frequency of about 1 per minute (usual range: frequency of $\frac{1}{2}$ to 2 per minute, amplitude of from 0 torr to 50 torr)
- *C-waves* (Fig. 9-6*C*): small rhythmic oscillations with a dominating

* Ladd, Burlington, Vermont.

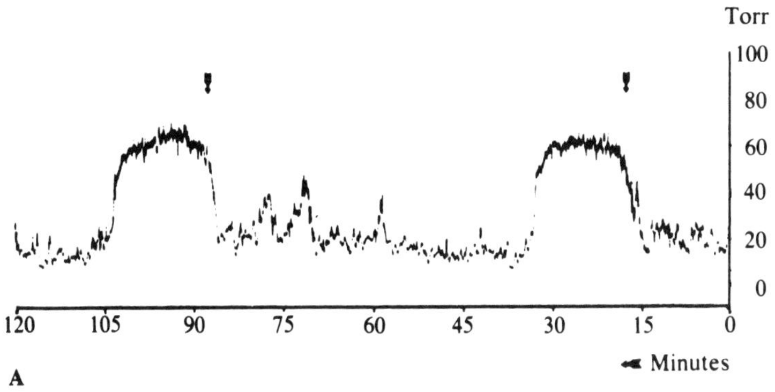

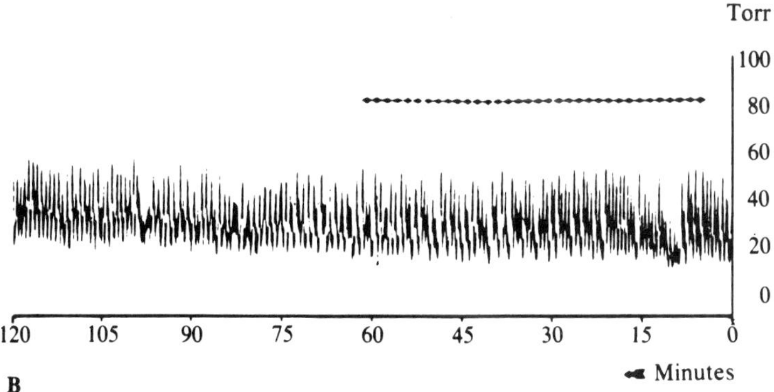

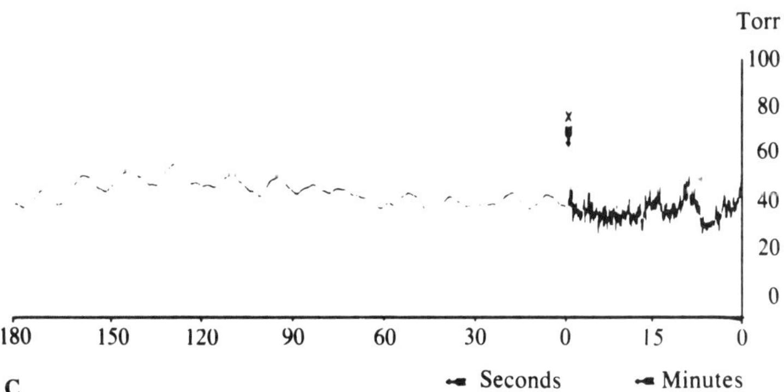

Figure 9-6. ICP waveforms. (*A*) A-waves. ICP usually rises to a level of 60 torr to 80 torr, where it persists for at least 2 minutes. Occurrence is irregular between every few minutes and several hours. (*B*) B-waves. Rhythmic ICP oscillations at a rate of $\frac{1}{2}$ to 2 per second usually associated with decreased wakefulness and Cheyne-Stokes respiration. (*C*) C-waves. These are sometimes difficult to discern, of relatively low amplitude with a frequency of 4 to 8 per minute. (Lundberg N: Continuous recording and control of ventricular fluid pressure in neurosurgical practice. Acta Psychiatr Scand [Suppl] 149:94, 1960)

frequency of about 6 per minute (usual range: frequency of 4 to 8 per minute, amplitude of 0 torr to 20 torr).

A-waves are premonitory signs of acutely rising pressures and are to be avoided if possible. These waves are caused by intrinsic vasomotor control of cerebral circulation. First, vasodilatation takes place, and with it an increasing intracranial blood volume and ICP. With subsequent vasoconstriction, volume and pressures return.

B-waves apparently reflect respiration of the Cheyne-Stokes type, and C-waves are related to rhythmic variations of the systemic arterial pressure or Traube–Hering waves. They are usually observed in patients with severe ICP elevation.[27]

REFERENCES

1. Shapiro K, Marmaron A: Clinical applications of the pressure–volume index in treatment of pediatric head injuries. J Neurosurg 56:819–825, 1982
2. Soul TG, Duclerr TB: Intracranial pressure monitoring in patients with severe head injury. Am Surg 48:477–480, 1982
3. Stuart GG, Merry GS, Smith JA, et al: Severe head injury managed without intracranial pressure monitoring. J Neurosurg 59:601–605, 1983
4. Guillaume J, Janny P: Monometrie intracranienne continue: Interet de la methode et premiers resultats. Rev Neurol (Paris) 84:131, 1951
5. Strandgaard S, Olesen J, Skinhoj E et al: Autoregulation of brain circulation in severe arterial hypertension. Br Med J 1:507, 1973
6. Morita H, Bleyaert AL, Stezoski SW et al: The effect of halothane anesthesia on cerebral blood flow, autoregulation and cerebral metabolism of oxygen and glucose. In: Abstracts of Scientific Papers, ASA Annual Meeting, p. 63. Park Ridge, IL, American Society of Anesthesiologists, 1974
7. Turner JM, McDowall DG: The measurement of intracranial pressure. Br J Anaesth 48:735, 1976
8. Sullivan HG, Becker DP: Intracranial pressure monitoring and interpretation. In Cottrell JE, Turndorf H (eds): Anesthesia and Neurosurgery, p 58. St Louis, CV Mosby, 1980
9. Moore MT, Stern K: Vascular lesions in brain-stem and occipital lobe occurring in association with brain tumors. Brain 61:70, 1938
10. Rockoff MA: Does lumbar CSF pressure accurately reflect intracranial pressure? (letter to the editor). Pediatrics 67:746, 1981
11. Miller JD: Intracranial pressure monitoring. Br J Hosp Med 19:497, 1978
12. Friedman WA, Vries JK: Percutaneous tunnel ventriculostomy. J Neurosurg 53:662, 1980
13. Levin AB, Braun SR, Grossman JE: Physiological monitoring of the head injured patient. Clin Neurosurg 29:240–287, 1982
14. Wyler AR, Kelly WA: Use of antibiotics with external ventriculostomies. J Neurosurg 37:185, 1972
15. Dorsch NWC, Symon L: The validity of extradural measurement of the in-

tracranial pressure. In Lundberg N, Ponten U, Brock M (eds): Intracranial Pressure, Vol II, p 403. Heidelberg, Springer-Verlag, 1975

16. Turner JM, Gibson RM, McDowall DG, et al: Further experiences with extradural pressure monitoring. In Lundberg N, Ponten U, Brock M (eds): Intracranial Pressure, Vol II, p 397. Heidelberg, Springer-Verlag, 1975
17. Shields CB, McGraw CP, Garretson HD: Accurate intracranial pressure monitoring (technical note). Neurosurgery 14:592–593, 1984
18. Wilkinson HA: The intracranial pressure monitoring cup catheter (technical note). Neurosurgery 1:139, 1977
19. Goitein KJ, Amit Y: Percutaneous placement of subdural catheter for measurement of intracranial pressure in small children. Crit Care Med 10:46–48, 1982
20. Villanueva: Simplified technique for subdural pressure monitoring (technical note). Neurosurgery 16:238–240, 1985
21. Numoto M, Wallman JK, Donaghy RMP: Pressure indicating bag for monitoring intracranial pressure. J Neurosurg 39.784, 1973
22. Davidoff LM, Chanlin M: "The Fontanometer." Adaptation of the Schiøtz tonometer for the determination of intracranial pressure in the neonatal and early periods of infancy. Pediatrics 24:1065, 1959
23. Epstein F, Wald A, Hochwald GM: Intracranial pressure during compressive head wrapping in treatment of neonatal hydrocephalus. Pediatrics (Suppl) 54:786, 1974
24. Hill A, Volpe JJ: Measurement of intracranial pressure using the Ladd intracranial pressure monitor. J Pediatr 98:974, 1981
25. Key A, Retzius G: Studien in der Anatomie des Nervensystems und des Bindegewebes. Stockholm, Samson and Wallin, 1875
26. Lundberg N: Continuous recording and control of ventricular fluid pressure in neurosurgical practice. Acta Psychiat Neurol Scand (Suppl) 361:149, 1960
27. Moss E, McDowall DG: Monitoring of intracranial pressure. In Trubuhovich RV (ed): Management of Acute Intracranial Disasters. International Anesthesiology Clinics, Vol 17, Nos 2 and 3, p 375, Boston, Little, Brown & Co, 1979

CHAPTER 10

Depth of Anesthesia, Electroencephalography, and Evoked Potentials

"I just had the weirdest trip" . . . "I wanted to move but couldn't" . . . "I heard them say I looked blue" . . . "They said I had a boy."

Such accounts of awareness during anesthesia are uncommon. The overall incidence of sporadic awareness during the lack of amnesia after general anesthesia is estimated to be 1%. For patients undergoing cesarean section it is roughly 10%.[1] A traumatic neurotic reaction may result from intraoperative awareness.

We urgently need to monitor the degree of analgesia, the level of consciousness, and the extent of amnesia, but we often cannot. In addition, we must be able to detect ischemia in the central nervous system, whether it be a patient undergoing carotid endarterectomy, or intracranial, spinal, or cardiac surgery.

GAUGING ANESTHETIC DEPTH

Analgesia and level of consciousness can be assessed only if the patient can respond to questions, complain, or give signals, all of which require motor control. During light, general anesthesia, we worry about the level of analgesia, consciousness, and amnesia, especially because, in these instances, muscle relaxants are frequently used. Thus, our patients are not able to communicate with us, although sometimes a patient can still wrinkle the forehead, lift an eyebrow, or shrug a shoulder.

To guard against total loss of motor function, one limb can be excluded from the effect of the muscle relaxant by applying a blood pressure cuff to that extremity and inflating the cuff to well above systolic pressure before the relaxant is administered.[2] In this way, the patient can use that hand to signal. When this technique is employed, the anesthesiologist should arrange with the patient in advance a code of signals indicating pain, discomfort, and "yes" or "no" responses to questions.

Amnesia cannot be assessed in advance because a patient may be able to perceive and identify a stimulus, yet cannot recall it. For example, patients under the influence of thiopental can name an object held up for inspection, but later may be incapable of recalling having seen the object. This phase of the effect of thiopental is marked by nystagmus. Thus, nystagmus suggests, but does not guarantee, amnesia, even though the patient is responding to stimuli.

Respiratory Signs

Depth of anesthesia is assessed from respiratory patterns (see also Chap. 2), eyeball motion, pupillary size, conjunctival injection, and tearing. The classic stages of ether anesthesia relied much on pupillary size. Coarse, coordinated rotation of the eyeballs denotes very light anesthesia or excitation (Stage I or II). Tearing and conjunctival injection betray light anesthesia. Conjunctival injection also occurs during normal sleep.

With newer anesthetic agents, and particularly with the use of muscle relaxants, these signs are no longer reliable except for these extremes: spontaneous movement of the eyes indicates light anesthesia and fixed, dilated pupils imply excessively deep anesthesia. However, with halothane, a patient may have a fixed, centered stare with constricted pupils that, under ether anesthesia, would indicate a level of surgical anesthesia. However, this sign is unreliable: the patient may move on incision or may tolerate the surgical operation.

Respiratory patterns are no longer entirely reliable because the newer anesthetic agents, such as halothane, enflurane, and isoflurane, are all respiratory depressants. Few anesthesiologists allow their patients to breathe spontaneously when anesthesia has to be deep enough for abdominal procedures and when one of the new halogenated anesthetics is being used. Nevertheless, the classic signs of respiratory patterns in the spontaneously breathing patient are still valuable.

Active Expiration

The abdominal muscles tighten during expiration, so that the abdomen may rise during that time. Gently resting a hand on the patient's abdomen detects tensing of the abdominal wall with every expiration when anesthesia is light.

Jerky Inspiration

During inspiration, the diaphragm contracts rapidly, rather than in smooth coordination, and the abdominal contents are pushed down. The abdomen may rise during inspiration without the abdominal walls tightening. A laryngeal tug may develop simultaneously. This classic picture of deep ether anesthesia is often associated with a paradoxical "rocking the boat" chest motion: the upper chest falls during inspiration, while the abdomen rises. In the modern anesthetic picture (without ether use), this is usually associated with respiratory insufficiency, deep anesthesia, muscle weakness, or respiratory obstruction. This ominous respiratory pattern cannot be treated with deeper anesthesia or relaxants, but with appropriate ventilatory support and, perhaps, lightening of anesthesia.

Cardiovascular Signs

Heart rate and blood pressure are frequently monitored to gauge the level of anesthesia. Under very light anesthesia, painful stimuli lead to tachycardia and hypertension. Deep anesthesia, however, brings about hypotension (and bradycardia in infants). It is helpful to monitor these vital signs and to observe the responses to the surgical incision. A brisk elevation in blood pressure under a halogenated anesthethetic, upon surgical incision, rules out excessively deep anesthesia. However, awareness and recall sometimes occur to patients who have no marked changes in blood pressure and heart rate. Pain may provoke a vagal response manifested by hypotension and bradycardia. Thus, monitoring blood pressure and heart rate is insufficient to judge the level of anesthesia.

Esophageal Contractions

The autonomic nervous system affects not only the cardiovascular system, but also intestinal motility. Evans and co-workers have monitored the contractions of smooth muscle—hence, immune to neuromuscular blocking drugs—of the lower third of the esophagus.[3] A water-filled balloon was placed in the lower third of the esophagus and a pressure transducer and recording system sensed and plotted the slow contractions that lasted about 5 seconds in the awake patient. With deepening anesthesia, these contractions slowed and their amplitude diminished. The method is still new and experience must show how frequently false negative and false positive findings might mislead the clinician. It must be anticipated that drugs and diseases that affect the autonomic nervous system and smooth muscle without altering consciousness will lead to misinterpretations of changes in esophageal motility.

ELECTROENCEPHALOGRAPHIC MONITORING

Deducing the degree of anesthesia, amnesia, and oxygenation from the electrical activity of the brain is an enticing possibility. Unfortunately, much work needs to be done before this can become a clinical routine. Although several studies have attempted to correlate electroencephalogram (EEG) levels with amnesia and analgesia, for the present time the clinician must settle for the more modest goals served by electroencephalography.

Caton in 1875, observed electrical signals emanating from the animal brain.[4] Later, von Marxow observed an alteration of animal brain waves with chloroform anesthesia.[5] Hans Berger first placed surface electrodes on the scalps of humans and, in 1933, he studied brain-wave patterns during chloroform anesthesia. Gibbs and colleagues foresaw that "a practical application of the observations might be the use of the EEG as a measure of the depth of anesthesia during surgical operations. The anesthetist and the surgeon could have before them, on tape or screen, a continuous record of the electrical activity of both heart and brain.[6]

Carrying this to the operating room, Penfield and Jasper used the EEG during craniotomies. Gradually, the effects of several anesthetics on the EEG were studied and catalogued, which led Verzeano in the 1950s, to use a rectified EEG signal in a closed-loop system to govern the administration of intravenous anesthetics.[7] Later, Bellville also did this for gaseous agents.[8] Excellent reviews of the EEG and general anesthetics can be found in many articles.[9–11]

Principles of Electroencephalography

The EEG is a continuous recording of the voltage and amplitude of signals obtained by scalp electrodes. The electrical signals emanating from the brain are tiny compared to those recorded on an electrocardiogram. The voltages detected between two arbitrary points on the scalp appear to be generated by neurons in the cerebral cortex. Because the signal of interest is so small, a bit of manipulation becomes necessary. When the voltage between points A and B on the scalp is to be determined, a reference point (R), on the neck, for example, is also chosen. The voltages between R and A, as well as those between R and B, are now fed into a differential amplifier. Physiologic potentials not of interest to the electroencephalographer, such as the electrocardiac signals, are common (*common mode*) to both R–A and R–B. By taking the difference between the two inputs, the common mode is eliminated (*common mode rejection*), leaving only the EEG signal. Typical EEG wave forms and electrode placement and labeling are shown in Figure 10-1.[10,12]

Electronic filters further reduce the noise. In standard clinical EEG signal processing, signals with frequencies below 0.3 Hz and above 70 Hz are attenuated. In the operating room, with its greater electrical noise, signals of less than 0.5 Hz and more than 30 Hz are often filtered out.

During periods of active mentation, the EEG demonstrates a desynchronized pattern with no obvious underlying frequency. When a patient is relaxed, but awake, the neurons' electrical activities become somewhat more coordinated and the waves assume a more synchronous pattern of varying amplitudes and frequencies. During sleep, the brain waves become even more synchronized, as if neurons were working in unison, and the resultant wave pattern appears still more regular.

In the interpretation of the EEG patterns, certain characteristics are identified. Although many aspects can, and are, analyzed, three are most important: frequency, amplitude, and symmetry.

Frequency

Subdivisions of the synchronized EEG are based on the frequency of the synchronized electrical waveforms, where frequency is defined as the number of repetitive waveforms in 1 second. The frequency band usually analyzed lies between 1 Hz and 30 Hz. The several subdivisions, along with the usual physiologic state, are[13]

Delta: 0 Hz to 3 Hz

Theta: 4 Hz to 7 Hz

Alpha: 8 Hz to 13 Hz (typical for a subject who is relaxed with eyes closed.)

Beta: 14 Hz to 30 Hz (typical for a subject who is awake and alert.)

Amplitude

Amplitude refers to the height of the EEG wave as measured in microvolts (μV). The classification is

Low amplitude: <20 μV

Medium amplitude: 20 μV to 50 μV

High amplitude: >50 μV

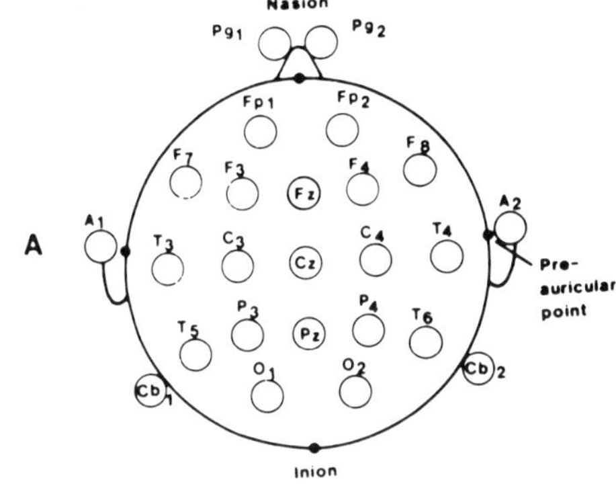

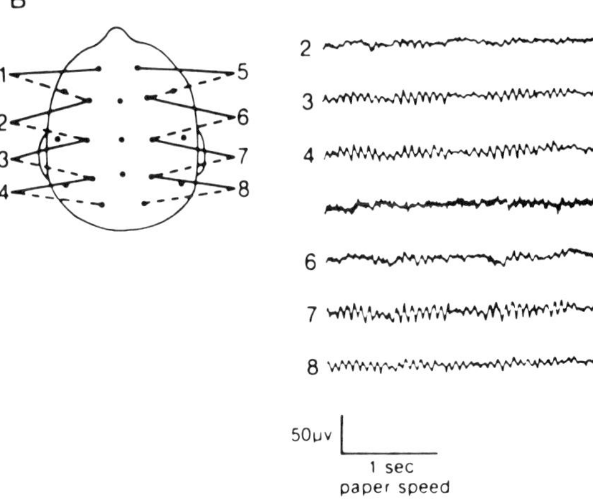

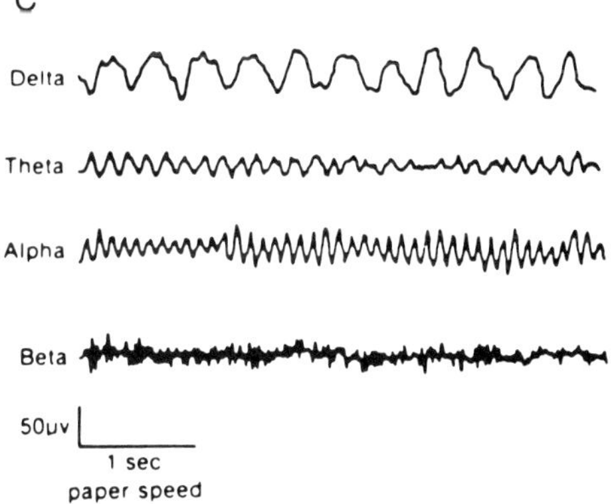

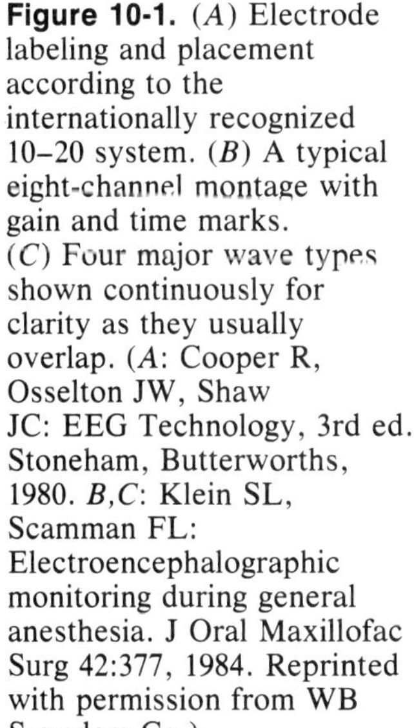
Figure 10-1. (*A*) Electrode labeling and placement according to the internationally recognized 10–20 system. (*B*) A typical eight-channel montage with gain and time marks. (*C*) Four major wave types shown continuously for clarity as they usually overlap. (*A*: Cooper R, Osselton JW, Shaw JC: EEG Technology, 3rd ed. Stoneham, Butterworths, 1980. *B,C*: Klein SL, Scamman FL: Electroencephalographic monitoring during general anesthesia. J Oral Maxillofac Surg 42:377, 1984. Reprinted with permission from WB Saunders Co.)

Symmetry

In health, the EEG signal is symmetrical at about the mid-saggital line. Asymmetry, particularly of an acute nature, usually signifies an alarming event, for instance, inadequate perfusion of part of the brain, as might occur during carotid endarterectomy.

Brain waves are very weak signals, about 20 μV to 200 μV, that must be amplified to provide a waveform large enough for us to analyze. Two types of brain waves are recognized: spontaneous and evoked. *Spontaneous brain waves* are intrinsic to cerebral electrophysiology and occur even if no external stimulus can be identified. *Evoked brain waves* occur in response to external stimuli. Peripheral sensory inputs stimulate certain parts of the brain and culminate in an electrical signal from that portion of the brain. For example, a light flashed before the eye causes a signal to be sent to the occipital region of the brain. In turn, a signal is emitted by the occipital lobe. A wave (cortical evoked potential) typical for its shape, frequency, and amplitude is generated.

Anesthetic Effects on the EEG

Alpha rhythm typifies the conscious state. The alpha pattern has a great deal of variability, influenced, for instance, by opening and closing the

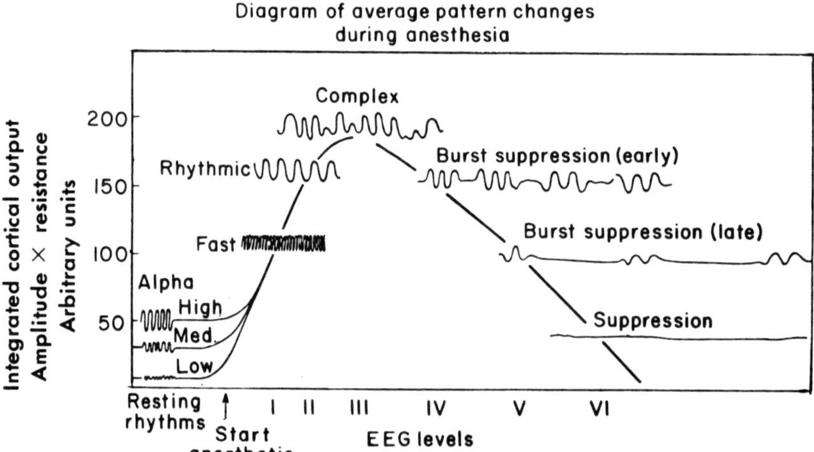

Figure 10-2. Changes in electroencephalogram are shown with increasing depths of anesthesia. Note that the alpha rhythm amplitude range decreases as anesthesia is administered. (Martin JT, et al: Electroencephalography in anesthesiology. Anesthesiology 20:360, 1959)

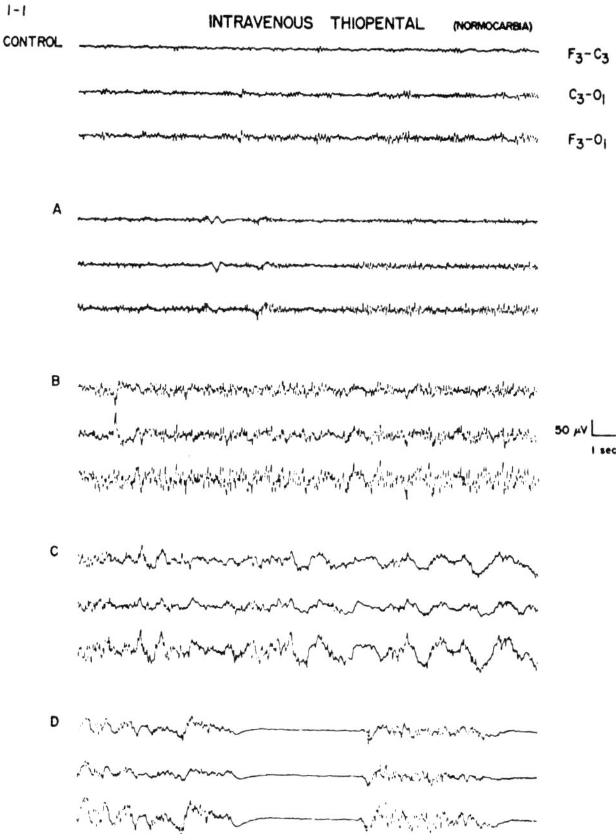

Figure 10-3. Electroencephalographic levels of thiopental anesthesia in humans. (Clark DL, Rosner BS: Neurophysiologic effects of anesthesia. Anesthesiology 38:566, 1973)

eyes. Although each anesthetic agent produces a characteristic pattern, a few general statements can be made on anesthesia and EEG patterns. First, with light levels of anesthesia, the alpha rhythm gives way to a faster rhythm in the beta range. As the depth of anesthesia is increased and the excitement stage is passed, wave frequency decreases and a delta rhythm supervenes. If the central nervous system is further depressed, the waveform becomes more complex; slow waves persist, but amplitude and frequency become variable. At even deeper anesthetic levels, occasional cessation of activity known as "burst suppression" occurs. Eventually, total electrical silence is reached (Fig. 10-2).

In Figure 10-3, EEG tracings obtained during anesthesia with thio-

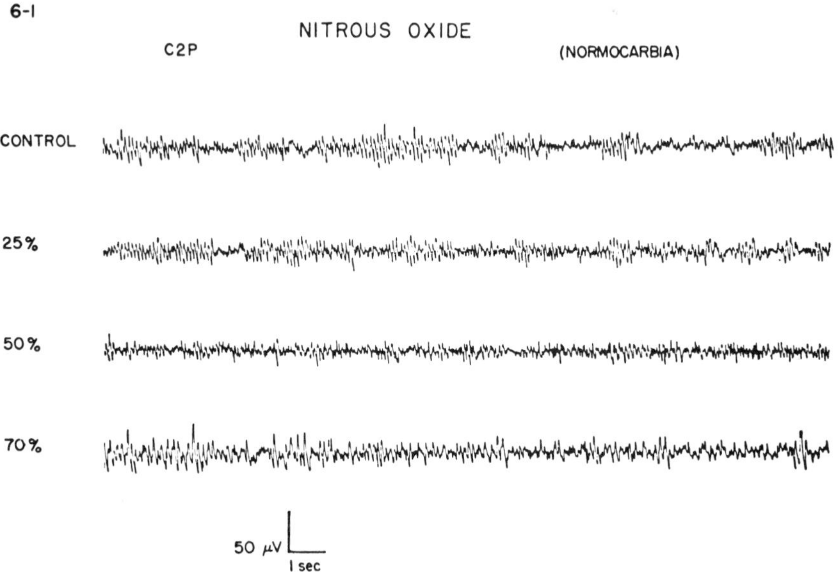

Figure 10-4. Electroencephalographic levels of nitrous oxide anesthesia in humans. Burst suppression is not attained. (Clark DL, Rosner BS: Neurophysiologic effects of anesthesia. Anesthesiology 38:573, 1973)

pental are reproduced. Observe the increasing amplitude and the decreasing frequency as anesthesia is deepened. Burst suppression, with electrical silence interrupted by slow wave (2–8 Hz) activity, is clearly seen. With nitrous oxide, the picture is quite different (Fig. 10-4). Even with 70% N_2O, burst suppression is not reached at atmospheric pressure. The EEG first shows loss of alpha waves, then progressive slowing. In Figure 10-5, we see not only the effects of increasing concentrations of enflurane, but also the effect of altering P_aCO_2. On the left, somatic, sensory-evoked potentials are recorded. Age also plays a role in the EEG changes seen under anesthesia. For example, Oshima et al[14] found different EEG responses to noxious stimuli under halothane anesthesia, which depended on the age of the patient. Adults showed a low-voltage, fast wave response, whereas a high-voltage, slow wave response was characteristic of children less than 8 years old. It can easily be imagined how difficult it is to separate the effects on the EEG of thiopental from those of N_2O and enflurane. Mixing various agents, as in routine anesthetic practice, makes the correlation of the anesthetic state with the brain-wave activity difficult or impossible.

Sebel and colleagues[15] reported typical EEG changes in patients an-

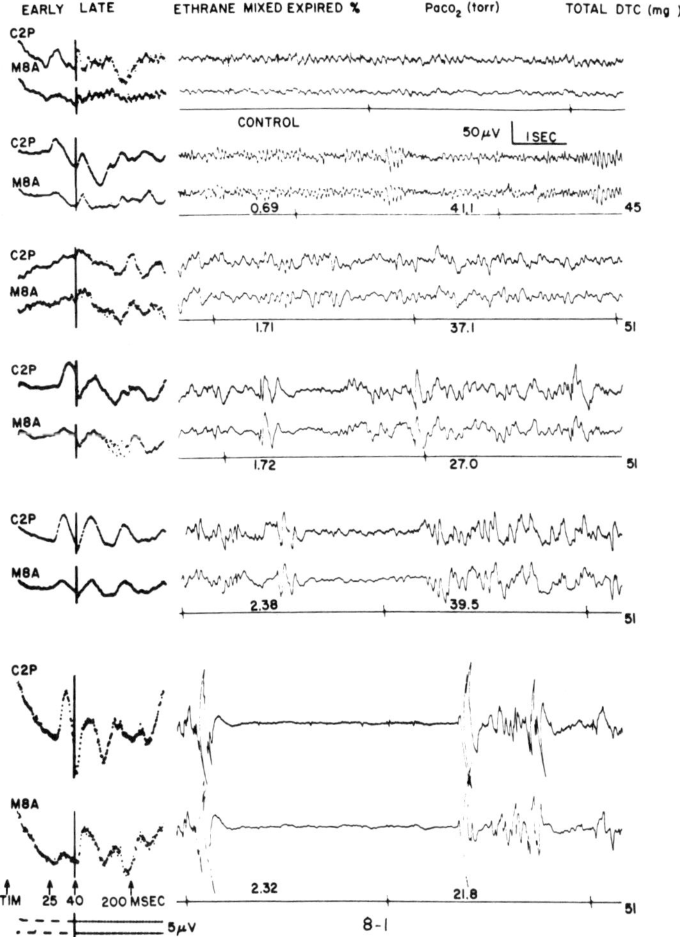

Figure 10-5. Somatic-evoked response (*left*) and EEG (*right*) as affected by various concentrations of enflurane and CO_2 measured at two points (*C2P* and *M8A*). (Clark DL, et al: Neurophysiological effects of different anesthetics in unconscious man. Anesthesiology 38:675, 1973)

esthetized with high doses (up to 70 μg/kg) of fentanyl. Under the influence of rising fentanyl levels the EEG rhythms progressed from alpha waves (9–13 Hz) over diffuse theta waves (4–8 Hz) to diffuse delta waves (less than 3 Hz). The authors claim good correlation between EEG levels and amnesia and analgesia. Similar results were found in a study for high-dose sufentanil (15 mg/kg; Fig. 10-6), which also showed that the effect on EEG was different for adults, children, and babies.[16]

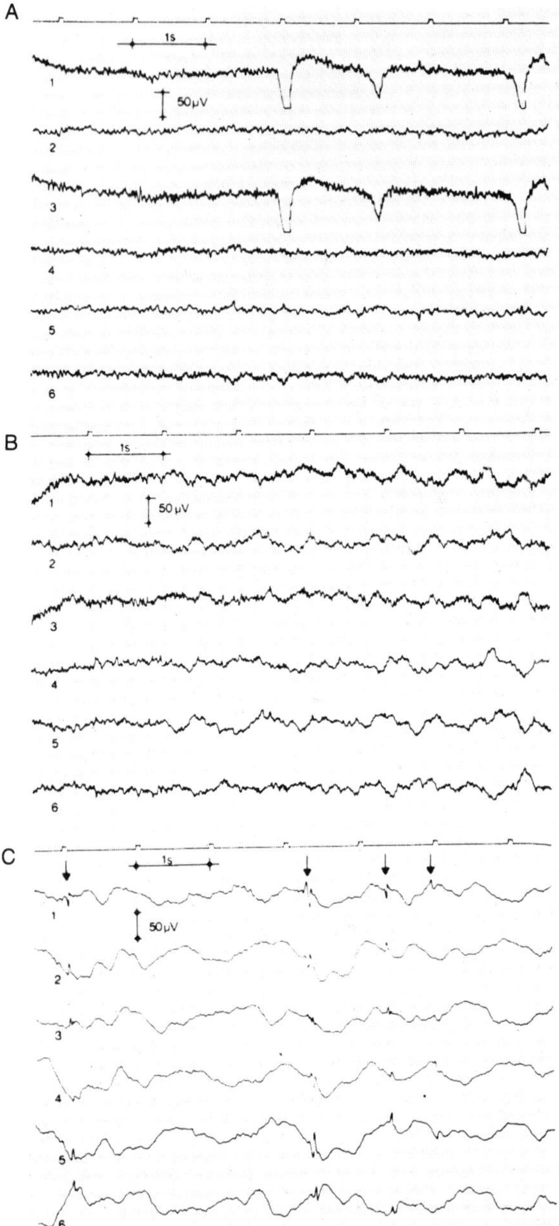

Figure 10-6. (*A*) EEG after premedication. (*B*) EEG 1 minute after start of induction with sufentanil. Note the slowing. (*C*) EEG 3 minutes after start of induction with sufentanil. Most activity is in the delta range. *Arrows* indicate sharp waves. (Bovill JG, et al: Electroencephalographic effects of sufentanil anaesthesia in man. Br J Anaesth 54:45–52, 1982. Reproduced with permission.)

THRESHOLD FOR CHANGES
IN BRAIN ELECTRICAL FUNCTIONS

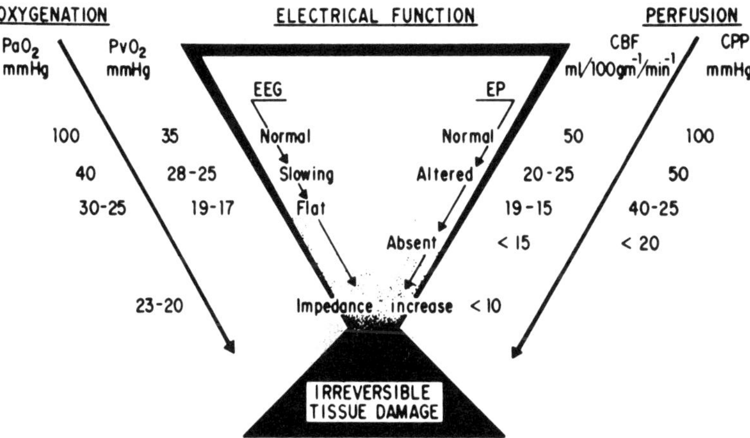

Figure 10-7. A considerable gap exists between irreversible tissue damage and the absence of detected electrical activity. Hypoxia and decreased cerebral perfusion are both seen to diminish measurable electrical potential. (Shapiro HM: The cerebral circulation. ASA 1978 Annual Refresher Course Lectures, p 12. Park Ridge, IL, American Society of Anesthesiologists, 1978)

Effects of Physiologic Changes on the EEG

Physiologic changes also affect brain waves. By monitoring the EEG, some inferences can be made about the hemodynamic and respiratory status of the patient. Remember, anesthetic drugs will modify these effects in an unpredictable fashion.

Hypoxemia

Hypoxemia with a hemoglobin saturation of less than 65%, or P_aO_2 less than 40 torr, decreases the high energy phosphates (ATP) present in the brain and may be recognized by significant changes in the EEG. Alpha waves give way to delta waves as consciousness is lost. The predominant frequency shifts from between 8 Hz and 13 Hz to less than 4 Hz during hypoxia. The EEG, as shown in Figure 10-7, is not useful in detecting moderate hypoxia.

Hypocarbia

Hypocarbia is also associated with slowing but increasing amplitude of the EEG. The dominant frequency occurs in the 4 Hz to 6 Hz range or theta range. The changes are reduced by increased oxygen concentration and obliterated by amyl nitrite; implying that vasoconstriction is the responsible mechanism.

Hypercarbia

An arousal pattern is seen initially with hypercarbia. If the CO_2 pressure exceeds 190 torr, rapid EEG activity slows until it finally disappears. At higher levels, delta activity dominates at relatively high amplitude. At carbon dioxide levels of 600 torr, for 2 min to 5 min, the EEG becomes isoelectric.

Hypotension

If cerebral blood flow falls to less than 50% of normal, EEG changes similar to those of hypoxia take place. The waves flatten and slow as blood flow decreases (Fig. 10-7).

Hypoglycemia

Hypoglycemia can result in a loss of consciousness and a loss of the EEG alpha rhythm. The EEG slows and delta activity is observed. Unfortunately, these effects are difficult to separate from the effects of general anesthesia, which also hides the clinical signs of hypoglycemia. Hyperglycemia does not alter the EEG.

Physiologic changes and resultant EEG changes are summarized in Figure 10-7. The thresholds for changes in brain function are shown. It is obvious where our present state of technology leaves a gap. With currently available technology, we cannot tell from the EEG whether irreversible tissue damage has occurred. The EEG can be flat, but the brain may be either intact or irreversibly damaged.

Recording the EEG

Location of Electrodes

Electrode placement is usually based on the 10–20 system, which is internationally recognized (Fig. 10-1).[17] It is based upon four standard points on the head—the nasion, the inion, and the left and right pre-auricular points. To make the measurements, Cooper and colleagues suggest the following procedure, using a tape measure and a marking pencil for precise electrode location.[17]

(1) Measure the distance from nasion to inion along the midline through the vertex and make a preliminary mark at the midpoint, C_z.

(2) Ensure that this point is midway between the pre-auricular points (each of which can be felt as a depression at the root of the zygoma just anterior to the tragus) by applying the tape transversely.
(3) Reapply the tape along the midline through C_z and mark points at 10, 20, 20, 20, 20, and 10% of the total nasion–inion distance. These are the positions of F_{pz}, F_z, C_z, P_z, and O_z.
(4) Reapply the tape transversely through C_z and mark points at 10, 20,20, 20, 20, and 10% of the total distance between the pre-auricular points. These are positions of T_3, C_3, C_z, C_4, and T_4. Note that odd-numbered positions are always on the left.
(5) Measure the distance between F_{pz} and O_z by applying the tape along the great circle passing through T_3 and mark points at 10, 20, 20, 20, 20, and 10% of this length. These are the positions of F_{p1}, F_7, T_3, T_5, and O_1.
(6) Repeat this procedure on the right side and mark the positions of F_{p2}, F_8, T_4, T_6, and O_2.
(7) Measure the distance between F_{p1} and O_1 by applying the tape along the great circle passing through C_3 and mark points at 25% intervals. These give the positions of F_3, C_3, and P_3.
(8) Repeat this procedure on the right side and mark the positions of F_4, C_4, and P_4.
(9) Check that F_7, F_3, F_z, F_4, and F_8 are equidistant by applying the tape transversely along the great circle passing through F_7, F_z, and F_8.
(10) Check that T_5, P_3, P_z, P_4, and T_6 are equidistant in a similar manner.

All of the electrode locations are usually not used simultaneously. Instead, electrode pairs are selected for study depending upon the clinical situation. Electrode pairs chosen are called *derivations*. The grouping of the derivations selected for study is called *electrode montage* (Fig. 10-8).[17]

Application of Electrodes

1. Select a location and part the patient's hair at that location.
2. Clean the area thoroughly with acetone and let dry. ***Caution***: Be careful when using alcohol, acetone, or collodion on or near the patient as these substances are flammable. Allow vapors to dissipate before using an ECG, EEG amplifier, or any other electrical device.
3. Saturate a gauze square with collodion. Hold the electrode in place and place collodion-saturated gauze over it. Do not place electrodes on areas where the surface of the scalp is broken. ***Note***: Electrode surfaces must be clean, the lead firmly attached to the electrode disc, and all plugs firmly connected. Frayed wires and electrodes that are scratched, bent, or have metal showing should be discarded.

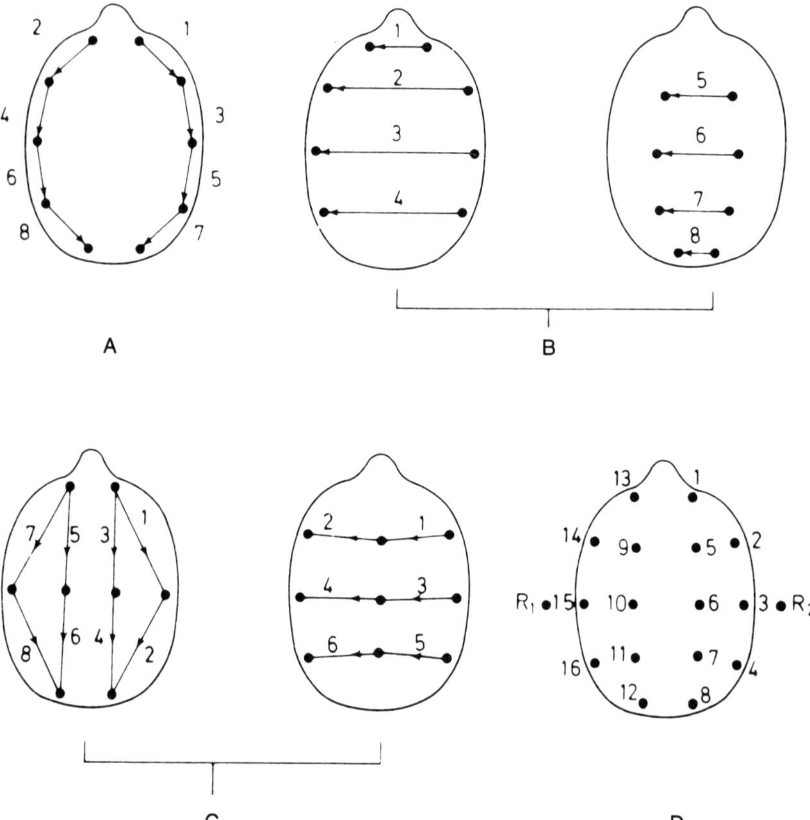

Figure 10-8. (*A*) Bipolar montage made up of alternating anteroposterior derivations. (*B*) Bipolar montage made up of transverse derivations between pairs of symmetrically placed electrodes. (*C*) Bipolar montages made up of anteroposterior and transverse derivations from widely spaced electrodes. (*D*) Common reference montage. Channels 1 to 8 are referred to as R_1: channels 9 to 16 are referred to as R_2. (Cooper R, et al: EEG Technology, 3rd ed. Stoneham, Butterworths, 1980)

4. Hold electrode and gauze in place, allowing 30 seconds until gauze has dried.
5. With a blunted cannula, dilate the opening in the electrode. Gently rub the skin beneath the electrode with the cannula, then inject enough electrolyte to fill the space between the electrode and the skin. ***Caution***: Do not overfill.

To record a full EEG entails many hurdles that preclude its routine use in the operating room. Unless the EEG machine is accompanied by one or more technicians, it is seldom seen in the operating theater or intensive care unit. The reasons are many:

- The location of electrodes is critical. For a quantitative analysis, a full montage with 16 or more electrodes is required. Correct location of electrodes is quite important, but the landmarks are difficult to locate and untrained personnel obtain poor results.
- The machine is bulky.
- Information from many channels is recorded at approximately 300 pages per hour. The anesthesiologist cannot cope with so much data if he is to monitor other aspects of the patient besides the EEG.
- Electrically, the operating room is a rather hostile environment. Electrocautery, other monitoring devices, pumps, television, and videotape make for much electrical noise in the operating room.
- Individual variability of the EEG makes interpretation difficult.
- Anesthetic depth is not easily deduced from the EEG.
- Low cardiac output, hypoxia, and hypercarbia can be monitored more reliably and easily by other methods.

When we require an EEG, for instance, during microneurosurgical vascular procedures, we recruit the help of an electroencephalographer who brings a technician and applies 16 leads. In order to overcome some of the systematic difficulties, several attempts have been made to simplify the presentation of electroencephalographic data. Some use a single-lead EEG. Although this simplifies interpretation, much information is lost. The two-electrode EEG can be implemented by attaching one electrode over the left half of the forehead and the other behind and slightly inferior to the right ear.

We occasionally use a three-electrode EEG system during cardiopulmonary bypass. The location we use is shown in Figure 10-9. Whichever electrode system is employed, a reference or ground electrode must also be used. It may be placed anywhere on the body as long as good contact is maintained. If the same monitor is used for ECG and EEG, one ground will suffice for both.

Limiting the number of EEG channels to one or two is but one way to facilitate EEG monitoring in the operating room and intensive care unit. An alternative is to process the EEG signals and then generate a compact display. Various methods have been marketed.

Simplification of EEG Monitoring

Cerebral Function Monitor

One of the first techniques used to simplify EEG monitoring was the Cerebral Function Monitor.[18] Rather than multiple electrodes, a single

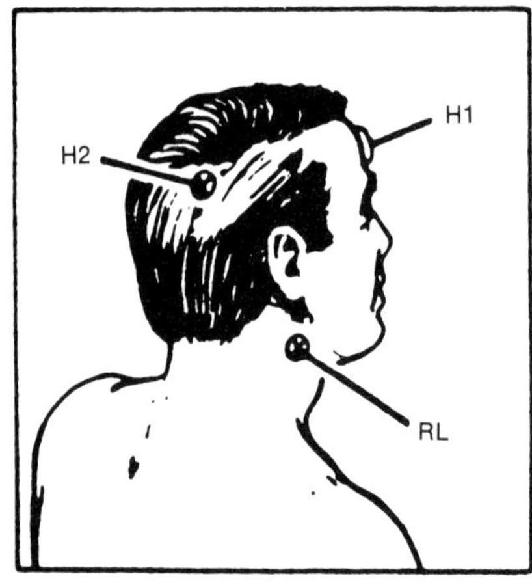

Right side

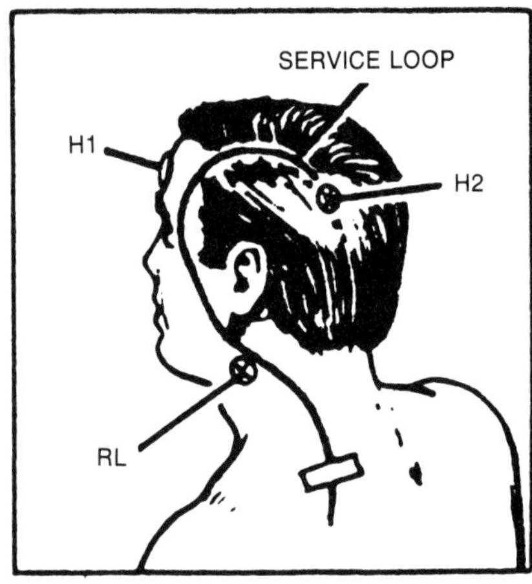

Left side

Figure 10-9. To determine levels of cerebral electrical activity, position electrodes over the patient's dominant hemisphere. Choose the side of the head to be monitored and attach electrodes as shown. *H1*, on midline of forehead above the eye on dominant side of the head. *H2*, in the upper parietal area on the dominant side of the head. *R1*, on the flat portion of the neck directly below the ear and jaw on the dominant side of the head. (Reprinted with permission from Hewlett-Packard Operator's Manual 78208-91999)

bipolar lead is used. Generally, it is placed in the biparietal position. By use of filters, signals below 2 Hz and those above 15 Hz are cut off sharply. In this way, the frequency spectrum is markedly narrowed. By manipulating the signal through semilogarithmic compression, integration, and rectification, a smooth line is drawn between the peaks of the signal. It represents a voltage that varies both with amplitude and with frequency of the cerebral waves. On semilogarithmic paper, at a very slow speed, the output generates a thick band (Fig. 10-10). The lower edge of the band represents the lowest peak-to-peak amplitude. The band's upper edge reflects the upper peak-to-peak amplitude. Therefore, the thickness of the band indicates the amount of variability inherent in the signal. The closer the band is to the baseline, the less cerebral activity there is. A second channel continuously monitors the impedance between the two electrodes. This helps to determine artifacts and deterioration of electrode contact. Dubois and co-workers have reported on the clinical use of this equipment.[19]

Several authors have found the Cerebral Function Monitor useful in the resuscitation of patients after cardiac arrest or during open heart surgery, after drug overdose in postoperative conditions, or in clinical anesthesia. Induction of anesthesia corresponds to increased activity of the

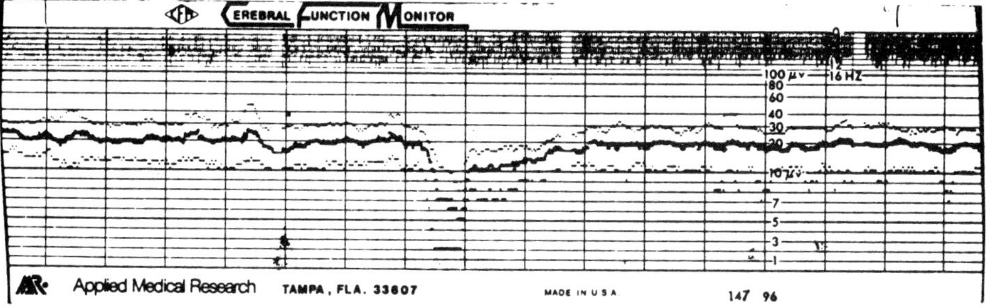

Figure 10-10. Traces obtained with a Cerebral Function Monitor (Critikon, Inc., Tampa, FL) from a patient undergoing a carotid endarterectomy. The scale on the upper border is calibrated in hertz and represents the predominant EEG frequency, with cutoffs below 2 Hz and above 15 Hz. The tracing is interrupted every 10 minutes. The heavy line in the middle of the record gives the mean cortical activity in microvolts. The thinner lines above and below represent maximal and minimal voltages. The drop in voltage in the middle of the panel occurred when the carotid artery was clamped. (Courtesy of R. F. Cucchiara, MD, Mayo Clinic, Rochester, MN)

trace with an elevation of the baseline. If anesthesia is continued, the band returns toward baseline and broadens as variation in activity increases. Further deepening of anesthesia is indicated by closer approximation of the band to the baseline. With burst suppression, the variability increases greatly and band width dramatically increases. Awakening narrows and elevates the band width. Even devotees to this machine admit that inhalation anesthesia is difficult to manage with this method, but the monitor can indicate general seizure activity.

An advanced version of the Cerebral Function Monitor is the Cerebral Function Analyzing Monitor. It presents a more detailed plot of the amplitude distribution and also gives a frequency analysis of the EEG. Figure 10-11 shows the output scheme, and Figure 10-12 shows a trace from a patient.[20]

EEG Combined with EMG

Electromyography has been combined with the EEG in the anesthesia and brain activity monitor (ABM), which uses a single-channel EEG as does the Cerebral Function Monitor. It has been shown by Harmel and colleagues that the resting tone of skeletal muscles is related to anesthetic levels if neuromuscular blocking agents are not present.[21] Edmonds and Paloheimo evaluated this system for intraoperative monitoring and reported that "alone or in combination changes in thc EEG and EMG displays do not necessarily accompany changes in the common clinical signs

(Text continues on p. 262)

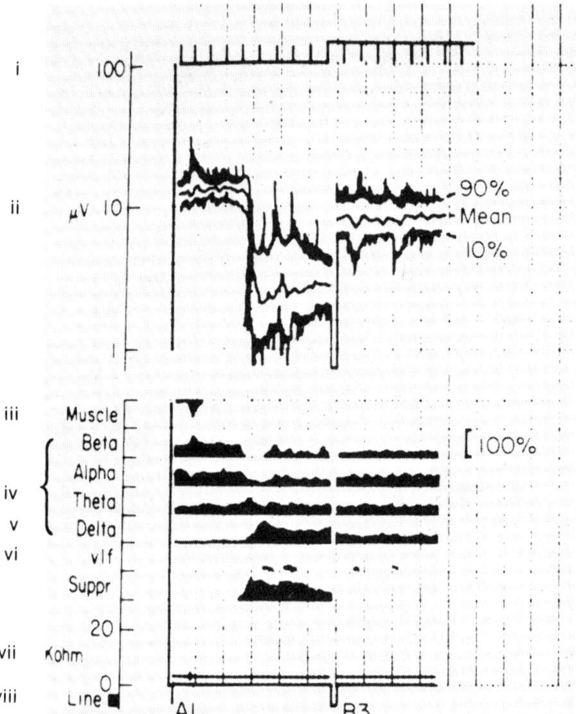

Figure 10-11. Simulated Cerebral Function Analyzing Monitor trace. *From top to bottom,* the traces are as follows: (i) Time marker at 1-minute intervals. (ii) The 90th centile, the mean, and the tenth centile of the weighted amplitude distribution with maximum and minimum excursions in any 2-second epoch. (iii) Muscle activity. (iv) Percentage of weighted EEG activity in the beta, alpha, theta, and delta bands. (v) Percentage of very low frequency activity (less than 1 Hz). (vi) Suppression band: percentage time the weighted EEG is below a preset amplitude (adjustable from 1.0 μV to 10.5 μV). (vii) Electrode impedance in kilohms (kΩ). (viii) Marker. Data are analyzed from either of two pairs of electrodes, channel A or B. Amplitude may be displayed on a scale of 1 μV to 100 μV, or 3 μV to 300 μV. *A1* is printed on the trace to indicate analysis from channel A on the 1 μV to 100 μV scale, and *B3* indicates analysis from channel B on the 3 μV to 300 μV scale. The amplitude and frequency plots cut out to below their baselines when the input channel overloads and also for 12 seconds when the input channel is automatically changed, as at *B3*. A further trace (not shown here) is written below the impedance trace to indicate the presence of 50-Hz line interference at the recording electrodes. (Maynard DE, Jenkinson JL: The cerebral function analysing monitor. Anaesthesia 39:678–690, 1984)

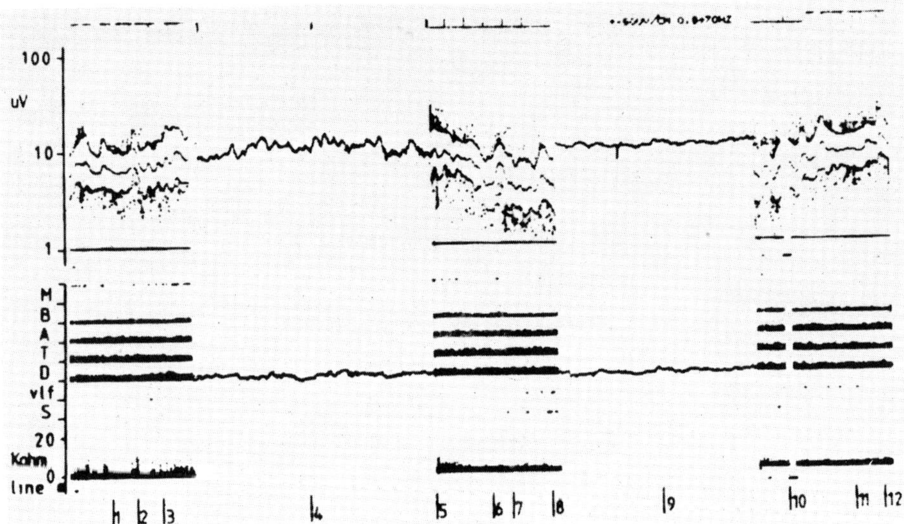

Figure 10-12. Induced hypotension. At the start of the example, anesthesia was being maintained with 60% nitrous oxide in oxygen and 0.5% halothane. At *2*, 2% halothane was introduced to produce hypotension. This was followed by an initial rise of amplitude and subsequently a fall. At *7*, halothane was withdrawn and this was followed by a gradual recovery of amplitude to its initial level. Throughout the recording frequency shifts were minimal. Mean arterial pressures (in millimeters of mercury) were *1* = 70; *2* = 65; *3* = 60; *5* = 58; *6* = 53; *8* = 60; *10* = 70; *11* = 68; *12* = 75. The EEG before and during the period of EEG amplitude depression is shown at *4* and *9*. The impedance trace indicates at times frequent electrode artifacts. One of these is visible in the second EEG sample as downward spike deflection. (Maynard DE, Jenkinson JL: The cerebral function analysing monitor. Anaesthesia 39:678–690, 1984)

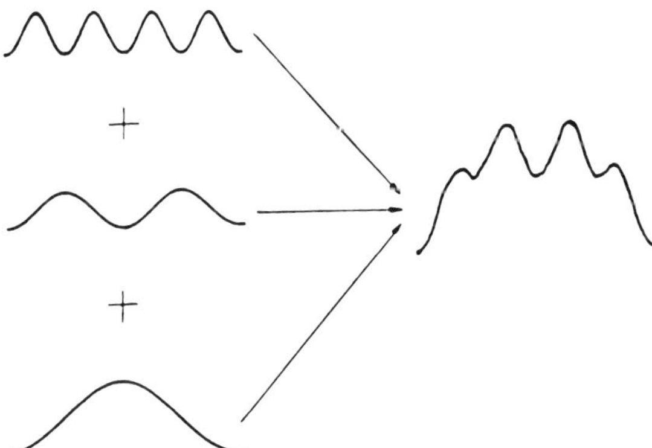

Figure 10-13. Waveform summation using waves of various amplitudes and frequencies to produce a complex waveform. (Interspec: EEG and Evoked Potential Monitoring, 3rd rev, 1985. Compliments of Interspec, Inc., Conshohocken, PA.)

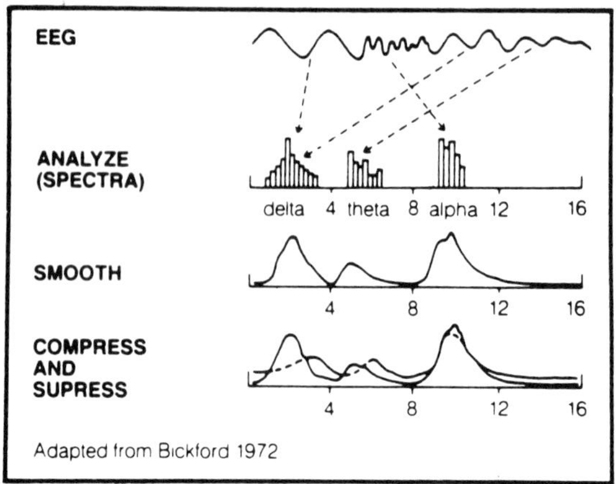

Figure 10-14. EEG processing to produce the compressed spectral array. (Interspec: EEG and Evoked Potential Monitoring, 3rd rev, 1985. Compliments of Interspec, Inc, Conshohocken, PA.)

of anesthetic depth and adequacy,'' such as heart rate, blood pressure, and motion of the patient.[22] Although the unit has its limitations, it has proved useful to warn the clinician of decreased cerebral activity.

Power and Frequency Analysis

An additional way to process the EEG is by frequency analysis. Here the complex EEG waveform is mathematically scrutinized and dissected. The complex waveforms are reduced to the sum of simple sine waves of different amplitudes and frequencies. This is shown in Figure 10-13.[12] The mathematical method used most frequently is called the fast Fourier transform. Once the EEG signal has been analyzed for its frequency and power (the square of the amplitude) content, it can be displayed in many different ways. One of these is the *compressed spectral array,* which is a three-dimensional display of frequency and power over time, popularized by Bickford and colleagues.[23] Figure 10-14 shows schematically how this is done for each time interval.

With frequency on the x axis, power on the z axis, and time on the y axis, a smooth line can be plotted. By moving the paper slightly at each interval, the plot eventually resembles a topographic map (Fig. 10-15). In this manner, the patient's EEG activity over many minutes is recorded on one sheet of paper or displayed on a screen. Changes in the EEG become very apparent even to the layman. The compressed spectral array (CSA) does have some disadvantages, however. A persistent high peak in the plot may obscure other data behind the peak; a dominant peak may

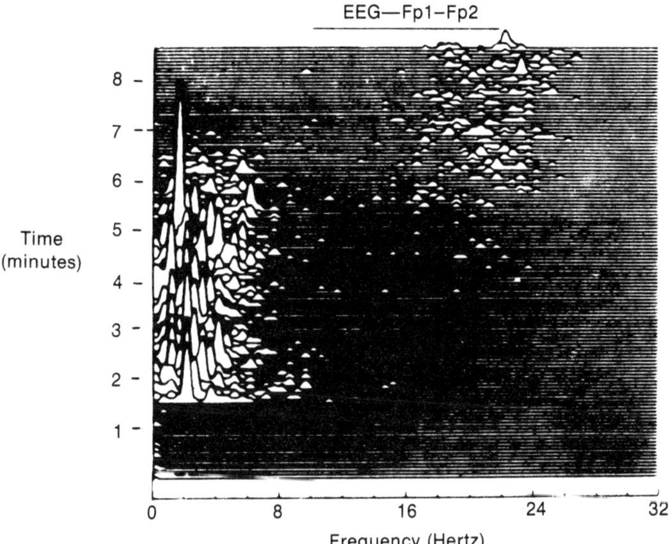

Figure 10-15. After an injection of thiopental (150 mg), it does not require an expert electroencephalographer to detect the changes in the EEG. (Gravenstein JS, et al: Monitoring Surgical Patients in the Operating Room, p 127. Springfield, IL, Charles C Thomas, 1979)

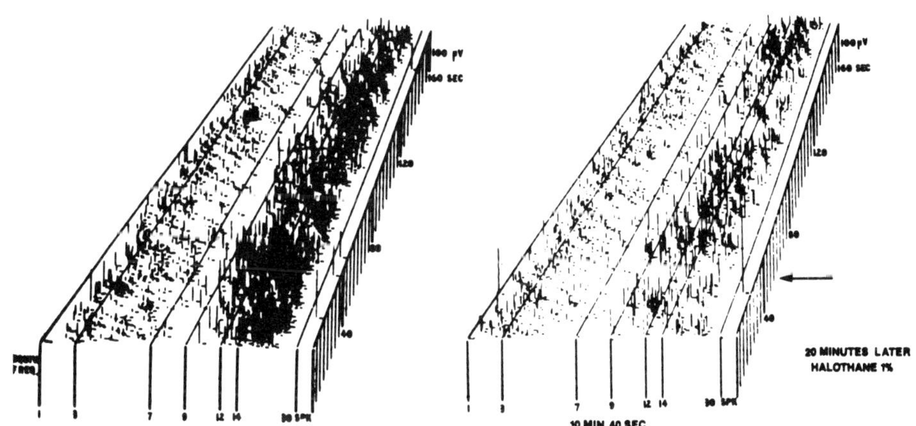

Figure 10-16. The EEG analytic method of Demetrescu is shown. Note the three-dimensional effect produced by perspective. The *left panel* represents the EEG during light halothane and residual thiopental anesthesia. In the *right panel,* the patient is "too light" and moved about 1 minute after this EEG warning was given. (Gravenstein JS, et al: Monitoring Surgical Patients in the Operating Room, p 134. Springfield, IL, Charles C Thomas, 1979)

imply a high degree of activity but, in point of fact, the patient's EEG may have become flat.

Demetrescu[24] has approached EEG recording and analysis by retaining more of the traditionally used techniques. An isometric projection of a three-dimensional plot is used (Fig. 10-16). The EEG is scanned continuously. Each wave is analyzed for frequency and amplitude. The frequency is recorded by placing a vertical line in the proper place on the frequency axis, and its amplitude is noted by the height of the vertical line. Spikes are also represented.

To simplify the EEG, more specific aspects of the CSA can be displayed. For example, the frequency where half the power lies above and half below, the *median power frequency,* can be identified. The frequency at which the highest power is found is called the *peak power frequency.* The frequency at which 97% or so of the power occurs at lower frequencies is called the *spectral edge frequency.* Displays of the CSA can be enhanced by identifying the locations of these various frequencies (Fig. 10-17).[12]

Density Modulated Spectral Array

Loss of data behind the peaks has been a criticism of the CSA method. Fleming and Smith developed a method by which the processed EEG is represented in a dot matrix form.[25] Frequency is on the horizontal scale. The size of the dots or the density of dots on a horizontal line is a function of the frequency content of the EEG at the particular frequency. Each line represents data gathered over a finite period of time known as an

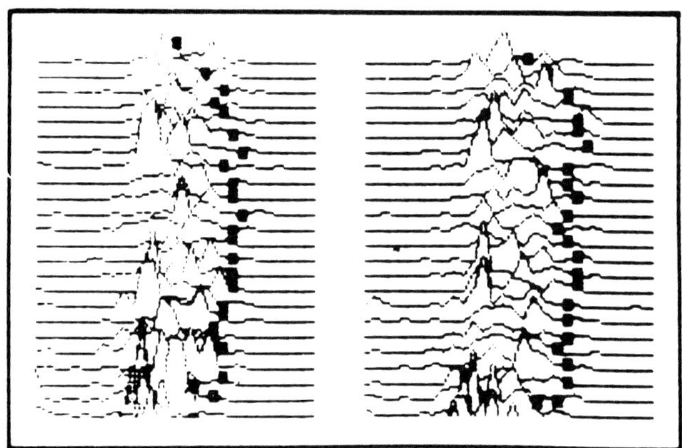

Figure 10-17. Compressed spectral array with the spectral edge indicated by the squares. (Interspec: EEG and Evoked Potential Monitoring, 3rd rev, 1985. Compliments of Interspec, Inc, Conshohocken, PA.)

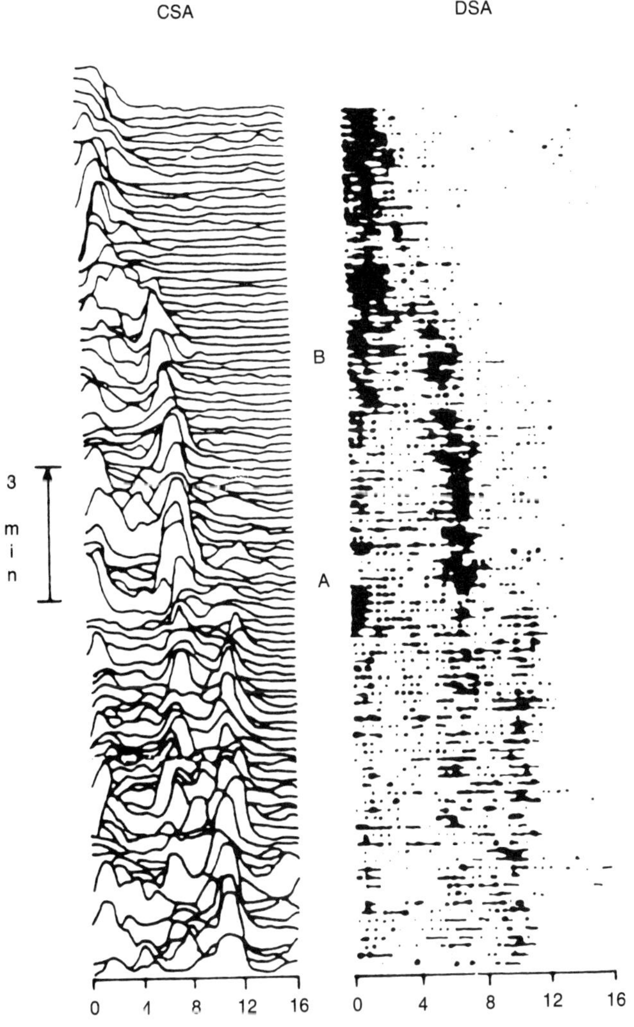

Figure 10-18. CSA and DSA display comparison. A patient under deepening halothane N_2O anesthesia. Note at time *B* to *A* the greater 4 Hz to 8 Hz activity, and at time *A* the greater 8 Hz to 12 Hz activity. (Levy WJ, et al: Automated EEG processing for intraoperative monitoring: A comparison of techniques. Anesthesiology 53:229, 1980)

epoch. Time then appears on the vertical axis. The so-called *density modulated spectral array* (DSA) has less resolution than the CSA, but color rather than the use of shades of grey may improve this. A comparison of CSA and DSA plots is shown in Figure 10-18.[25]

Zero-Crossing Frequency

Known more generally as period analysis than as zero-crossing frequency (ZXF), this early method analyzes one of the most fundamental properties of the EEG (voltage) signal, namely its oscillations between positive and negative.[26] By calculating the rate at which the EEG crosses the zero voltage line (the isoelectric point) we can establish the ZXF. Unfortunately, two EEG signals may be quite different but have the same ZXF, because the complex EEG signal contains high and low frequencies that are superimposed. Small changes in a higher amplitude component may force a lower amplitude component out of or into the zero-crossing range, causing large changes in the ZXF.

Power Plus Frequency Analysis

Attempts to further simplify EEG monitoring by power spectrum analysis are exemplified in devices using one channel on each hemisphere. This display consists of four bar graphs, two for each channel, which shows power on one graph and frequency on the other.

EVOKED POTENTIALS

The EEG is the random, continuous electrical output (10–200 μV) of the outer layers of the cerebral cortex. If, instead, we are interested in a specific sensory function, we must extract information from the EEG. For example, if we want to monitor function of the spinal cord at T10, a cortical response can be evoked by stimulation of a sensory nerve distal to T10. The response is called an *evoked response* or, because of its electrical nature, an *evoked potential*.

The evoked potentials are very small, 1 μV to 5 μV, and tend to get buried in the EEG signal. To extract the evoked potential from the EEG, the sensory pathway of interest is stimulated repetitively. The response is measured through electrodes precisely located and the signal averaged to strip away the "EEG noise."

To date, three types of evoked potentials are of clinical interest both for diagnosis and clinical monitoring. By stimulating the auditory nerve with sound, an auditory evoked potential (AEP) is generated. The early part of the AEP is called the brain-stem auditory evoked potential (BAEP), monitored during operations in the posterior cranial fossa. By stimulating the retina with flashes of light, the visual evoked potential (VEP) is obtained, which is helpful during operations encroaching on the optic nerve or chiasm. Electrical stimulation of a sensory nerve of an extremity leads to somatosensory evoked potentials (SEPs). We monitor SEPs during operations on spine, spinal cord, and thoracic aorta to guard against ischemia of the spinal cord. Of course, since the evoked potentials travel from periphery to center on sensory nerves, only effects on ascending sensory tracts can be detected. In some instances, subtle changes limited to the motor tracts have been missed when SEPs were monitored.

Principles of Evoked Potentials

The small potentials evoked in the spinal cord, brain stem, or cortex by stimulation in the periphery call for sophisticated electronic techniques. Because the small evoked potentials are buried in the background of the EEG, many responses are averaged and the averages are replicated to make sure that a valid evoked potential is recorded. In Figure 10-19, the posterior tibial nerve of a patient was stimulated 1024 times with 5.1 stimuli per second. All cortical responses were averaged. In order to suppress extraneous signals, a filter was used to eliminate all frequencies below 30 Hz and above 250 Hz. The numbers attached to the positive and negative potentials represent the milliseconds that elapsed after stimulation, also called the latency. Thus, all recorded potentials arose with a latency of less than 100 msec. Such potentials are called near-field potentials, and are assumed to arise in nervous tissue near the scalp electrode, that is, in the cortex of the patient's brain. The figure shows how isoflurane increases the latency and decreases the amplitude of the near-field SEP.

Far-field potentials arise from neural generators that lie relatively far from the scalp electrodes, often in the brain stem. A peripheral stimulus thus reaches the neural generator of a far-field potential in the brain stem before it has worked its way to the near field in the cortex. Since the far-field potential can be conducted through brain tissue as if it were an electrolyte solution, the far-field potential will arrive under the scalp electrode before the stimulus that will trigger the near-field potential has had time to work its way through multiple synapses into the cortex. Far-field potentials arise, therefore, with a latency of less than 45 msec and, because they travel further from the neural generator to the electrode, have less voltage; they thus require more amplification. For the far-field potentials shown in Figure 10-20, all frequencies below 150 Hz and above 1000 Hz were filtered out. Because the far-field potentials have a shorter latency, it is possible to use more rapid rates of stimulation, and because they have less voltage, more stimuli are usually averaged; here 2048 replicated stimuli were given at a rate of 15.1 per second.

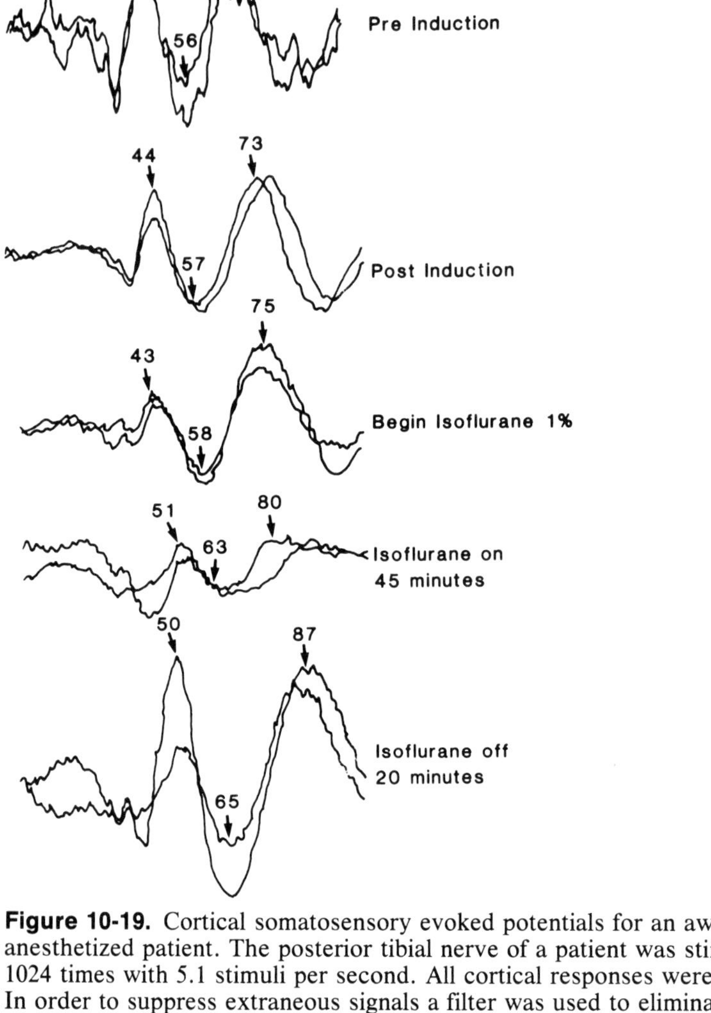

Figure 10-19. Cortical somatosensory evoked potentials for an awake and an anesthetized patient. The posterior tibial nerve of a patient was stimulated 1024 times with 5.1 stimuli per second. All cortical responses were averaged. In order to suppress extraneous signals a filter was used to eliminate all frequencies below 30 Hz and above 250 Hz. The numbers attached to the positive and negative potentials represent the time (in milliseconds) that elapsed after the stimulation, also called the latency. Thus all recorded potentials arose with a latency of less than 100 msec. Such potentials are called near field potentials. These are assumed to arise in nervous tissue near the scalp electrode, in other words, in the cortex of the patient's brain. The figure shows how isoflurane increases the latency and decreases the amplitude of the near field evoked somatosensory evoked potential. (Courtesy of Maryann Gravenstein, MD)

HUMAN FAR-FIELD SEP

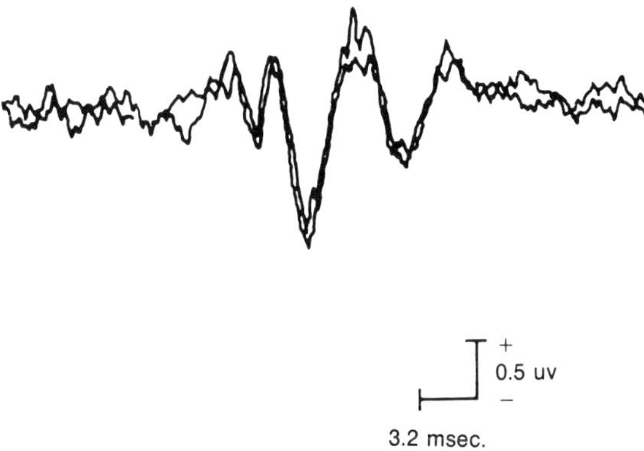

Figure 10-20. A far-field potential. In this figure frequencies below 150 Hz and above 1000 Hz were filtered out. Two thousand forty-eight replicated stimuli were given at a rate of 15.1 per second to the posterior tibial nerve of a patient. (Courtesy of Maryann Gravenstein, MD)

Types of Evoked Potentials

Somatosensory Evoked Potentials

In recording SEPs at least two channels are used, each of which consists of a pair of electrodes. One electrode is placed along the anatomic pathway of the sensory nerve and the second serves as a reference electrode. For surgery, we monitor the two sites along the anatomic pathway. For example, as shown in Figure 10-21, the median nerve and posterior tibial nerve are stimulated sequentially. The nerve-action potential is measured at Erb's point and the popliteal fossa, respectively. The response time and voltage are measured over the contralateral cortex for the stimulation of the posterior tibial nerve and the median nerve. If the spinal cord at the thoracic or lumbar level is insulted, the cortical and cervical SEP from posterior tibial nerve stimulation may be altered. The median nerve SEPs should not be affected since the entrance to the spinal cord lies above the potential lesion. Figure 10-22 shows posterior tibial nerve SEPs recorded during an operation involving stretching of the spinal cord. As can be seen, the potentials were not markedly reduced after distraction. Many experts in the field will consider reductions in amplitude of up to 50%, and increases in latency of up to 20%, as clinically acceptable.

We monitor evoked potentials from both upper and lower extremities during aortic coarctation surgery to guard against spinal cord ischemia while the aorta is cross clamped. Thoracic spinal cord ischemia will even-

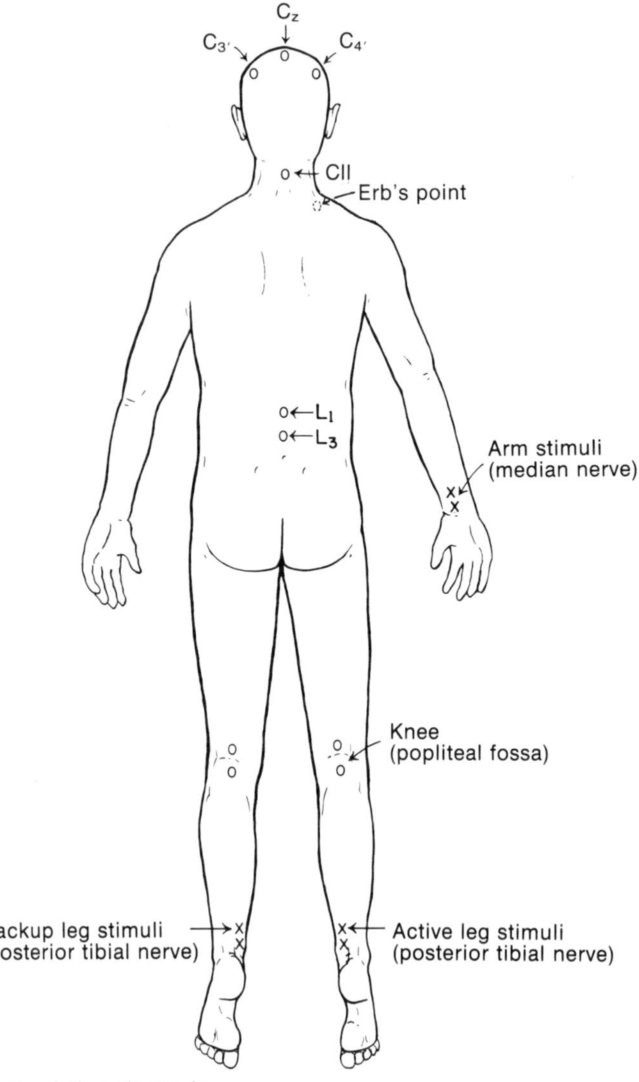

Figure 10-21. The median nerve and posterior tibial nerve of a patient are stimulated. Electrode locations for both stimulating and sensing are shown (patient is prone). $C_{3'}$ is located centralateral to the site of stimulation, 3 cm posterior to C_3. $C_{4'}$ is ipsilateral to the stimulation; it is 3 cm posterior to C_4.

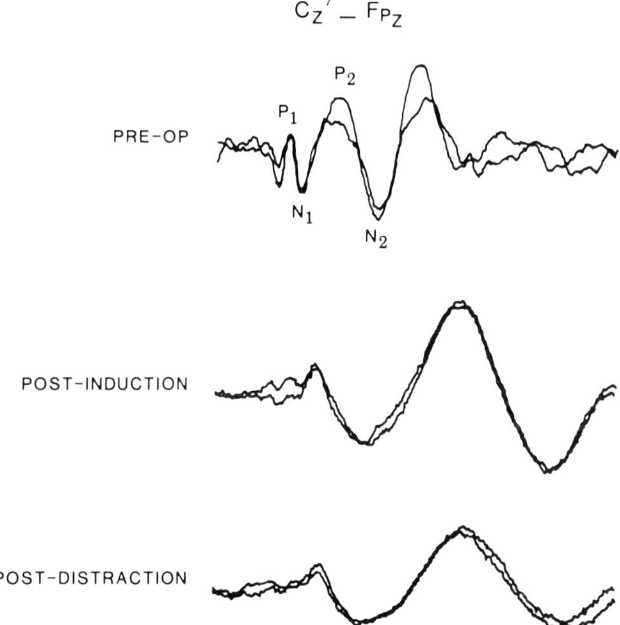

Figure 10-22. Somatosensory (posterior tibial nerve) evoked potentials during intraoperative spinal cord stretching. (Courtesy of Maryann Gravenstein, MD)

tually cause lower extremity SEP changes, whereas upper extremity SEPs will not be affected by the ischemia, but will be effected by metabolic and electrical factors. Since the cervical potentials are much less influenced by metabolic parameters, including halogenated anesthetic agents, we rely on them heavily during surgery.[27] As can be seen in the series of SEPs (Fig. 10-23), ischemia initiated during aortic cross clamping caused loss of the lower extremity SEP. Cessation of the aortic cross clamping led to reappearance of the cervical and cortical SEPs.

Visual Evoked Potentials

Visual evoked potentials (VEPs) are measured by studying a peak voltage called P100 at occipital scalp locations. Flashes of light presented monocularly through the closed lid by an array of light-emitting diodes trigger the VEP. Intraoperative measurement of VEP is in its infancy.

Brain-Stem Auditory Evoked Potentials

An audible click is delivered to one ear at a time. This activates the eighth nerve, which stimulates the related brain-stem structures. A cascade of

(Text continues on p. 279)

A

	MSEC/DIV	uVLT/DIV
A8 A4 A7 A3	4.000	1.25
A6 A2	4.000	5.00
A5 A1	4.000	12.50
B8 B4	6.000	0.50
B7 B3	6.000	1.25
B6 B2	6.000	2.50
B5 B1	6.000	25.00

A1 908 POST INDUCTION INCISION
A5 912 RIBS SPREAD

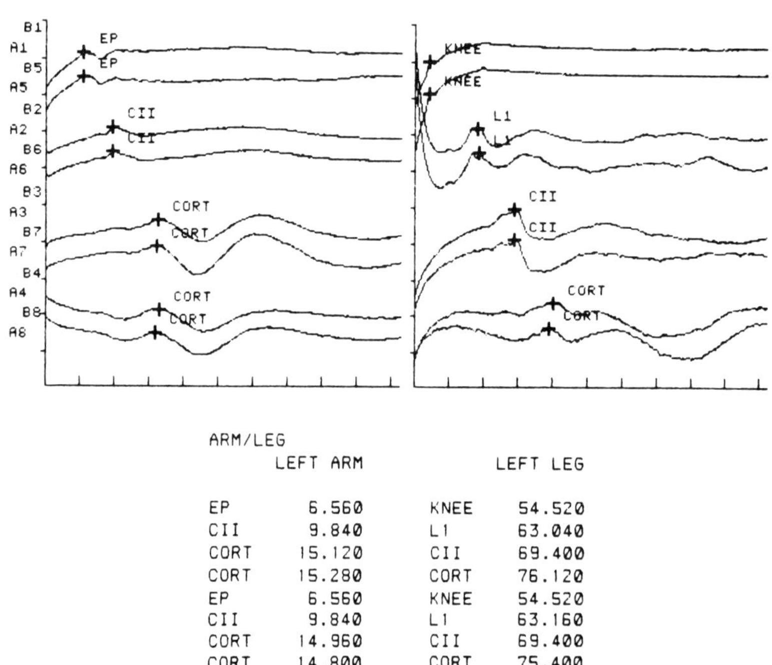

ARM/LEG

LEFT ARM		LEFT LEG	
EP	6.560	KNEE	54.520
CII	9.840	L1	63.040
CORT	15.120	CII	69.400
CORT	15.280	CORT	76.120
EP	6.560	KNEE	54.520
CII	9.840	L1	63.160
CORT	14.960	CII	69.400
CORT	14.800	CORT	75.400

Figure 10-23. Sequential somatosensory evoked potentials (SEPs) during aortic surgery. SEPs for two times using both the arm and leg are shown, as well as latencies. (*EP*, Erb's point potential; *CII,* cervical potential; *LI,* lumbar potential; *cort,* cortical potential.) (*A*) SEPs at start of surgery after induction of anesthesia. (*B*) SEPs immediately prior to and after 5-minute test cross clamping of the aorta. No changes seen. (*C*) SEPs after 8 and 10 minutes of cross clamping. No changes. (*D*) SEPs after 13 and 15 minutes of cross clamping. The cortical potentials are abolished and the cervical potentials are lessened while the leg CII latency has increased. (*E*) SEPs after 18 and 21 minutes of cross clamping. The cortical cervical and lumbar potentials are lost. (*F*) Shortly after the cross clamping is removed, potentials and latencies have returned to pre-cross clamping levels. (Courtesy of William Friedman, MD)

B

	MSEC/DIV	uVLT/DIV
A8 A4 A7 A3	4.000	1.25
A6 A2	4.000	5.00
A5 A1	4.000	12.50
B8 B4	6.000	0.50
B7 B3	6.000	1.25
B6 B2	6.000	2.50
B5 B1	6.000	25.00

A1 917 PRE-TEST CLAMP
A5 924 5 MIN TEST CLAMP

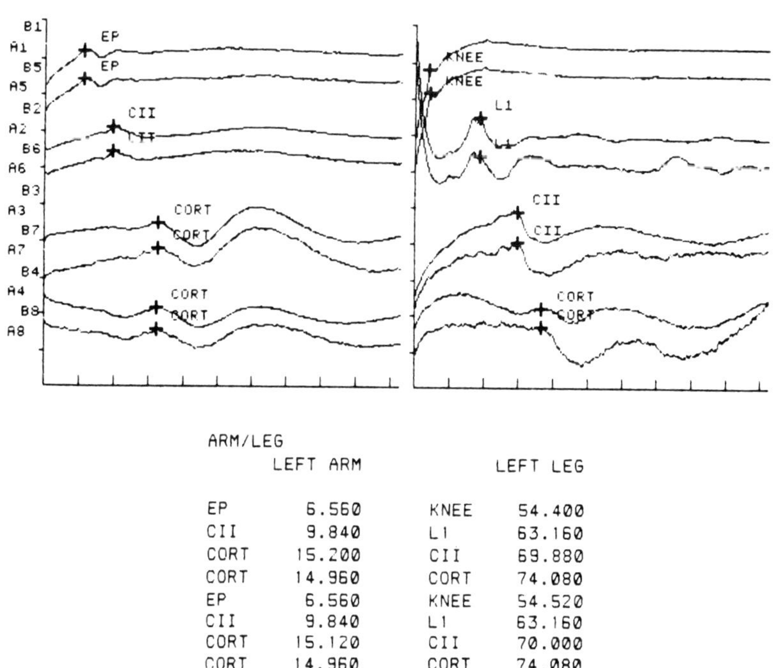

ARM/LEG

LEFT ARM		LEFT LEG	
EP	6.560	KNEE	54.400
CII	9.840	L1	63.160
CORT	15.200	CII	69.880
CORT	14.960	CORT	74.080
EP	6.560	KNEE	54.520
CII	9.840	L1	63.160
CORT	15.120	CII	70.000
CORT	14.960	CORT	74.080

Figure 10-23. *(continued)*

C

	MSEC/DIV	uVLT/DIV
A8 A4 A7 A3	4.000	1.25
A6 A2	4.000	5.00
A5 A1	4.000	12.50
B8 B4	6.000	0.50
B7 B3	6.000	1.25
B6 B2	6.000	2.50
B5 B1	6.000	25.00

A1 934 8 MIN CLAMP
A5 936 10 MIN CLAMP

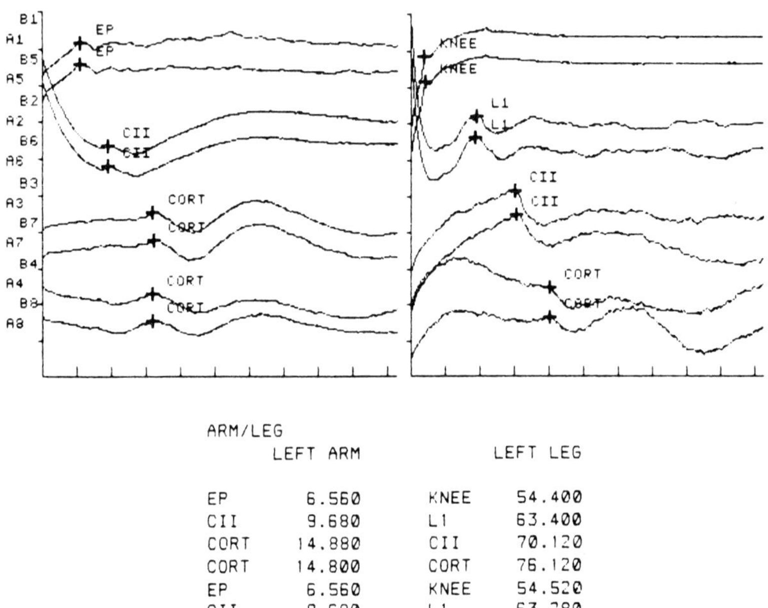

ARM/LEG

LEFT ARM		LEFT LEG	
EP	6.560	KNEE	54.400
CII	9.680	L1	63.400
CORT	14.880	CII	70.120
CORT	14.800	CORT	76.120
EP	6.560	KNEE	54.520
CII	9.680	L1	63.280
CORT	14.960	CII	70.360
CORT	14.800	CORT	76.120

Figure 10-23. (*continued*)

D

	MSEC/DIV	uVLT/DIV
A8 A4 A7 A3	4.000	1.25
A6 A2	4.000	5.00
A5 A1	4.000	12.50
B8 B4	6.000	0.50
B7 B3	6.000	1.25
B6 B2	6.000	2.50
B5 B1	6.000	25.00

A1 939 13 MIN CLAMP
A5 941 15 MIN CLAMP

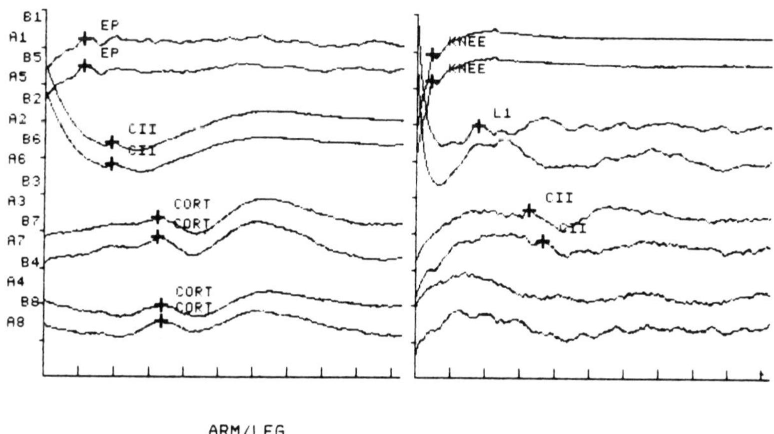

ARM/LEG

LEFT ARM		LEFT LEG	
EP	6.560	KNEE	54.640
CII	9.760	L1	62.680
CORT	15.040	CII	71.680
CORT	15.440	CORT	
EP	6.560	KNEE	54.640
CII	9.760	L1	
CORT	15.040	CII	74.080
CORT	15.440	CORT	

Figure 10-23. *(continued)*

E

	MSEC/DIV	uVLT/DIV
A8 A4 A7 A3	4.000	1.25
A6 A2	4.000	5.00
A5 A1	4.000	12.50
B8 B4	6.000	0.50
B7 B3	6.000	1.25
B6 B2	6.000	2.50
B5 B1	6.000	25.00

A1 944 18 MIN CLAMP
A5 947 21 MIN CLAMP

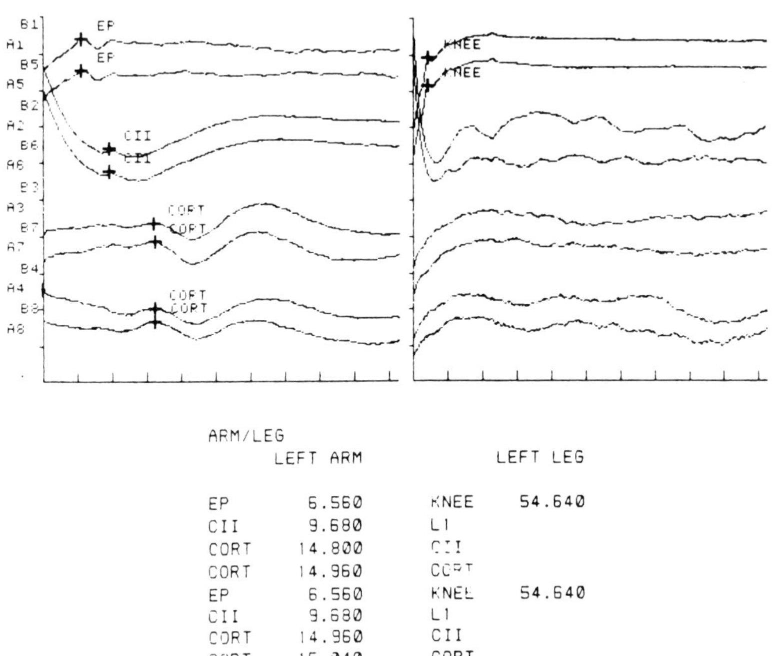

ARM/LEG

	LEFT ARM		LEFT LEG
EP	6.560	KNEE	54.640
CII	9.680	L1	
CORT	14.800	CII	
CORT	14.960	CORT	
EP	6.560	KNEE	54.640
CII	9.680	L1	
CORT	14.960	CII	
CORT	15.040	CORT	

Figure 10-23. (*continued*)

F

	MSEC/DIV	uVLT/DIV
A8 A4 A7 A3	4.000	1.25
A6 A2	4.000	5.00
A5 A1	4.000	12.50
B8 B4	6.000	0.50
B7 B3	6.000	1.25
B6 B2	6.000	2.50
B5 B1	6.000	25.00

A1 950 2 MIN POST CLAMP REMOVED
A5 956 8 MIN POST

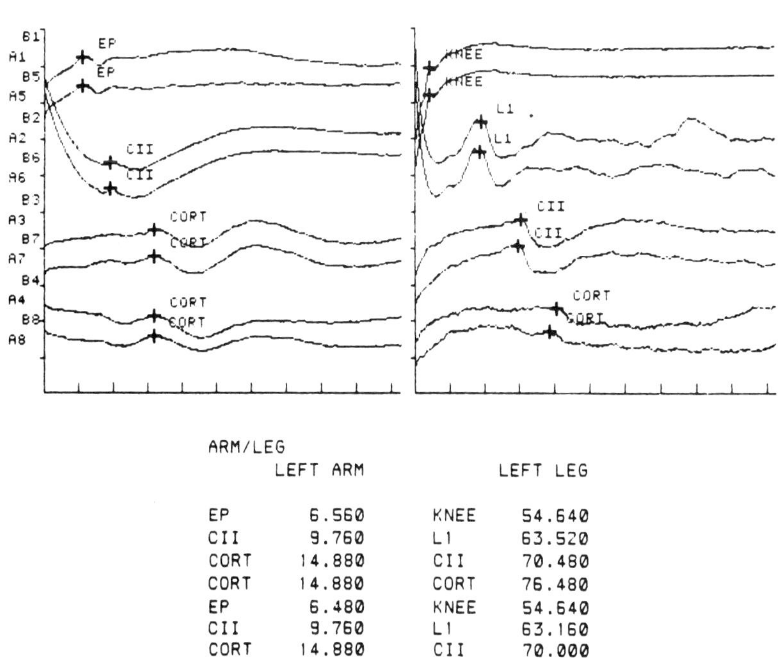

ARM/LEG

LEFT ARM		LEFT LEG	
EP	6.560	KNEE	54.640
CII	9.760	L1	63.520
CORT	14.880	CII	70.480
CORT	14.880	CORT	76.480
EP	6.480	KNEE	54.640
CII	9.760	L1	63.160
CORT	14.880	CII	70.000
CORT	14.800	CORT	75.280

Figure 10-23. *(continued)*

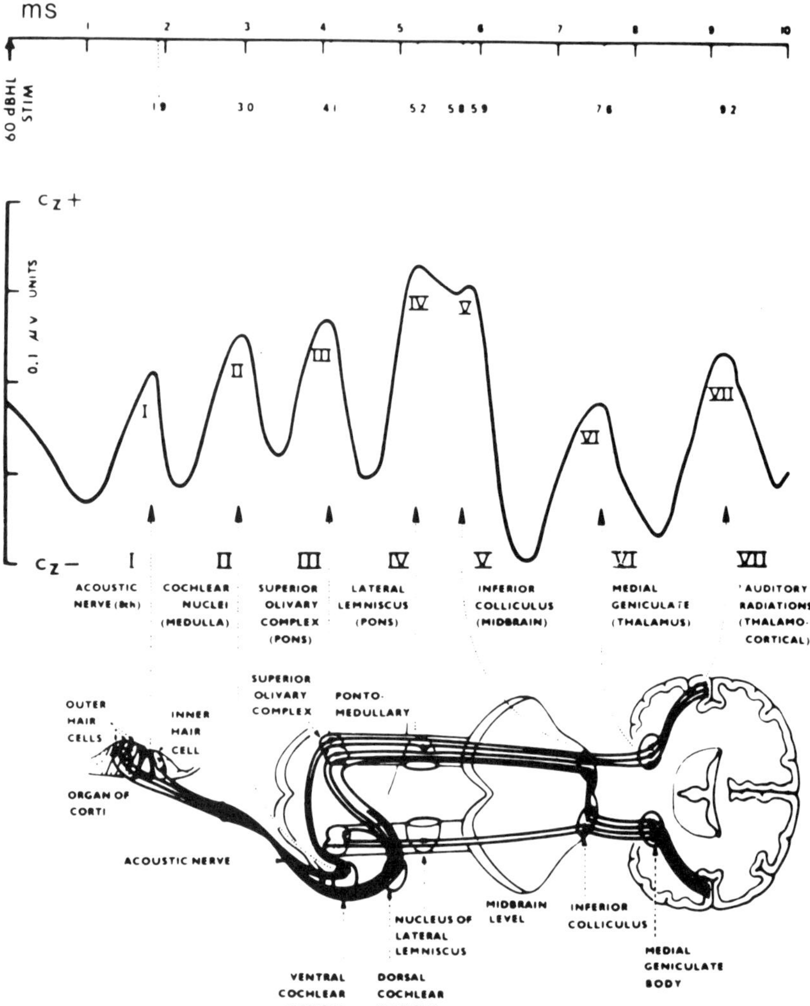

Figure 10-24. Diagram of normal latencies for vertex-positive brain-stem auditory potentials. Waves I through VII are evoked by clicks of 60 dBHL (60 dB above normal hearing threshold) at a rate of 10 per second. Lesions at different levels of auditory pathway tend to produce response abnormalities beginning with indicated components, although this does not specify the precise generators of the response; the relative contributions of synaptic and axonal activity to the response are as yet unknown. Intermediate latency (5.8 msec) between those of waves IV and V is mean peak latency of fused wave IV/V when present. C_z+, C_z- = vertex positivity, represented by an upward pen deflection, and vertex negativity, represented by a downward pen deflection. (Courtesy of Ellen Grass and modified with her permission and that of Stockard JJ, et al: Detection and localization of occult lesions with brainstem auditory responses. Mayo Clin Proc 52:761–769, 1977)

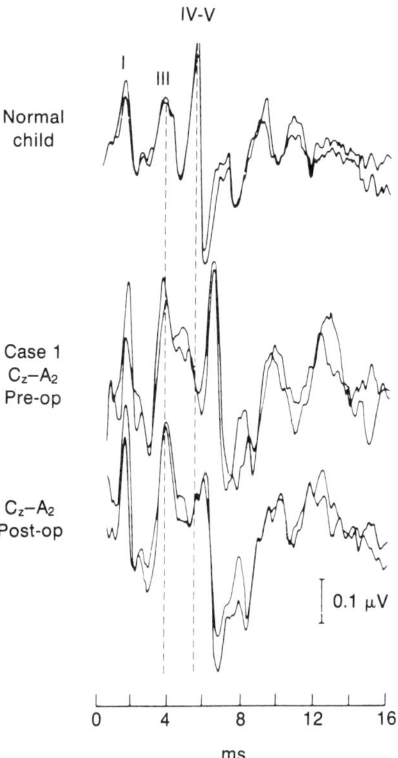

Figure 10-25. *Upper tracing:* Normal brain-stem auditory responses (note wave III) in child evoked by monaural stimulation of 60 dBHL with III–IV/V interwave latency of 1.8 msec. Two separate averages of responses to 2000 clicks at 10 per second are superimposed in this to demonstrate response reliability. *Middle Tracing:* Preoperative brain-stem auditory responses evoked by right monaural stimulation in case 1 with prolonged III–V interwave latency of 2.9 msec. *Lower tracing:* Postoperative brain-stem auditory response evoked by right monaural stimulation, showing decrease in III–IV/V interwave latency to 2.4 msec (still abnormal) and normalization of morphology and duration of wave III. C_z–A_2 = vertex to right mastoid recording. (Stockard JJ, et al: Detection and localization of occult lesions with brainstem auditory responses. Mayo Clin Proc 52:761–769, 1977)

waves is seen through scalp electrodes. The sequence is reproducible enough so that anatomic structural lesions can be well localized. We can identify the location of the lesion by examining the waveform and measuring the peak-to-peak distance (Figs. 10-24 and 10-25).[28] BAEPs are the most useful tool for detecting acoustic neuromas. Intraoperatively, changes in BAEPs lead to repositioning retractors, refining operative manipulation, and altering blood pressure.

Pitfalls and Controversies of Evoked Potentials

To date, evoked potential monitoring requires sophisticated, expensive equipment, and personnel must be well trained and experienced to properly interpret results. Anesthetic agents can affect evoked potentials, and it sometimes becomes a difficult decision whether anesthetic agents or surgical manipulation have altered evoked potentials. Some anesthetic agents introduce difficulties because of directly opposite effects on VEPs and SEPs.[29]

REFERENCES

1. Schultetus RR, Hill CR, Dharamraj CM, et al: Wakefulness during cesarean section after anesthetic induction with ketamine, thiopental or ketamine and thiopental combined. Anesth Analg 65:723–728, 1986
2. Tunstall ME: Detecting wakefulness during anaesthesia for cesarean section. Br Med J 1:1321, 1977
3. Evans JM, Davies WL: Monitoring anaesthesia. Clin Anaesth 2:243–262, 1984
4. Caton R: The electrical currents of the brain. Br Med J 2:278, 1875
5. von Marxow EF: Mitheilung, betreffend die Physiologie der Hirnrinde. Zentralbl Physiol 4:537, 1890
6. Gibbs FA, Giffs EL, Lennox WG: Effect on the electro-encephalogram of certain drugs which influence nervous activity. Arch Intern Med 60:154, 1937
7. Verzeano M: Servo-motor integration of the electrical activity of the brain and its applications to the automatic control of narcosis. Electroencephalogr Clin Neurophysiol 3:25, 1951
8. Bellville JW, Artusio JF Jr: Electroencephalographic pattern and frequency spectrum analysis during diethyl ether analgesia. Anesthesiology 16:379, 1955
9. Clark DL, Rosner BS: Neurophysiologic effects of general anesthetics: I. The electroencephalogram and sensory evoked responses in man. Anesthesiology 38:564, 1973
10. Klein SL, Scamman FL: Electroencephalographic monitoring during general anesthesia. J Oral Maxillofac Surg 42:376, 1984
11. Frost EAM: Inhalation anaesthetic agents in neurosurgery. Br J Anaesth 56:47S, 1984
12. EEG and Evoked Potential Monitoring, 3rd rev. Conshohocken, PA, Interspec, Inc., 1985
13. Levy WJ: Intraoperative EEG patterns: Implications for EEG monitoring. Anesthesiology 60:430–434, 1984
14. Oshima E, Shingu K, Mori K: EEG activity during halothane anaesthesia in man. Br J Anaesth 53:65, 1981
15. Sebel PS, Bovill JG, Wauquier A, et al: Effects of high-dose fentanyl anesthesia on the electroencephalogram. Anesthesiology 55:203, 1981
16. Bovill JG, Sebel PS, Wauquier A, et al: Electroencephalographic effects of sufentanil anaesthesia in man. Br J Anaesth 54:45–52, 1982
17. Cooper R, Osselton JW, Shaw JC: EEG Technology, 3rd ed, pp 93–97. Stoneham, Butterworths, 1980

18. Homberg G: The electroencephalogram during hypoxia and hyperventilation. Electroencephalogr Clin Neurophysiol 5:371, 1953
19. Dubois M, Savege TM, O'Carroll TM, et al: General anaesthesia and changes on the cerebral function monitor. Anaesthesia 3:157, 1978
20. Maynard DE, Jenkinson JL: The cerebral function analysis monitor. Anesthesia 39:678–690, 1984
21. Harmel MH, Klein FF, Davis DA: The EEMG—a practical index of cortical activity and muscular relaxation. Acta Anaesth Scand 70(suppl):97–102, 1978
22. Edmonds HL, Paloheimo M: Computerized monitoring of the EMG and EEG during anesthesia. Int J Clin Monit Comput 1:201–210, 1984
23. Bickford RG, Billinger TW, Fleming NI, et al: The compressed spectral array—a pictorial EEG. Proc San Diego Biomed Symp 11:365, 1975
24. Demetrescu M: The aperiodic character of the electroencephalogram (EEG): A new approach to data analysis and condensation. Physiologist 18:189, 1975
25. Fleming RA, Smith NT: An inexpensive device for analyzing and monitoring the electroencephalogram. Anesthesiology 50:456–460, 1979
26. Levy WJ, Shapiro HM, Maruchak A, et al: Automated EEG processing for intraoperative monitoring: A comparison of techniques. Anesthesiology 53:223–236, 1980
27. Kaplan BJ, Friedman WA, Alexander JA, et al: Somatosensory evoked potential monitoring of spinal cord ischemia during aortic surgery. Neurosurgery 19:82–90, 1986.
28. Stockard JJ, Stockard JE, Sharbrough FW: Detection and localization of occult lesions with brainstem auditory responses. Mayo Clin Proc 52:761–769, 1977
29. Editorial: The depth of anaesthesia. Lancet 1:553–554, 1986

CHAPTER 11

Air Embolism

DEFINING THE PROBLEM OF AIR EMBOLISM

Distended veins bleed when cut. Veins that are not full may collapse and, when cut, they do not bleed much nor are they likely to admit air. Some veins cannot collapse when not full because they are encased in bone or supported by fibrous tissue. When cut, they may admit air, which is then swept along to the right side of the heart, giving rise to air embolism.

Air embolism can be prevented by causing the veins in the operative field to be engorged. This can be accomplished by positioning the patient so that the surgical field is at or below the level of the right atrium or by compressing the veins before they enter the thorax. These maneuvers increase venous bleeding in the operative field.

In the past it was also thought helpful to increase intrathoracic pressure by applying positive end-expiratory pressure (PEEP) to the airway or by using the Valsalva maneuver. This is now discouraged because any maneuver that raises airway and thus intrathoracic pressure will also raise atrial pressure.[1] While this would increase venous pressure and lessen the risk of air entrainment into an open vein, it can work to the disadvantage of the patient: an increased right atrial pressure may reverse the usual situation in which the left atrial pressure exceeds that of the right (Fig. 11-1). Increased intrathoracic pressure may elevate the right atrial pressure above that of the left atrium; in patients with a potentially patent foramen ovale, the valve may now swing open and entrained air can enter the left atrium and, thus, gain access to the cerebral and coronary circulation.

About 30% of all people have a potentially patent foramen ovale. Before birth, the foramen ovale, a hole in the atrial septum, provides a means of communication between the left atrium and the right atrium. At birth, this hole is closed by a membrane. In some 30%, it may open if conditions are propitious. Then, during venous air embolization, air may enter directly from the right side into the left side of the heart and, hence, into the arterial circulation, with access to coronary and cerebral vessels. Air embolism itself can cause this potential valve between the right atrium and left atrium to swing open. Air in the pulmonary artery obstructs blood flow, with a subsequent rise in pulmonary arterial, right ventricular, and right atrial pressure. Then, the valve opens and air enters the left atrium. Once on the left side, small bubbles of air can devastate the brain. When air enters the coronary arteries it can cause arrhythmias, ischemia, and myocardial failure.

Of interest is the observation that right atrial pressure may also exceed left atrial pressure without evidence of either air embolism or increased intrathoracic pressure. Thus, Perkins-Pearson and colleagues have measured right and estimated left atrial pressure in patients in the supine and sitting positions and have found that, after sitting up 1 hour, the left atrial pressure can fall more than the right, often leading to a pressure gradient, with the right being higher than the left atrial pressure.[2] This has led Cucchiara and co-workers to question whether or not the sitting position should be abandoned in all patients in whom air embolism is a possibility.[3] While presumably not all air gaining access to the systemic arterial circulation becomes symptomatic, the danger of cerebral lesions looms large for the up to 30% of patients with a potential open foramen ovale. If these concerns are substantiated by future studies, the preoperative diagnosis of a potentially patent foramen ovale with the help of echocardiographic studies may recommend itself. However, before adopting additional studies as routines we must also learn whether other factors may allow air to pass from the pulmonary artery to the systemic side without a patent foramen ovale. Butler and Hills suggest that small bubbles can pass through pulmonary capillaries, particularly after the administration of drugs that dilate the pulmonary vascular bed.[4]

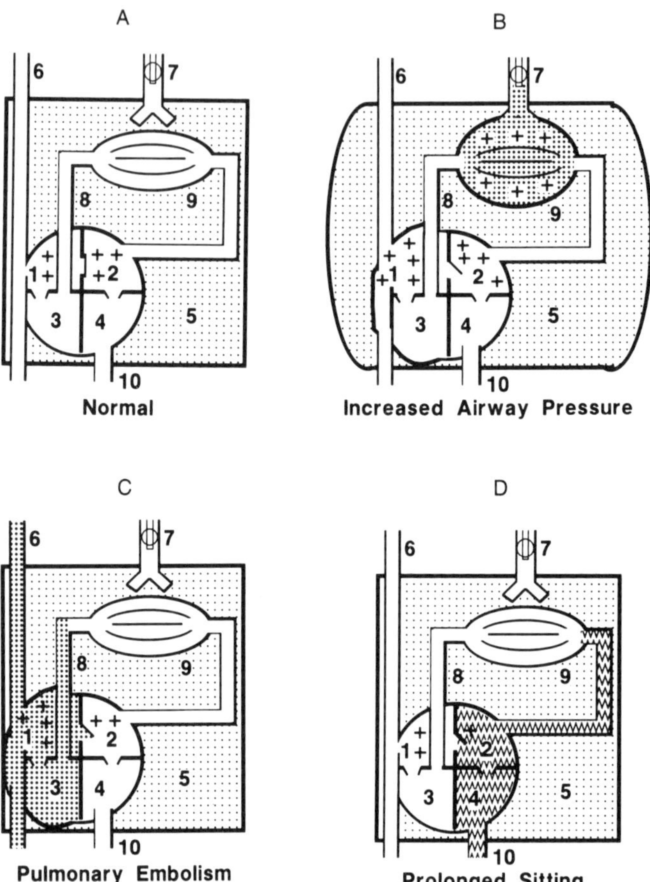

Figure 11-1. Diagrammatic representation of conditions leading to paradoxical embolism. The diagram represents the chest with heart, lung and vena cava. "1" indicates the right atrium and "2" the left atrium separated from the right one by a septum with a valve that may open when right atrial pressure exceeds left atrial pressure. The pressure is indicated by plus signs. "3" and "4" are right and left ventricle. "5" is the intrathoracic volume which increases with increased airway pressure. "6" is the vena cava, "7" the trachea with an endotracheal tube, "8" the pulmonary artery, "9" the pulmonary capillary system leading into the pulmonary vein and "10" the aorta. Under normal conditions (*A*), the valve between left and right atrium is closed. Three conditions are shown: (*B*) increased airway pressure (the lungs are shaded); (*C*) pulmonary embolism (area proximal to obstruction in pulmonary artery is shaded); and (*D*) prolonged sitting (pressure in left atrium, ventricle, and aorta is assumed to have decreased). In all situations, right atrial pressure may exceed left atrial pressure. When the right atrial pressure increases, the valve may open and allow emboli, for instance air, to pass from right to left, and thus into the systemic circulation.

Aspiration of air is made more likely by positioning the patient so that the wound is well above the right atrium (the sitting position), or enhancing negative pressures in the chest either with spontaneous inspiration—especially vigorous gasping inspiration—or with a negative phase in the respiratory cycle of the ventilator. According to some statistics, patients in the sitting position for a posterior fossa or cervical spine operation face the threat of air embolism, which occurs in up to 30% of the cases.[5] Well recognized by now is the chance for air embolism through holes often not readily inspected during operation on the head, namely where the surgeon attaches the head holder. Its pointed and heavy bolts are drilled into the outer table of the calvarium and thus, may broach veins that are well above the heart level during neurosurgical operations. If air embolism is detected as soon as these pins are placed, the diagnosis can be made easily. Often, however, just a trickle of air gains access, and only as it accumulates does it become symptomatic, perhaps after the head holder has been draped out of the field and the head is opened. A search of the operative field may now fail to reveal a site for air embolism, while the small hole around one of the head-holder pins may be hidden from inspection. Of course air embolism can also occur in other operations. Among these are all operations in which the operative field is higher than the right atrium. Catheterization of the great veins with large bore cannulae for the monitoring of central venous, pulmonary arterial, or wedge pressures provides a ready and dangerous opportunity for air embolism.[6]

Air embolism has been reported in operations on the head, neck, thorax, abdomen, pelvis, heart, liver, and hip.[7] It has also been reported in two clinical situations

- Parturition with placenta previa
- Abortion by vacuum extraction

and in several procedures

- Vaginal or tubal insufflation
- Pneumoencephalography
- Angiocardiography
- Pneumoarthrography
- Perinephric pneumography
- Insufflation of air into the sinuses
- Induced pneumoperitoneum
- Hyperbaric therapy for lung cysts or emphysema
- Positive pressure to the airway
- Subclavian or internal jugular venous puncture
- Insufflation of air into the ear canal
- Pneumorbitography

In many of these procedures, air or CO_2 under pressure is applied. Gas embolization, of course, can easily occur, if a vein is entered. Air embolism is also possible with intravenous fluid therapy, if air under pressure is used to force the fluid from the intravenous fluid container.

SYMPTOMS OF AIR EMBOLISM

The symptoms of air embolism are readily explained by *how much* air went in and *where* it went. Where the air goes depends on the anatomical circumstances. During general anesthesia, small air emboli in the brain are difficult or impossible to detect. Postoperatively, however, they become quite manifest when the patient fails to regain consciousness or is found to have a neurologic deficit.

When air is confined to the right side, it is flushed into the pulmonary artery and its branches. With a small amount, for example, a few milliliters in an adult, the air does no harm and is slowly absorbed. If too much air enters the right side of the heart or the pulmonary arterial system, the air blocks the outflow from the right ventricle. As output falls, hypotension and arrhythmias develop. Gasping inspirations are a late and dangerous sign of air embolism; dangerous because each gasp lowers intrathoracic pressure, which facilitates aspiration of more air! Ultimately, cardiac arrest will supervene.

Nitrous oxide in blood worsens the effect of air embolism. The anesthetic gas diffuses into the air bubble, which contains no N_2O and expands the bubble. Given enough time and the opportunity to equilibrate, an air bubble may grow twofold to fivefold if surrounded by tissue and blood containing in equilibrium with 50% to 80% N_2O.

MONITORING FOR AIR EMBOLISM

Monitoring for air embolism can be divided into basic, routine monitoring, which applies whether air embolism is feared or not, and special monitoring efforts that are designed to detect air.

The Basic System

Blood Pressure

Blood pressure monitoring is mandatory during anesthesia and invasive monitoring is justified for patients at risk of air embolization. With embolization of large amounts of air, cardiac output and blood pressure will fall. However, monitoring blood pressure does not detect *early* symptoms of air embolism. Blood pressure is monitored to detect and treat significant hypotension that occurs concomitantly with air embolization.

Monitoring blood pressure to assess mean cerebral perfusion pressure of a patient who sits on the operating-room table for a posterior craniotomy is particularly important. A mean pressure measured at the level of the heart will not portray the mean pressure in the head. Perfusion pressure in the brain will be less than mean arterial pressure in the chest by the weight of the column of blood between the heart and the brain (see Chap. 4).

Electrocardiography

With air embolization, arrhythmias, particularly ventricular extrasystoles, occur frequently. However, they may be rather late signs of significant air embolizations. These extrasystoles should be considered alarming and treatment of air embolism should begin at once.

When embolism has progressed even further, the ST segment and P-waves may also change. All changes must be viewed in the context of the patient's physical condition. Clearly, a patient with existing heart disease will develop ECG changes with less provocation than a healthy patient.

Auscultation

The mill wheel murmur (*bruit de moulin*) heard over the heart has often been described. It has been compared to the sound of water and air shaken in a plastic bag, an analogy more easily appreciated by those who have never seen an old mill and never heard water murmur as it runs over and under the mill wheel. The murmur is continuous; heard during systole and diastole. Brechner and Bethune[8] say that when circulatory collapse occurs after the embolization of massive amounts of air, the murmur assumes a sound resembling the squeezing and releasing of a wet sponge. Auscultation of the precordium is often more likely to detect the mill wheel murmur than auscultation using the esophageal stethoscope. However, murmurs are not early signs of air embolism.

While blood pressure, ECG monitoring, and auscultation are essential routines for all patients, as well as those at risk of air embolization, these routines are not specific enough when air embolism is feared. Therefore, special monitoring techniques are employed.

Specific Monitoring for the Detection of Air Embolism

These procedures can be divided into noninvasive and invasive methods.

Noninvasive Methods

MONITORING NITROGEN

Some atmospheric air trapped in venous blood will dissolve and increase the partial pressure of nitrogen in blood. If the patient was previously denitrogenated and is not breathing air, but an anesthetic mixture without nitrogen, the appearance of nitrogen in expired air is pathognomonic for air embolism. Mass spectrometers will allow nitrogen tensions in respired air to be followed. However, this technique is not an established routine.[9]

MONITORING EXPIRED CO_2

Under normal circumstances, the venous system delivers CO_2 to the right heart, pulmonary artery and, hence, to the lungs to be exhaled. When CO_2 production stays constant but pulmonary blood flow decreases, as with air embolism, the amount of CO_2 delivered to the lungs also decreases. By monitoring end-expired CO_2, a downward trend of CO_2 can be discovered, and this is quite helpful.

For CO_2 monitoring, a number of analyzers are on the market. Most aspirate gas from the breathing circuit or the endotracheal tube. Some have a sensing unit that is inserted directly into the breathing circuit.

Most CO_2 monitors employ the infrared technique. A few new systems are based on mass spectrometry. See Chapter 6 for a discussion of these devices.

MONITORING O_2

When reduced pulmonary blood flow diminishes the appearance of CO_2 in the expired air, it also causes less oxygen to be taken up. Therefore, the end-expired oxygen tension will rise as CO_2 tension falls, if ventilation is not changed (Fig. 11-2). Without mass spectrometry, it is difficult to observe this phenomenon. The mass spectrometer allows the rapid, simultaneous analysis of several gases and will make it possible to watch a fall in CO_2, and then corroborate that it was caused by a change in pulmonary flow by observing a rise in end-expired O_2. If expired N_2 also rises, the diagnosis of air embolism is assured.

USING THE DOPPLER EFFECT

In 1968, Maroon and co-workers[10] reported on the use of ultrasound employing the Doppler phenomenon to detect venous air embolism. The term *Doppler method* is based on Doppler's observation, in 1842, that sound changes its pitch when the source of the sound approaches and then recedes from the listener. Ultrasound waves or sound frequencies too high to be detected by the human ear are beamed at a target (arteries, the fetus *in utero*, or, with monitoring for air, the heart). The sound waves

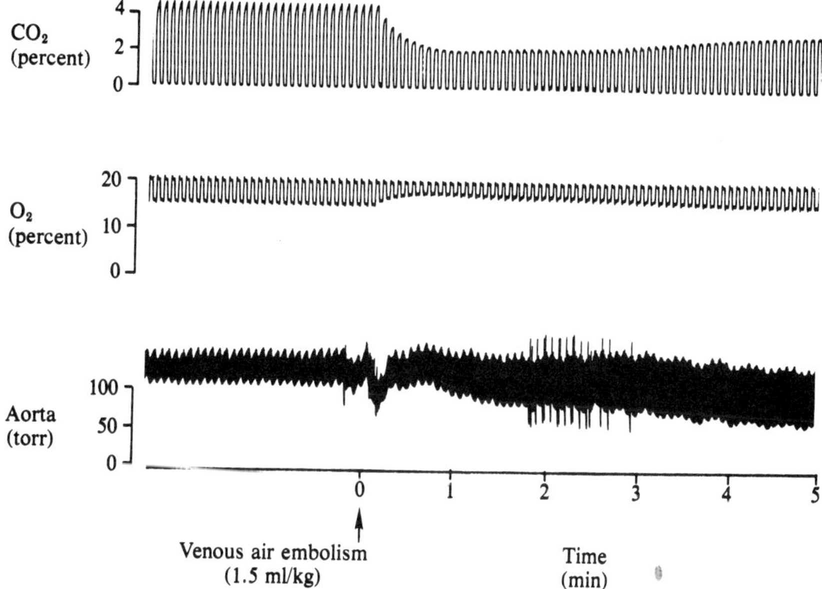

Figure 11-2. Carbon dioxide and oxygen were monitored continuously at the endotracheal tube of an anesthetized dog. Baseline inspired CO_2 (*top panel*) was zero and end-expired CO_2 about 4.5%; inspired O_2 (*middle panel*) 21% and end-expired O_2 about 16%. *Bottom panel* shows arterial blood pressure. After the rapid intravenous injection of much air, the blood pressure became unstable briefly but then stabilized for over a minute while end-expired CO_2 fell and end-expired O_2 rose. A trend recording makes these changes quite visible. (Courtesy of E. S. Munson, MD).

are reflected and either measured or transduced into audible sound. From a stationary object, all sound waves would return at the same time. A moving object will cause the Doppler phenomenon. The presence of oscillations or movement of blood flow, moving valves, and heart muscle, for example, can be ascertained in this way. When air (as little as 0.5 ml air injected as a bolus) instead of, or in addition to, blood is detected, the reflection of ultrasound is quite markedly altered. It is assumed that the change in pitch and loudness is caused by air. Theoretically, it could be anything that differs enough from blood that causes the sound waves to be distorted. An injection of a bolus of saline, for instance, will give a Doppler signal. Indeed, a rapid injection of 3 ml to 5 ml of saline into a right atrial catheter will help to ascertain that an ultrasound Doppler probe over the precordium works and that it is placed correctly. This technique does *not* assure us that the central venous catheter lies in the right atrium or close to it. Saline injected into the subclavion or axillary vein will also produce a Doppler signal in a probe placed over the right atrium.[11] We

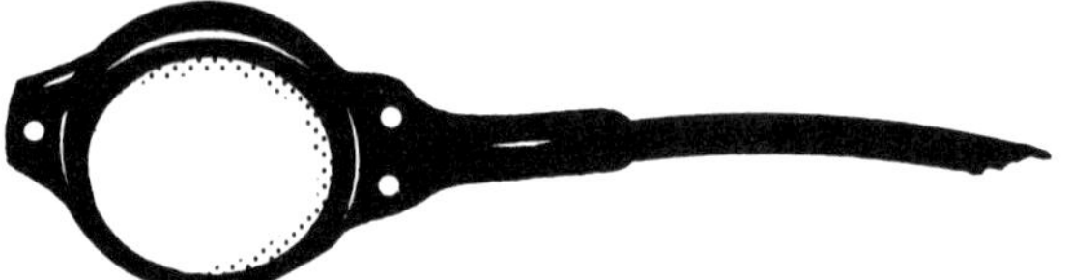

Figure 11-3. A flat Doppler probe fashioned for application to be applied to the chest over the right atrium. The probe transmits and receives the reflected ultrasound of about 2.4 MHz. The same probe can be used to monitor fetal heart activity.

prefer putting the probe just to the right of the sternum in the third or fourth intercostal space.

The units available on the market today offer different probes for applications to arteries, uterus, and fetus, as well as to the heart. On some units, the frequency of the ultrasound is adjusted for optimal results; high frequencies (5–20 MHz) for the detection of blood flow, and low frequencies (2–2.5 MHz) for the monitoring of the heart and fetus. The probes themselves are sized to facilitate their application (small for arteries and large for fetal or cardiac monitoring). Some large probes for precordial application have two or three transmitting and one or two receiving crystals (Fig. 11-3).

Ultrasound does not easily penetrate air. Therefore, a special jelly, a light oil, or a soapy solution must bathe the skin and the head of the probe to eliminate an air interface. Do not use electrocardiogram paste, which damages the probe. Also, all bubbles must be removed.

The output of the instrument usually has audible, swooshing sounds. These are easily monitored because they are monotonous. Any change in monotony, as is heard when air appears under the probe, is readily discerned by the human ear. In addition to monitoring by ear, the output can also be recorded on paper or watched on an oscilloscope. Not only are we incapable of watching the scope or the paper record for hours without wavering in our attention, but we also have to take our eyes off the record to attend to other chores. An audible signal is, therefore, better. Even while engaged in other tasks, we can hear and can notice a change in pitch.

Unfortunately, the ultrasound units are sensitive to the surgeon's electrocautery unit. Therefore, many manufacturers use shielded cables and switches to turn off the ultrasound equipment for however long the surgeon buzzes with the electrocautery unit. These switches are either incorporated into the foot pedal operated by thc surgeon or work automatically by means of electronic receivers sensitive to the powerful ratio frequency of the cautery unit.

Invasive Methods

MONITORING BLOOD PRESSURE

Continuous invasive monitoring of arterial blood pressure is justified in patients at risk for air embolism.

Venous air embolism may also be detected by measuring changes in airway pressure. Sloan and Kimovec have reported that air embolism (and embolism with other substances) can result within a matter of seconds in bronchoconstriction perhaps triggered by the release of a number of mediators.[12] The authors describe a patient experiencing air embolism during a neurosurgical operation. Concurrent with changes in the Doppler signal, an increase in central venous pressure and a decrease in expired CO_2, the peak airway pressure increased from a stable baseline of 19 torr to 25 torr.

Transesophageal echocardiography (see Chap. 5) may also offer a sensitive method of detecting small air emboli, being as sensitive or perhaps even more sensitive than a precordial Doppler according to experiments in animals performed by Michenfelder and his co-workers.[13] Transesophageal echocardiography can also demonstrate the passage of a paradoxical air embolism from right atrium to left atrium.[14] More experience with these devices is needed.

USE OF A TRANSCUTANEOUS VENOUS CATHETER

The insertion of a transcutaneous central venous catheter (CVP) is useful for two reasons: to assess right atrial pressure and to aspirate air in case of air embolism. Methods of placing a CVC are found in Chapter 5, Cardiac Function.

The catheter can be connected to a water manometer. This is simple and inexpensive, and has the advantage of being open to the outside. In one case of a sudden increase in right atrial pressure with infusion of air under pressure, the catheter functioned as a relief valve, venting the air through the manometer and, thus, relieving the right atrial pressure. However, we prefer to connect the catheter to a transducer. Without recordings, trends are not readily detected and a slowly rising pressure, as occurs with repeated, small air emboli, may go undiscovered longer than desirable. Simultaneously rising CVP, falling arterial pressure, and the occurrence of arrhythmias are quite apparent on a polygraph record but are not that easily correlated without a paper record.

The CVP catheters inserted transcutaneously are small; usually no larger than 16 gauge. Though it is possible to aspirate air through such a catheter, the experience of many indicates that much air escapes aspiration and that, with massive air embolism, the air cannot be aspirated fast enough to prevent major changes in the cardiovascular system.

If flow through the pulmonary artery system is blocked by air, pulmonary artery pressures will rise. This will eventually affect the right

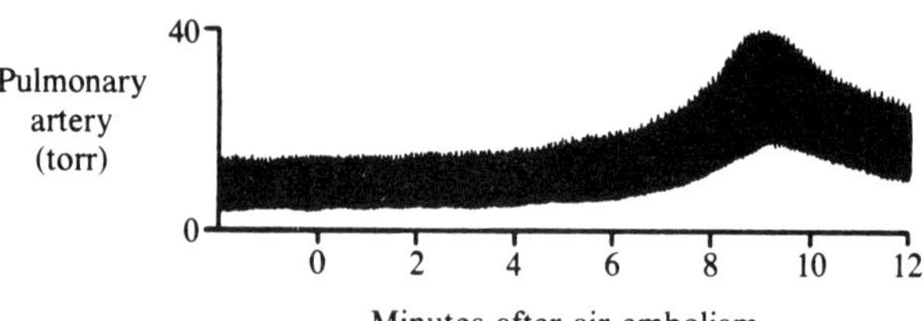

Figure 11-4. Pulmonary arterial pressure rises with air embolism. These changes occur early, with small amounts of air. They are as dramatic as shown here. Recording pulmonary arterial pressure is a sensitive but highly invasive monitoring technique when air embolism is feared.

ventricle and the right atrium. Thus, right atrial pressure may not rise initially with a constant trickle of air, but only after significant disturbances in cardiac hemodynamics have occurred. Right atrial pressure will rise quickly and steeply if a large bolus of air has lodged in the right atrium, the right ventricle, or the pulmonary artery.

The technique of inserting a pulmonary artery catheter is discussed in Chapter 5. Monitoring the pulmonary artery pressure of patients at risk for air embolism is a highly invasive but sensitive method of detecting air that has been flushed into the pulmonary artery and has not escaped through a patent foramen ovale. The typical record of pulmonary air embolism shows a sudden increase in pulmonary artery pressure secondary to outflow obstruction produced by air (Fig. 11-4).

In summary, patients sitting for craniotomies or cervical operations are at great risk of air embolism. A typical monitoring protocol includes ECG monitoring for arrhythmias and arterial pressure monitoring. The latter means the continuous monitoring of invasive blood pressures and their recording on a strip chart to facilitate the detection of trends. It is useful to adjust the pressure transducer to the level of the patient's head and to determine, in advance, what mean arterial blood pressure to accept. Should the pressure fall below this predetermined limit, the arterial pressure should be raised with IV fluids, drugs, decreased depth of anesthesia, or a combination of these.

Specific monitoring for air embolism should include a Doppler probe, which is recognized to be a very sensitive instrument for the detection of air. A right atrial catheter is helpful primarily in the diagnosis but can also aid in the treatment of air embolism. Expired CO_2 monitoring is advisable, and a pulmonary artery catheter can complement the other systems.

REFERENCES

1. Albin MS: The paradox of paradoxic air embolism—PEEP, Valsalva, and patent foramen ovale. Should the sitting position be abandoned? (letter to the editor). Anesthesiology 61:222–223, 1984
2. Perkins-Pearson NAK, Marshall WK, Bedford RF: Atrial pressure in the seated position. Anesthesiology 57:493–497, 1982
3. Cucchiara RF, Nugent M, Seward JB, et al: Air embolism in upright neurosurgical patients: Detection and localization by two-dimensional transesophageal echocardiography. Anesthesiology 60:353–355, 1984
4. Butler BD, Hills BA: The lung as a filter for microbubbles. J Appl Physiol 47:537–543, 1979
5. Michenfelder JD, Miller RH, Grovert GA: Evaluation of an ultrasonic device (Doppler) for the diagnosis of venous air embolism. Anesthesiology 36:164, 1972
6. Kondo K, O'Reily LP, Chiota J: Air embolism associated with an introducer for pulmonary arterial catheters. Anesth Analg 63:871–872, 1984
7. Geevarghese KP: Anesthetic management of patients undergoing surgery for posterior fossa lesions. Int Anesthesiol Clin 15:165, 1977
8. Brechner VL, Bethune RWM: Recent advances in monitoring pulmonary air embolism. Anesth Analg 50:255, 1971
9. Matjasko MJ, Hellman JH, Mackenzie CF, et al: The sensitivity of end-tidal nitrogen in the detection of large bolus venous air embolism in dogs. Anesth Analg 64:253, 1985
10. Maroon JC, Goodman JM, Horner TG et al: Detection of minute venous air emboli with ultrasound. Surg Gynecol Obstet 127:1236, 1968
11. Colley PS, Pavlin EG, Groepper J: Assessment of a saline injection test for location of a right atrial catheter. Anesthesiology 50:258, 1978
12. Sloan TB, Kimovec MA: Detection of venous air embolism by airway pressure monitoring. Anesthesiology 64:645–647, 1986
13. Glenski JA, Cucchiari RF, Michenfelder JD: Transesophageal echocardiography and transcutaneous O_2 and CO_2 monitoring for detection of venous air embolism. Anesthesiology 64:541–545, 1986
14. Furuya H, Okumura F: Detection of paradoxical air embolism by transesophageal echocardiography. Anesthesiology 60:374–377, 1984

CHAPTER 12

Acid–Base and Blood Gas Measurements

INDICATIONS FOR MONITORING ACID–BASE VALUES AND ARTERIAL BLOOD GASES

Acid–base and blood gas parameters are now frequently monitored in patients in intensive care units and operating rooms because respiratory and metabolic disturbances in these patients are common and the consequences of not recognizing them grave. In addition to the well-known shift in arterial carbon dioxide with hyper- or hypoventilation, endogenous metabolic factors (renal disease, diabetes, hypoxic or toxic lactic acidosis, hormonal abnormalities) and exogenous factors (ingestion of acid, methyl alcohol, ethylene glycol, sulfur) can powerfully affect blood carbon dioxide levels and hydrogen ion concentrations.

The only variables regularly assessed for an analysis of acid–base disturbances are hydrogen ions and carbon dioxide. Because carbon dioxide readings make powerful statements about respiration, the other important respiratory gas, namely oxygen, is usually also reported when the acid–base status is determined. Even though we are dealing with only three variables, $[H^+]$, CO_2, and O_2, the terminology used to describe acid–base disturbances is complex and confusing. Several schools use different terms. Acidity can be reported as *p*H or hydrogen ion concentration, and CO_2 and oxygen levels in terms of partial pressure or blood gas content. To makes matters worse, additional variables can be derived without direct measurement. These include bicarbonate, standard bicarbonate, buffer base, base deficit or base excess, and, finally, standard base. Older texts still use other words and concepts, and various modern schools report their results in terms not universally used. It is, therefore, necessary to present some background and to explain the basic facts, so that the reader can apply the laboratory data regardless of which particular terminology was used to report them.

DEFINITIONS

In an aqueous medium, acids donate protons, and bases accept protons. A simpler, clinical definition describes the action of hydrogen ions instead of protons. Thus, an acid donates and a base accepts H^+ (Fig. 12-1). A common example is carbonic acid which, after donating H^+, becomes bicarbonate (Table 12-1). Bicarbonate has a negative charge and can accept positively charged hydrogen. Bicarbonate behaves like a base (hydrogen acceptor) and is called a *conjugate base*.

A predictable relationship exists between the hydrogen ion concentration, $[H^+]$, and the ratio of carbonic acid to bicarbonate. Henderson's formula describes this relationship:

$$[H^+] = K \times \frac{[H_2CO_3]}{[HCO_3^-]}$$

K is a *constant*. When $[H^+] = K$, the amounts of H_2CO_3 and of HCO_3^- must be equal. For example, if $K = 800$ for the carbonic acid

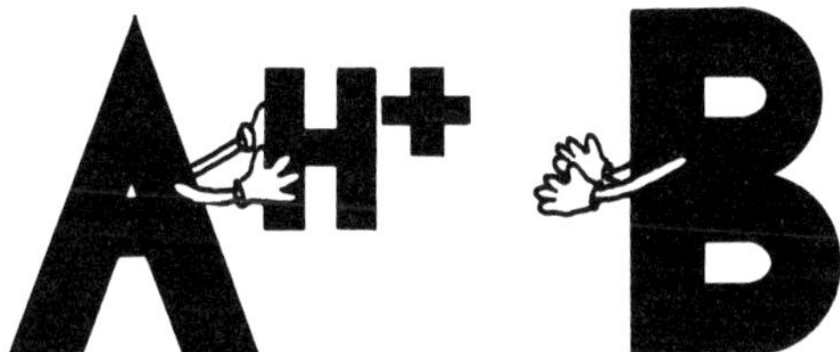

Figure 12-1. Acids are hydrogen donors. Bases are hydrogen acceptors. An acid that has donated its hydrogen is no longer a full blooded acid; it can accept the hydrogen back. It is, therefore, called a conjugate base as long as it is lacking its hydrogen. Conversely, the base, after having accepted a hydrogen, is called a conjugate acid.

Table 12-1. CARBONIC ACID AND ITS CONJUGATE BASE*

$HO{-}\underset{\underset{O}{\|}}{C}{-}OH \rightleftharpoons$	$HO{-}\underset{\underset{O}{\|}}{C}{-}O^{-}\ H^{+}$
Carbonic acid = H_2CO_3 undissociated	Bicarbonate and hydrogen ion = HCO_3^- and H^+ dissociated

* Carbonic acid can dissociate into a hydrogen ion, H^+, and bicarbonate. Bicarbonate is a conjugate base because it can accept an H^+ and thereby turn into carbonic acid.

and bicarbonate system, the equation (arbitrarily assuming 50 units of carbonic acid) is

$$800 = 800 \times \frac{50\ H_2CO_3}{50\ HCO_3^-}$$

If we now add hydrogen ions, for example, we increase the concentration of hydrogen ions by a factor of two (*i.e.*, from 800 to 1600), and nothing else, the formula must rearrange itself. The constant stays the same:

$$1600 = 800 \times \frac{66.66665\ H_2CO_3}{33.33335\ H_2CO_3^-}$$

The sum of the carbonic acid–bicarbonate pair is still 100, but their new ratio has accommodated the change in hydrogen ion concentration. This process is fundamental to all acid–base disturbances. It illustrates why one must know the values of the constant K and two of the other variables to calculate the third. Usually, the CO_2 level and the hydrogen ion concentration are given and the bicarbonate concentration is calculated.

K is also called the *dissociation constant*. It gives the $[H^+]$ in an acid that is 50% dissociated. Every acid–conjugate base pair has a K value. For clinical purposes, this constant is assumed to be immutable, although it is actually influenced by temperature (which is kept at 37°C in modern analyzers) and large shifts of *p*H.

Instead of expressing acid–base balance in terms of the Henderson formula, a logarithmic version, the Henderson–Hasselbalch equation, is most often used:

$$\log \frac{1}{[H^+]} = \log \frac{1}{K} + \log \frac{[HCO_3^-]}{[H_2CO_3]}$$

Observe that:

- The ratio of carbonic acid to bicarbonate has been inverted to match the inversion of $[H^+]$ into $1/[H^+]$.

- Instead of multiplying K × [H_2CO_3]/[HCO_3^-], add log 1/K to log [HCO_3^-]/[H_2CO_3] with the same results.
- In Henderson's formula, [H^+] is expressed in nanomoles (nmol).

$$1 \text{ mol} = 10^3 \text{ mmol} = 10^9 \text{ nmol}$$

Now the convention of writing *p*H instead of log [1/H^+] and *p*K instead of log 1/K can be introduced. The Henderson–Hasselbalch formula, therefore, becomes:

$$pH = pK + \log \frac{[HCO_3^-]}{[H_2CO_3]}$$

CO_2, CARBONIC ACID, AND CO_2 CONTENT

In clinical practice, we do not reckon carbonic acid in terms of H_2CO_3. Instead, the partial pressure of CO_2 (the P_{CO_2}) is measured in torr (mm Hg). Torr is then converted into millimoles of H_2CO_3 by assuming that for every torr of P_{CO_2} at 37°C, there is 0.03 mmol of H_2CO_3. With normal values of

$$pH = 7.4$$

$$pK = 6.1$$

$$[HCO_3^-] = 24 \text{ mmol}$$

$$P_{CO_2} = 40 \text{ torr}$$

the equation

$$pH = pK + \log \frac{[HCO_3^-]}{P_{CO_2} \times 0.03}$$

becomes

$$7.4 = 6.1 + \log \frac{24}{1.2}$$

The sum of bicarbonate and carbonic acid (24 + 1.2) is the CO_2 content.

CONVERSION OF [H^+] TO *p*H

Values of *p*H can be converted into nanomoles of hydrogen ions. This conversion can be done accurately with the help of tables or calculations, or it can be estimated. In the clinical setting, estimates are often sufficient and there are numerous ways to arrive at them. We outline one of them (in Fig. 12-2 and the accompanying exhibit) not only for the sake of estimating these variables without the use of a table or calculator or computer, but also to make the point that small changes in *p*H represent large changes in hydrogen ion concentration.

The conversion is based on the simple fact that each change of an everyday arithmetic number (*e.g.*, the concentration of hydrogen ion or the ratio of bicarbonate to carbonic acid) by a factor of two entails a shift of 0.3 log units. For example, when $[H^+]$ doubles from 40 nmol to 80 nmol, the *p*H changes only from 7.4 to 7.1. Conversely, when *p*H changes from 7.0 to 7.3, $[H^+]$ changes from 100 nmol to 50 nmol. The same principle pertains to

$$\log \frac{[HCO_3^-]}{[H_2CO_3]}$$

Assume a normal ration of

$$\frac{24 \text{ mEq } HCO_3^-}{1.2 \text{ nmol } H_2CO_3}$$

The log ratio of 20 (24/1.2) is 1.3. Changing the ratio to 24/2.4 (doubling

ESTIMATION OF VALUES OF BICARBONATE CONCENTRATION OR *p*H

To estimate *p*H values for different ratios of bicarbonate or concentrations of hydrogen ions, follow the arrows in Figure 12-2. All values can be estimated if you know the starting point stippled in the figure.

Knowledge of the relationships between the arithmetic number and the log base 10 system, to which *p*H belongs, makes for easy computation of the values shown in Figure 12-2.

In order to estimate the approximate ratio of bicarbonate to carbonic acid, $[HCO_3^-]/[H_2CO_3]$, observe that:

1. The ratio is 20/1 for *p*H 7.4 at 37°C.
2. Any change of *p*H by 0.3 units will result in a twofold change in ratio (short arrows; Fig. 12-2).
3. Any change of *p*H by 1 unit will result in a tenfold change in ratio (long arrows; Fig. 12-2).
4. Knowing the ratio of bicarbonate to P_{CO_2} will permit an estimation of *p*H.

Figure 12-2 shows how the ratios were obtained. If you only remember that the ratio of HCO_3^- to H_2CO_3 is 20/1 at *p*H 7.4, with this knowledge you can fill in the cells by following the arrows as shown:

What is the bicarbonate if *p*H = 7.2 and P_{CO_2} = 40 torr?

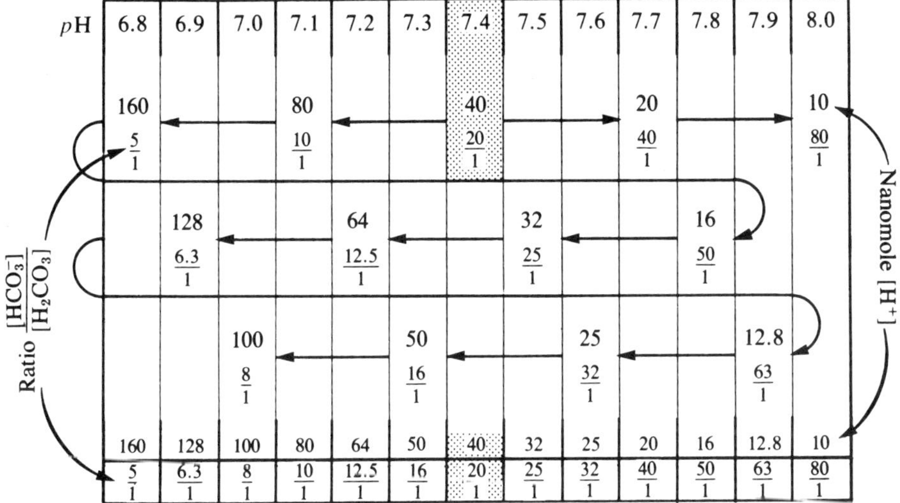

Figure 12-2. Visual aid to explanation of *p*H values for different ratios of bicarbonate or concentrations of hydrogen ions. All values may be obtained by working from a known starting point (*stippled*) and following the arrows as indicated. (See also displayed text example.)

At *p*H of 7.2, the ratio is 12.5/1, meaning that the bicarbonate concentration must be 12.5 times as large as the carbonic acid concentration. Therefore, 12.5 = $[HCO_3^-]/[H_2CO_3]$, but H_2CO_3 = $P_{CO_2} \times 0.03 = 40 \times 0.03 = 1.2$. Substituting: 12.5 = $[HCO_3^-]/1.2$, and so

$$[HCO_3^-] = (1.2) \times (12.5) = 15.$$

Answer: Bicarbonate is about 15 mEq/l.

What is the *p*H if P_{CO_2} = 40 torr and CO_2 content = 16.2 mmol?

Since $H_2CO_3 = (40 \times 0.03) = 1.2$ mmol, the bicarbonate concentration must be $16.2 - 1.2 = 15$ mEq/l. The ratio $[HCO_3^-]/[H_2CO_3]$ is 15/1.2 or 12.5/1.

Answer: The *p*H, then, must be approximately 7.2.

When values are presented that are intermediate to those shown in Figure 12-2, you can interpolate for an estimate. For example, *p*H is 7.15 and P_{CO_2} is 45 torr. What is the bicarbonate?

The ratio $[HCO_3^-]/[H_2CO_3]$ lies between 10/1 (*p*H 7.1) and 12.5/1 (*p*H 7.2). Through interpolation a ratio of 11.25/l is estimated. Using the calculation shown above, an approximate bicarbonate of 15.2 mEq/l is obtained. A nomogram would also give approximately 15 mmol/l for bicarbonate (see Fig. 12-6).

P_{CO_2}) changes the ratio from 20/1 to 10/1 and changes the logarithmic value by 0.3 units:

$$\log \frac{24}{2.4} = \log \frac{10}{1} = 1.0$$

The only other fact we need to know is that changes by a factor of 10 (*e.g.*, from an $[H^+]$ of 20 nmol to 200 nmol) cause the logarithmic expression, that is the *p*H, to change by a full unit. (In the example, *p*H would change from 7.7 to 6.7.) The same applies to the ratio of bicarbonate to carbonic acid; any change by a factor of 10 results in a change by one full unit (*e.g.*, 36/0.36 to 36/3.6, or 100/1 to 10/1 causes log 100 = 2 to change to log 10 = 1).

THE EFFECT OF BUFFERS ON *p*H

Buffers stabilize *p*H. Hemoglobin, bicarbonate, and protein are the principal buffers of blood. Extravascular spaces have no hemoglobin and hence their buffering capacity is less than that of blood. Because we have no measure of extra- and intracellular buffering capacity, it is difficult to predict how much *p*H will change when the concentration of acid or CO_2 changes. The expression

$$CO_2 + H_2O \rightleftarrows H_2CO_3 \rightleftarrows H^+ + HCO_3^-$$

shows that any addition or subtraction of H^+ or of HCO_3^- ions causes a change in CO_2 level. By changing ventilation, CO_2 concentration can be altered. The Henderson or Henderson–Hasselbalch equation can be used to calculate one variable *only if the other two are known*; for example, we can calculate $[HCO_3^-]$ if *p*H and $[H_2CO_3]$ are known. The equation *cannot* be used to predict what will happen if only one variable changes and if we know nothing about the other two. Buffers and ventilation also come into play. Although we can estimate what might happen

Table 12-2. THE EFFECTS OF ACUTE CHANGES IN RESPIRATORY AND METABOLIC VARIABLES

	*p*H	Bicarbonate	P_{CO_2}
Add H^+*	↓	↓	↑
Lose H^+ or add OH^-*	↑	↑	↓
Add bicarbonate*	↑	↑	↑
Lose bicarbonate*	↓	↓	↓
Add CO_2†	↓	↑	↑
Lose CO_2†	↑	↓	↓

* Does not take into account respiratory response to change in *p*H or P_{CO_2}.
† Does not take into account renal compensatory mechanisms.

in response to an acid-load or a ventilatory change, we cannot be accurate. Clinical rules of thumb are based on experience and not on a mathematical model of the extraordinarily complex system responsible for acid–base regulation.

The direction of acute shifts is shown in Table 12-2.

COMPENSATION FOR ACID–BASE IMBALANCES

When disturbances in acid–base balance persist, the body can call into play compensatory efforts through an organ not primarily affected; for example, pulmonary disturbances resulting in respiratory acidosis or alkalosis will lead to compensation by the kidney. Conversely, primary disturbances of renal function or metabolism with acid–base imbalance lead to compenation by the lungs. Table 12-3 summarizes these relationships.

The body's compensatory efforts are governed by complex intracellular and extracellular stimuli and responses. Assume that a respiratory acidosis triggers a renal compensatory effort. Compensation will return the abnormal *p*H toward normal, without being successful in reestablishing completely normal values. Were complete compensation and correction of a respiratory acidosis to succeed, the drive that sustains the compensatory effort would cease. Figure 12-3 illustrates this point.

The Mixed Disturbance

If a patient with respiratory insufficiency develops metabolic acidosis, he loses his ability to compensate and a mixed respiratory–metabolic acidosis supervenes. Correspondingly, a mixed respiratory–metabolic alkalosis is also possible (Table 12-4).

Table 12-3. THE DIRECTION OF COMPENSATORY MECHANISMS, BICARBONATE, AND P_{CO_2}

	*p*H	Bicarbonate	P_{CO_2}	Compensation*
Respiratory				
Acidosis	↓	↑ ↑	↑	Renal effect on bicarbonate
Alkalosis	↑	↓ ↓	↓	
Metabolic				
Acidosis	↓	↓	↓ ↓	Respiratory effect on CO_2
Alkalosis	↑	↑	↑ ↑	

* Double arrows show direction of compensation. The *p*H change will be less pronounced in the presence of compensatory mechanisms than in their absence.

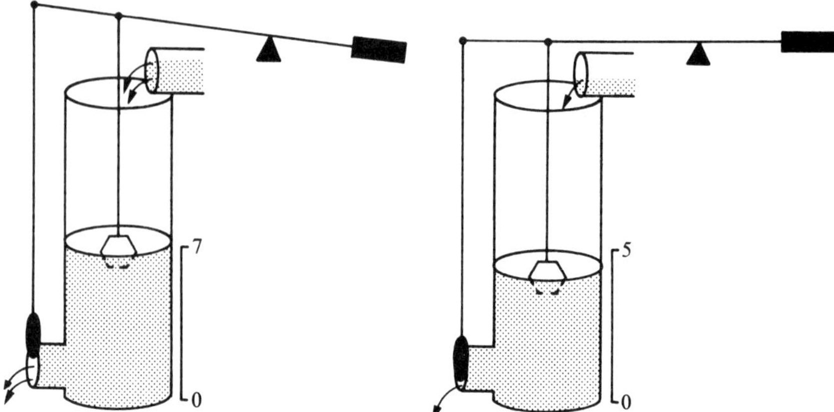

Figure 12-3. A simple servomechanism illustrates the principle of renal compensation of a respiratory acidosis. On the right, the system is at rest. Inflow equals outflow, the level of liquid in the reservoir stays constant. On the left, inflow has increased, the level in the reservoir rises, the float is lifted and the outflow gate is opened more than before. This accommodates increased outflow. The system again assumes steady state where increased inflow equals increased outflow. The new level of liquid in the reservoir is a little higher than before. The difference between the new and old level is small, the system is now fully or maximally compensated, yet the liquid level has not returned to control values.

MEASURING THE CO_2 CONTENT IN BLOOD

In modern laboratories, total CO_2 content is still determined (together with electrolytes) from venous blood and reported in milliequivalents per liter (mEq/l). In clinical practice, CO_2 content is assumed to be largely bicarbonate (which is usually true) and, therefore, to reflect a base excess (if CO_2 content is high) or deficit (if CO_2 content is low). Note that there

Table 12-4. MIXED DISTURBANCES*

	*p*H	Bicarbonate	P_{CO_2}
Mixed			
Acidosis	↓ ↓	↓	↑
Alkalosis	↑ ↑	↑	↓

* This table demonstrates that compensation cannot take place when respiratory and metabolic (renal) disturbances conspire. In mixed disturbances, both metabolic (bicarbonate) and respiratory (P_{CO_2}) factors pull in the same direction and *p*H changes are exaggerated (double arrows).

Table 12-5. CO_2 CONTENT CAN MISLEAD

	$[HCO_3^-]$	$P_{CO_2} \times 0.03$	*p*H
A	10	2	6.79
B	11.8	0.2	7.87

In *A* and *B*, the CO_2 content is 12 mmol/l. A CO_2 content of 12 mmol/l usually reflects metabolic acidosis, but the *p*H could be high or low, depending on how bicarbonate and P_{CO_2} are divided. *A* represents a mixed respiratory–metabolic acidosis, *B* is a respiratory alkalosis insufficiently compensated. CO_2 content—without additional data—can be quite misleading.

is a problem with this means of CO_2 measurement. Assume you get a report that the CO_2 content is 12 mEq/l. These 12 mEq/l are the sum of $[HCO_3^-]$ and $[H_2CO_3]$, the ratio of which will determine whether or not the patient is actually acidotic. For example, a CO_2 content of 12 mEq/l could come from either ratio shown in Table 12-5. A CO_2 content, therefore, has to be interpreted cautiously. A simultaneous determination of P_{CO_2} or *p*H eliminates the uncertainty. When arterial blood is analyzed, CO_2 content is often not reported, even though it is an easy matter to calculate it (the sum of $[HCO_3^-]$ and $P_{CO_2} \times 0.03$).

HOW TO ASSESS ACID–BASE CHANGES

Experience and uncounted experiments have taught us that during pure disturbances (those without compensation), certain ranges of values can be expected. If the data do not fall into such a range, we assume that either a degree of compensation or a mixed disturbance is occurring, depending on how *p*H, bicarbonate, and P_{CO_2} are distributed.

Several rules of thumb can be used to help the clinician make a quick assessment of the disturbance.

The CO_2-Up Rule

For every acute increase in arterial P_{CO_2} by 10 torr, there is an increase of bicarbonate by 1 mEq/l. Once the P_{CO_2} has remained elevated for over approximately 48 hours, the renal compensatory mechanisms have added another 2 mEq/l of bicarbonate for every 10 torr of CO_2 elevated above the normal baseline of 40 torr. Thus, in patients with chronic respiratory acidosis, one expects to see an increase of about 3 mEq/l for every 10 torr of elevated CO_2. If that is not present, additonal metabolic disturbances are suspected.

The CO_2-Down Rule

When CO_2 is reduced acutely below the normal 40 torr, the bicarbonate falls about 1.5 mEq/l for every 10 torr drop in P_{CO_2}. With chronic respiratory alkalosis, bicarbonate may fall by as much as 4.5 mEq/l for every 10 torr drop in P_{CO_2}.

The Metabolic Acidosis Rule

With metabolic acidosis the P_{CO_2} drops, frequently by 1.1 torr with every drop of bicarbonate by 1 mEq/l.

Nomograms

These convenient rules of thumb are enhanced either by plotting the data on nomograms or by reporting additional derived variables. The nomograms call for plotting the variables measured, namely *p*H and P_{CO_2}, and deriving bicarbonate concentrations from the plot. Ranges are then designated on the nomograms that correspond to pure (*i.e.*, uncompensated), compensated, and mixed disturbances. From many published presentations of these factors, we will present two:

1. *The triangular blood acid–base nomogram:* This method works with the familiar concepts P_{CO_2}, CO_2 content, and *p*H, and allows any easy visualization of the patient's acid–base disturbance (Fig. 12-4).
2. *The Siggaard–Andersen method:* This method allows plotting of the familiar variables, but also introduces new concepts.

The triangular blood acid–base nomogram (Fig. 12-4) allows the user to:

- Determine one of three variables, if the other two are known. For instance, if *p*H and CO_2 content are known, P_{CO_2} can be derived from the nomogram.
- Depict whether or not the values obtained represent a normal acid – base status (when they fall into the central hexagon) or a respiratory or metabolic disturbance, as shown.

The Siggaard–Andersen nomogram uses the term *base excess* or, if there is no excess of base, the awkward expression, *negative base excess* or—a little less convoluted—*base deficit*. The abbreviation BE (base excess) is entrenched and −BE or negative BE for base deficit is correspondingly well established.

The base excess allows an estimate of how much base (if BE is negative) or acid (if BE is positive) is necessary to bring a liter of blood to *p*H 7.4. These values (standard bicarbonate or base excess) do not ac-

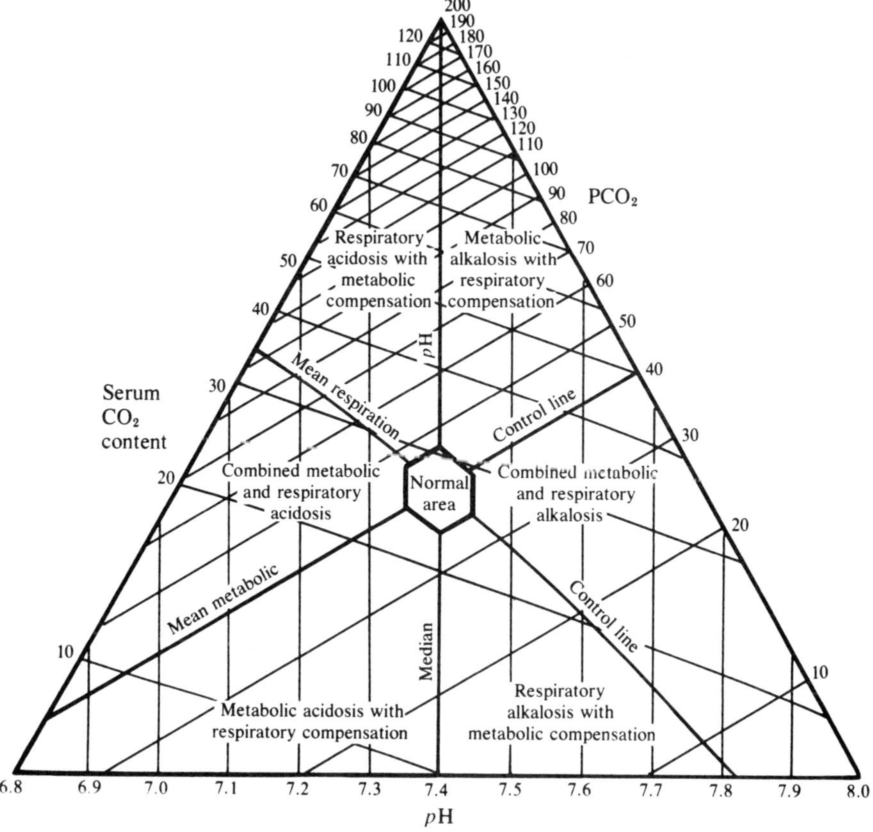

Figure 12-4. The acid–base nomogram (Instrumentation Laboratory, Andover, Massachusetts) is given. If two of the three variables (P_{CO_2}, pH, and CO_2 content) are known, the third one can be found at the corresponding intersection. Thus, a P_{CO_2} of 30 torr and a CO_2 content 20 mmol/l would correspond to a pH of about 7.4. The central hexagon describes normal ranges for the three variables. Diagnoses for different metabolic, respiratory, and mixed disturbances are shown.

curately depict the patient's requirement. Nor do they give information on the patient's buffering capacity. Standard bicarbonate makes no statement about buffering; base excess refers only to whole blood. Since the extracellular volume of the body contains about three times more extravascular (free of hemoglobin buffer) than intravascular (rich in hemoglobin buffer) volume, BE should not be used to calculate the dose of bicarbonate in case of an acidosis. Some clinicians like to report the *standard base excess,* a base excess assuming about 5 g hemoglobin/dl. This represents the average buffering capacity of the total extracellular volume. Intra-

USING THE SIGGAARD–ANDERSEN METHOD

The Siggaard–Andersen curve nomogram shows *p*H on the abscissa and a log P_{CO_2} scale on the ordinate (Fig. 12-5). When blood is titrated and increasing partial pressures of CO_2 and *p*H are measured, the data form a straight line on this nomogram (see line *A* in Fig. 12-5). Line *A* intersects the "buffer–base" curve at 48 mEq/l. Intuitively, we can appreciate that, if the blood were not buffered well, the slope of line *A* would not be as steep (as in line *B*). If P_{CO_2} were raised from 40 torr to 70 torr, the *p*H of the well-buffered blood would fall from 7.4 to 7.245 (line *A*), while the poorly buffered blood would have a *p*H of 7.225 (line *B*). It is, therefore, understandable how we can calibrate a curve to show the concentration of buffers per liter of blood. This is the *buffer-base curve*. For whole blood, the total buffer base equals approximately 48 mEq/l and, of these, hemoglobin accounts for about 0.45 mEq/g of hemoglobin.

If the buffer value is not normal, for example, if buffers have either combined with acid or been generated by extra base, a base deficit or excess exists. This will cause the titration line *A* or *B* to shift. With extra acid, line *A* shifts to the left and might assume the position of line *C*, which intersects the base excess curve at 10 mEq/l and the buffer-base curve at 38 mEq/l. Line *A* actually crossed the latter curve at 48 mEq/l, or 10 mEq/l higher than the intersection of line *C*. The buffer base (BB) *plus* the base excess

cellular buffers play an important role after a disturbance has persisted for some time, particularly in severe acid–base derangements. Then, standard base excess does not provide a useful guide to therapy; one has to titrate until the desired result is achieved.

Microprocessors in modern automated analyzers use algorithms that automatically calculate variables such as bicarbonate and standard base excess by deriving the blood's buffering capacity from known hemoglobin values.

If an apparatus displaying BE is not available, the Siggaard–Andersen alignment nomogram (Fig. 12-6) makes life easy. It allows us to use either CO_2 content with P_{CO_2} or *p*H, or *p*H and P_{CO_2} to find bicarbonate. Additionally, it can be used to determine a base excess for well- or poorly buffered systems.

It is simple to use. Just draw a straight line through any two of the known variables (*p*H, P_{CO_2}, CO_2 content) and read off not only the actual bicarbonate, but also BE for any appropriate hemoglobin concentration.

(−BE, in our example) is the normal buffer base (NBB). Therefore, NBB = BB − BE.

The curve nomogram in Figure 12-6 shows a scaled line going through a P_{CO_2} of 40 torr. With the Henderson–Hasselbalch equation and a constant P_{CO_2} of 40 torr, a bicarbonate value for every *p*H can be calculated. That has been done, and these bicarbonate values are entered on the P_{CO_2} 40 torr line. If the blood is fully oxygenated, the temperature is 37°C, and the P_{CO_2} is 40 torr, the bicarbonate is called *standard bicarbonate.*

Using the Siggaard–Andersen approach, we could report acid–base data by listing *p*H, P_{CO_2} standard bicarbonate, and base excess.

Note that it is no longer necessary to plot the data to see whether or not a metabolic acidosis (negative BE), alkalosis (positive BE), compensation for a respiratory acidosis (positive BE), or alkalosis (negative BE) exists.

If *p*H and P_{CO_2} are known, we could calculate easily enough the actual bicarbonate for that *p*H and P_{CO_2} (Fig. 12-2). In patients whose arterial P_{CO_2} is not close to 40 torr, the standard bicarbonate gives an idea, but, because of the unknown buffering capacity, it is not an accurate prediction of what bicarbonate we should expect if the arterial P_{CO_2} of the patient were 40 torr. The same holds true for *p*H. In patients with an arterial P_{CO_2} of 40 torr, the actual bicarbonate and the standard bicarbonate are identical.

For standard BE, use 5 g hemoglobin/dl blood, unless the patient is severely anemic.

OXYGENATED AND REDUCED HEMOGLOBIN

Since hemoglobin occurs in oxygenated and reduced forms and because oxyhemoglobin is a little more acidic than reduced hemoglobin, the state of oxygenation should be considered. The formula follows:

$$C = 0.3 \times \text{Hgb (g/dl)} \, \frac{100 - O_2\%\ \text{Sat.}}{100}$$

C gives the amount of base (in milliequivalents per liter) to add to the buffer base (BB) and the base excess (BE) if the hemoglobin (Hgb), *in vivo,* was not fully saturated, but, *in vitro,* was exposed to oxygen and saturated before being analyzed.

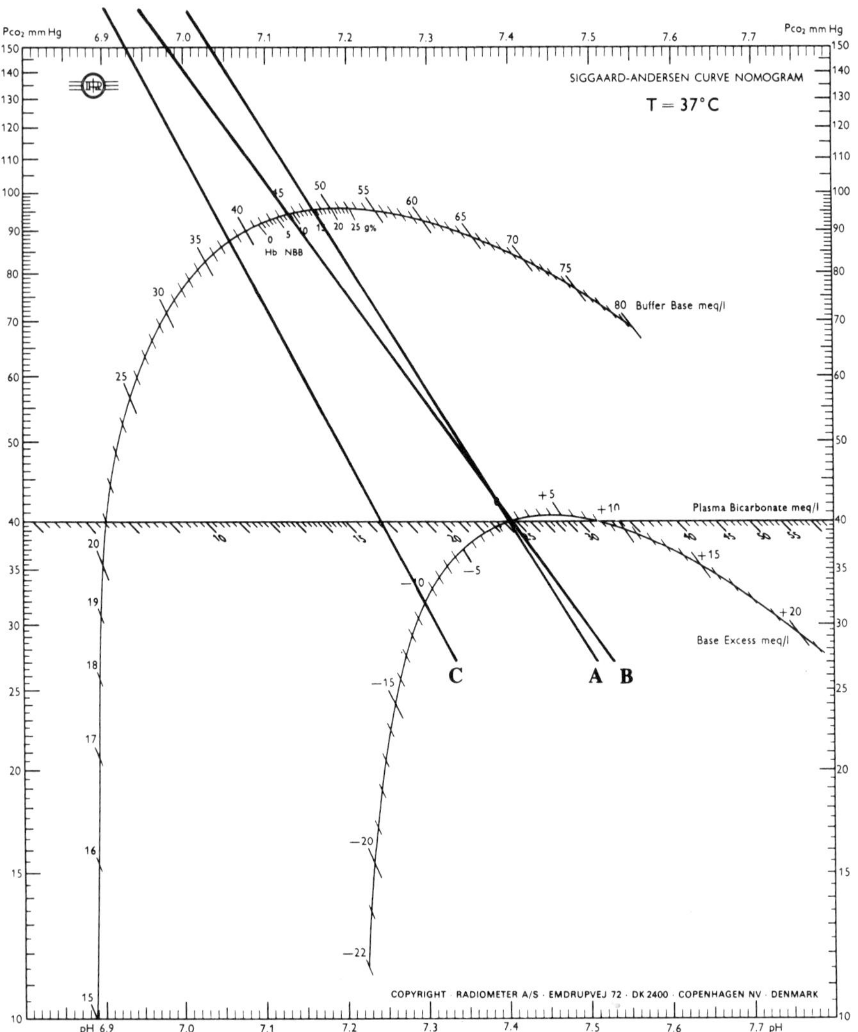

Figure 12-5. A Siggaard–Andersen curve nomogram. See explanation in displayed matter. (Siggaard–Andersen O, Engel K: A new acid–base nomogram: An improved method for the calculation of the relevant blood acid–base data. Scand J Clin Lab Invest 12:177, 1960)

VENOUS VERSUS ARTERIAL ACID–BASE DATA

In normal persons, the difference between arterial and venous P_{CO_2}, bicarbonate, and pH is not large. Table 12-6 shows representative data in round numbers. Of course, oxygen content or partial pressure is higher in arterial than venous blood.

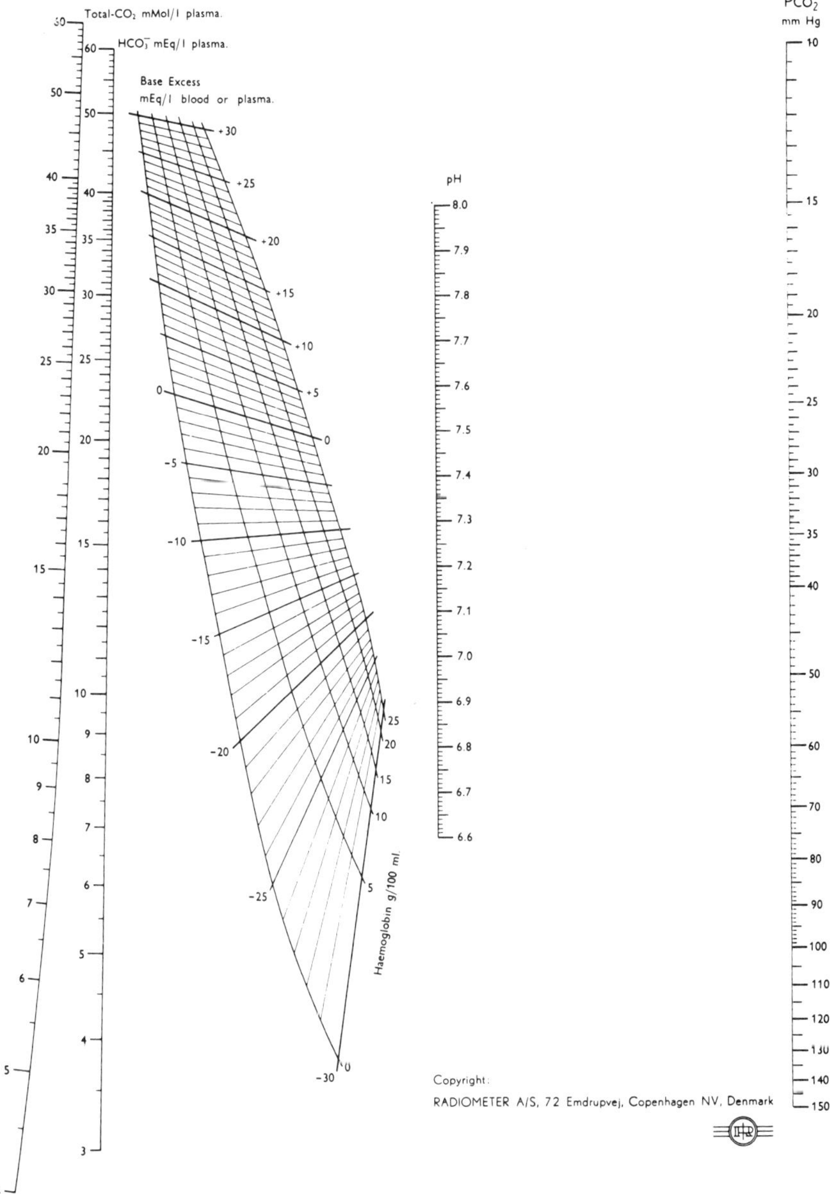

Figure 12-6. The Siggaard–Andersen alignment nomogram requires two measured variables. A straight line is drawn through these and the other variables can then be read. The base excess plot is subdivided for different hemoglobin values. It is, therefore, possible to determine the base excess for whole blood, the standard base excess (assuming a hemoglobin of 5 g/dl), and a base excess for fluid free of hemoglobin. (Siggaard–Andersen O: Blood acid–base alignment nomogram: Scales for pH, pCO_2, base excess of whole blood of different hemoglobin concentrations, plasma bicarbonate, and plasma total-CO_2. Scand J Clin Lab Invest 15:211, 1963)

Table 12-6. AVERAGE BLOOD GAS VALUES AT SEA LEVEL

	P_{CO_2} (torr)	*p*H	HCO_3^- (mEq/l)
Arterial	40	7.4	24
Venous	46	7.39	25

These differences in *p*H, produced by a higher P_{CO_2} in venous than in arterial blood, would be greater if it were not for hemoglobin. Reduced hemoglobin in venous blood shifts the system toward the alkaline side. Because the differences between venous and arterial *p*H are often small, some clinicians have advocated the use of venous rather than arterial blood for the assessment of acid–base parameters. Even closer than venous to arterial blood is capillary blood, which is often sampled in infants whose arterial or venous blood may be difficult to draw.

Sampling venous blood has drawbacks. It may be sampled from an area supplied by arterial shunts, for example, the back of the hand. During anesthesia, this site often yields venous blood with P_{O_2} and P_{CO_2} values close to those of arterial blood. True venous blood should be withdrawn from the mixing chambers in the right ventricle or the pulmonary artery; however, that procedure is more involved than an arterial puncture.

Sometimes venous blood is more venous than it should be. When blood is taken from a vein distal to a tourniquet that had been applied for minutes rather than seconds, for instance, the reading reflects local rather than systemic conditions.

Venous blood is often not handled anaerobically. Thus, gases in the blood have an opportunity to equilibrate with those in the ambient air. When this happens, P_{CO_2} and, consequently, $[HCO_3^-]$ fall. Under these circumstances, the drop in P_{CO_2} (equivalent to a respiratory alkalosis) causes the *p*H to rise and bicarbonate values to drop.

The assessment of P_{O_2} in venous blood does not reflect pulmonary oxygen dynamics. Venous blood for acid–base studies, therefore, has limited value. If the Siggaard–Andersen approach is used to calculate standard bicarbonate and BE, properly sampled venous blood will serve since these values are reckoned by assuming a P_{CO_2} of 40 torr and fully oxygenated blood.

AVERAGE *p*H

A controversy has developed surrounding the question of how to express an average of several *p*H measurements. If you have obtained a *p*H of 7.2, one of 7.3, and one of 7.4, what is the average? Some argue that these values should be converted into H^+ concentrations (in nanomoles), then the average should be calculated and reconverted into *p*H. Others suggest that to do so is to ignore some of the physiochemical relationships of the complex system described with *p*H and that to do anything else but to add 7.2 + 7.3 + 7.4 and divide by three is wrong.

A reasonable compromise between these two positions follows. When you take multiple readings from a patient and wish to know the average, add the *p*H values and get the average. The *p*H value reflects the millivolts of an electrical potential across a membrane. It is proper to average millivolts. If, however, you have titrated hydrogen ions per liter of fluid (in gastric juice, for example), and you wish to report the average output of hydrogen ions, it would be appropriate to do that in nanomoles of hydrogen ions.

THE EFFECT OF TEMPERATURE

The dissociation constant K (or *p*K), the solubility of O_2 and CO_2, and the O_2–hemoglobin dissociation, are affected by temperature. Therefore, the temperature of the patient's blood and the temperature of the system in which the blood was measured are important. If the *p*H electrode's temperature is not the same as the patient's, correction factors can be applied to bring the two into harmony. We advocate expressing all acid–base and gas values as if the patient's temperature were a normal 37°C. This makes it easier to compare values if the patient's temperature has changed from one acid–base assessment to the other. A disadvantage is that the clinician may fail to appreciate the degree of acidosis that develops with fever or the degree of alkalosis that develops with cooling. If you need to correct for changes in temperature, the following conversion factors can be applied to whole blood:

$$\Delta p\text{H} = -0.0146 \times \Delta \text{T}$$

If the temperature falls from 37°C to 27°C, the *p*H will *rise* by about 0.14 units using this equation. The effect on the solubility of CO_2 is

$$\Delta \log P\text{CO}_2 = +0.02 \times \Delta \text{T}$$

As temperature drops by 10°C, from 37°C to 27°C, a $P\text{CO}_2$ of 40 torr will *fall* to about 25 torr. These relationships are not entirely linear; however, for the ranges likely to occur in the operating room, the formulas are adequate.

Remember that these formulas apply to corrections that are to be calculated for whole blood. If a patient were to be cooled or warmed, the buffering capacity would be different and the correction factor for *p*H would be only about one-half of that listed above.

NORMAL VALUES IN ARTERIAL BLOOD

It is advisable to establish normal values for the hospital. These values may vary from place to place with altitude, equipment used, and, indeed, the population who seek care in the hospital. Some instruments, for instance, automatically use 14.5 g/dl (14.5 g%) as a normal hemoglobin. In many operating rooms, such "normal" values are rare, even in elective operations. In the first days of life, normal hemoglobin values are approximately 17 g/dl to 19 g/dl. By 3 months, they reach a normal low of approximately 10 g/dl, then they slowly rise in the first decade of life to approximately 12 g/dl.

Sometimes the Po_2 is measured at a point at which 50% of the blood is saturated. This is called the P_{50}. It starts at roughly 20 torr at birth and reaches 30 torr within a year, a little higher than the average adult level of 27 torr.

In the adult, average *p*H levels lie between 7.35 and 7.42. CO_2 tensions in arterial blood are usually 38 torr to 42 torr; often a little lower in women than in men. These sex-linked differences are clinically unimportant. During pregnancy, however, hyperventilation is common, with arterial Pco_2 values as low as 30 torr and *p*H up to 7.46.

At birth, the neonate's *p*H is low, from 7.2 to 7.25, but within 1 hour it rises to 7.3 or more. After 24 hours, it is practically normal. Also, remember that in infants with a patent ductus, particularly during crying, arteries of the left arm and body may contain admixtures of venous blood. The right arm, proximal to the ductus, may reflect lung functions more faithfully.

INDICATIONS FROM MONITORING ACID–BASE PARAMETERS IN THE OPERATING ROOM AND INTENSIVE CARE UNIT

Even if a patient is monitored with a pulse oximeter, it must be possible to check arterial blood to ascertain the level of oxygenation (a normal P_aO_2 is approximately 80 torr to 100 torr in patients breathing air) and CO_2 elimination (a normal P_aO_2 is approximately 40 torr). We analyze arterial blood whenever clinical signs raise the question of inadequate or excessive ventilation. Signs of inadequate oxygenation include a dusky hue to blood, mucous membranes, skin, and fingernails, and unusual trends in blood pressure (either decreasing or increasing pulse pressure, falling or rising mean pressures). A declining heart rate may be the ominous indicator of hypoxemia. Arrhythmias may be triggered by hypoxemia or hypercarbia. Sweating, wide pulse pressure, rising systolic pressure, and tachycardia are often seen with hypercarbia.

Whenever a conscious effort is made to alter resting values of arterial Po_2, Pco_2, or *p*H, blood gases and *p*H are monitored. Often an arterial catheter is used to facilitate repeated sampling. An example is induced hypocarbia in neurosurgical patients with intracranial masses.

Monitoring arterial or venous blood for evidence of a developing metabolic acidosis is indicated when cyanide poisoning is suspected; for instance, in the operating room and the intensive care unit when patients are receiving sodium nitroprusside infusions, particularly when larger than usual dosages have been given to control blood pressure or when the treatment has been prolonged. It is far quicker to check base excess (BE) than to obtain CN^- or lactate blood levels. Metabolic acidosis, the cardinal feature of cyanide toxicity, develops as the cyanide ion blocks mitochondrial oxygen consumption. When BE falls by 10 mEq/l or more, intravenous treatment with thiosulfate (150 mg/kg as repeated bolus) is initiated to tie up and convert the cyanide ions to thiocyanate. Inhalation of amyl nitrate or intravenous sodium nitrite (5 mg/kg) has been used to generate methemoglobin which binds cyanate. Nitrite can reduce the oxygen-carrying capacity of blood and cause hypotension.

Conditions that lead to a reduction of blood flow or arrest of the circulation (cardiopulmonary bypass or cardiac arrest) call for blood gas analysis. Not every patient with a cardiac arrest becomes acidotic. Vigorous treatment with bicarbonate without information on acid–base status can lead to severe alkalosis. In other circumstances, severe acidosis may supervene, and only monitoring of arterial acid–base data will provide a clue to how much treatment is needed and, later, how effective the treatment was.

A patient in shock with sepsis and severe respiratory or metabolic disturbance, of course, should have the benefit of acid–base monitoring.

AVAILABLE INSTRUMENTATION

Today, equipment is available to measure *p*H, Po_2, O_2 saturation of hemoglobin, and Pco_2. All other parameters, such as bicarbonate, standard bicarbonate, base excess, and standard base excess, have to be derived.

Measurement of *p*H

For complex physiochemical reasons, we do not actually measure $[H^+]$ or the concentration of protons or hydrogen ions in a solution, but we measure (H^+) or the *activity* of hydrogen ions. For this measurement, a *p*H electrode is used. This electrode functions as a little battery that generates a potential which can be measured by a voltmeter. The battery is made up of two compartments separated by a special glass membrane. In one compartment, a solution of known *p*H provides a reference. The other compartment accepts the solution to be measured. The formula, essentially the Nernst equation, that describes the distribution of ions in this electrode contains a logarithmic expression for (H^+). Therefore, it is reasonable to express the change of voltage read on the meter in logarithmic, pH units.

This electrode is quite sensitive to a change of temperature. During calibration and measurements, the temperature must be maintained at a constant level.

MEASUREMENT OF CO_2 CONTENT

The commonly used CO_2 electrode is known as a *Severinghaus electrode.* It resembles a pH electrode in many ways. The solution to be tested is exposed to the electrode. The dissolved CO_2 diffuses through a polymer membrane into an electrolyte solution which, in turn, lies next to the glass membrane that separates the test compartment from the reference compartment of the electrode. As CO_2 diffuses into the electrolyte solution, it causes the pH to change. This, in turn, changes the voltage. The voltmeter is calibrated in units of P_{CO_2} (partial pressure of CO_2 in millimeters of mercury or torr).

Temperature sensitivity of the electrode necessitates careful control of the temperature. With changes in barometric pressure, the partial pressure of CO_2 also changes. Five percent CO_2 (dry gas) at 760 torr would be 38 torr. At 600-torr ambient pressure (in the mountains), it would be 30 torr. Therefore, we need to correct for barometric pressure and calibrate the electrode against solutions containing known concentrations of CO_2. When alveolar water vapor pressure (47 torr at 37°C) is taken into account, these values drop to 35.7 torr and 27.7 torr, respectively.

Measurement of P_{O_2}

In the Clark electrode, liquid with dissolved or gaseous oxygen diffuses through a fine polypropylene membrane into a thin layer of an electrolyte solution covering a platinum wire. This wire is the cathode of an electrode to which a constant voltage is applied. As the oxygen is reduced at the platinum wire, a current is produced which is measured by an ammeter. The more oxygen, the greater the current. This current is compared to that generated by solutions with known oxygen tensions, and expressed as P_{O_2}. When gaseous O_2, rather than a liquid with dissolved O_2, is presented to the electrode, corrections have to be made as the calibration of the electrode differs for O_2 gas.

With changes in barometric pressure, the partial pressure of oxygen (P_{O_2}) changes just as it does for CO_2.

Instruments that Measure Acid–Base Variables

In the past, separate electrodes were used for pH and P_{CO_2}. Each had to be maintained and calibrated individually. The results obtained were then corrected for temperature and the necessary calculations of bicarbonate and base excess were carried out by hand.

Today, several companies have marketed marvelous instruments that comprise not just a *p*H electrode, but electrodes for the determination of P_{CO_2} and P_{O_2}, as well as automatic barometers. Some instruments provide a means of measuring hemoglobin content of blood. Microprocessors in these analyzers regulate all functions and carry out the necessary calculations. After a few moments of blinking and humming, the units display or print the requested data. It is an interesting phenomenon of our time that these new engineering gems no longer require highly trained personnel to operate them. These machines are not easily misused. Since in the past, analytical data from laboratories run by clinical services were often unreliable, regulatory agencies are now pressing for central control of all laboratory equipment. Today, however, the new robot analyzers and their microprocessors offer few opportunities for external control! They clean themselves. Some even ask questions of their human operators—not yet spoken—but displayed on a screen. The biggest opportunities for error exist in the preparation of the blood or gas sample, where little control from regulatory agencies can be exerted.

A new engineering development now offers indwelling arterial (or venous) catheters that come supplied with built-in sensors for *p*H, P_{CO_2}, and P_{O_2}. This is made possible by employing a technique that senses at the catheter tip changes in fluorescence sensitive to the variables to be measured. The fluorescences are transmitted fiberoptically to an analyzer that also calculates the other variables. The indwelling catheter still permits the measurement of blood pressure and withdrawal of blood. The response of these catheters does not permit the observation of breath-to-breath changes, but certainly offers acid–base data far faster than is possible with the fastest *in vitro* bench-bound analyzer.

BLOOD SAMPLING TECHNIQUE

Prepare a syringe; glass syringes are often preferred bcause they have a wide opening where the needle is attached. The plunger moves easily when moist so that arterial pressure can fill the syringe without need to aspirate. Plastic syringes have rubber-armed plungers that do not move as readily. Draw up a drop of heparin (1000 units/ml) solution to wet the inside of the syringe and expel all of the heparin. Too much heparin left in the syringe will affect the data.

For arterial blood, the radial, ulnar, or dorsalis pedis artery are the most accessible areas even during anesthesia. We use a 23-gauge needle. The dorsalis pedis artery is sometimes more readily entered when the needle is bent a little (Fig. 12-7) in order to compensate for the bulk of

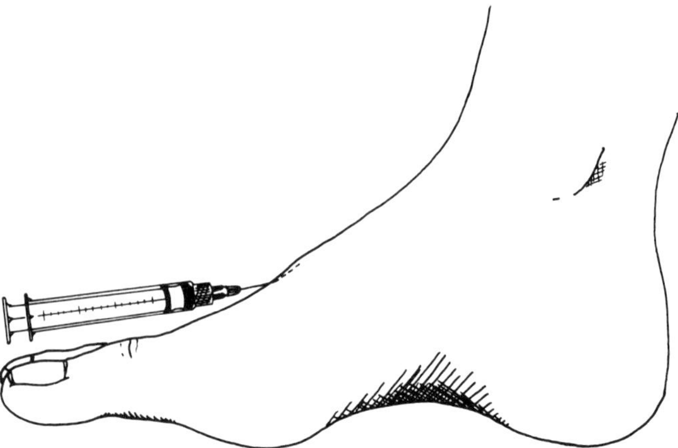

Figure 12-7. The bent needle. A bulky syringe makes it difficult to advance a straight needle into a superficial vein (or artery) that runs parallel to the skin. Bend the needle a little upon withdrawing it from its container to make it less likely that the needle will exit the vessel instead of staying inside.

the syringe, which makes it difficult to advance the needle into the artery. If the wrist cannot be sufficiently extended, the same trick helps.

Venous blood is easily drawn from hand, foot, or antecubital veins. Be sure not to obliterate the arterial pulse by applying the tourniquet too tightly. Check the pulse before you draw blood. In patients with narrow hand or foot veins, insert the needle so that it faces the stream (Fig. 12-8). This prevents collapse of the vein with the aspiration of blood.

When blood is collected from indwelling catheters, arterial or venous, make sure that no fluid other than blood is aspirated. It is a common mistake not to wait long enough until blood has washed out all solutions filling the tubing between needle or catheter and aspiration port. When in doubt, obtain simultaneously a *p*H and hematocrit from the indwelling catheter, as well as one from a fresh venipuncture. The two should be quite similar.

Capillary samples (*e.g.*, from the heel or finger pad of a baby) are obtained after rubbing or warming the tissue until it is quite pink, then lancing it, and waiting until a drop of blood appears. Avoid squeezing the tissue to hasten bleeding; it may give a falsely low hematocrit. Apply a capillary to the drop and allow capillary action to fill the capillary. Some capillaries come already heparinized and with a "metal flea." After capping the capillary, the flea can be moved up and down with a magnet to mix the blood. If blood has been collected in a syringe, expel the air, cap the syringe, and analyze it at once. If a delay is inevitable, place syringe or capillary in ice to reduce oxygen consumption and CO_2 production. Even a 10-minute delay will alter the reading if the blood is not cooled.

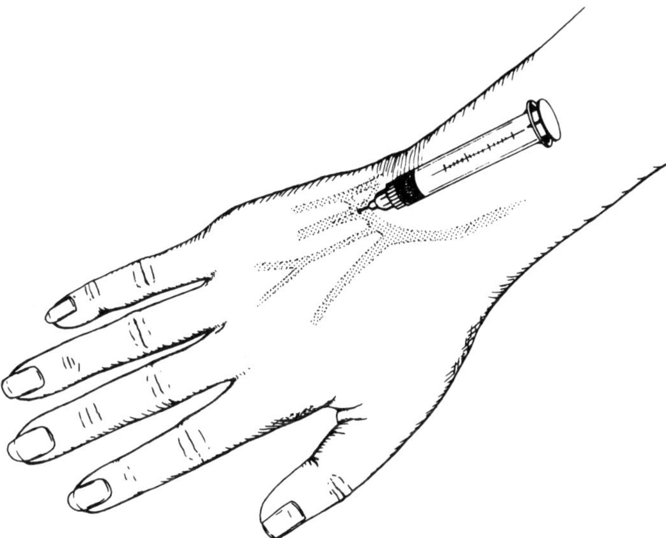

Figure 12-8. For collection of venous blood from patients with small veins, insert the needle so that it faces the stream. This makes aspiration of blood easier because the veins are not as likely to collapse.

With cooling, valid readings can be obtained 1 hour after sampling the blood. However, such a delay would be of little therapeutic benefit to the patient.

Before analyzing the blood, shake it well (or exercise the flea) so that the hemoglobin concentration will be read correctly. Because of a physicochemical phenomenon, the analyzers read the *p*H of whole blood a little lower (0.01 units) than that of plasma. This error is of no clinical significance.

CHAPTER 13

Fetal Monitoring

In many countries, continuous electronic monitoring of the fetal heart rate (FHR) during labor is used increasingly. The following statistics make the need for monitoring apparent: The perinatal death rate is 4 out of every 1000 births.[1] Intrapartum events account for approximately 30% of deaths that occur during birth and the early neonatal period. Furthermore, 20% to 40% of cerebral palsy, and 10% of severe mental retardation are also attributable to intrapartum factors.[2] As early as 1861, Little suspected a relationship between abnormal labor (perinatal adversities) and brain damage in infants.[3] Subsequently, risk scoring systems were developed.

Aubrey and associates developed a maternal and child health-care (MCHC) index and applied it to an obstetric population.[4] The results designated 23% of the total population to be at risk (Fig. 13-1). A labor index labeled 20% of the total population to be at risk, roughly one-half of whom had not been identified by the MCHC to be at risk. After correction for anomalies, it was found that the predicted high risk group

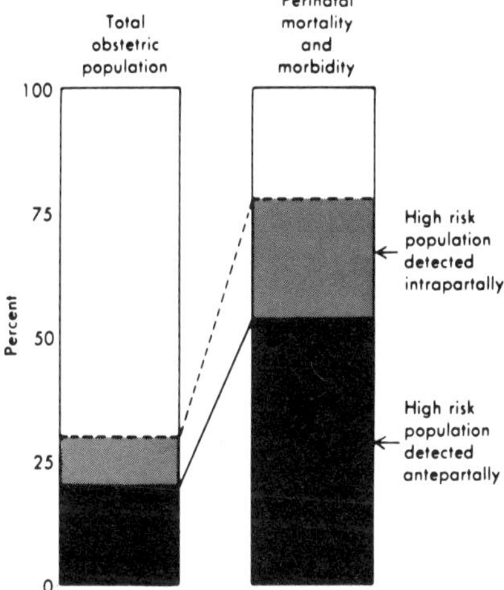

Figure 13-1. Identification of patients at risk by maternal and child health-care index (*area shaded black*). During labor, additional patients are identified (*stippled area*). Note that 25% of morbidity and mortality was not predicted by either antepartum or intrapartum indexes. (Aubrey R: Identification of the high-risk perinatal patient. In Aladjem S, Brown AK [eds]: Perinatal Intensive Care, p 68. St Louis, CV Mosby, 1977)

accounted for about 75% of all perinatal morbidity and mortality, leaving 25% unpredicted.

INDICATIONS FOR MONITORING

Unfortunately, antepartum and intrapartum risk prediction does not identify all patients subject to perinatal mortality and morbidity. Therefore, we cannot afford to exclude from careful monitoring those mothers not classified as representing high risk.

Many causes contribute to infant morbidity and mortality. Of greatest importance—because they are usually preventable—are diseases caused by the labor and delivery.

The American College of Obstetricians and Gynecologists has published a technical bulletin that recommends continuous monitoring of FHR and uterine activity during labor if one or more of the following conditions exist:[5]

Obstetrical History Factors
Age >35 or <16
Diabetes
Chronic hypertension

Cardiac disease
Rh-sensitization
Sickle-cell disease or trait
Previous cesarean section

PRENATAL EARLY INTRAPARTUM FACTORS
Anemia
Pre-eclampsia
Post-term >42 weeks
Polyhydramnios
Clinical evidence of intrauterine growth retardation
Vaginal bleeding
Abnormal fetal–placental tests
Induction of labor
Premature rupture of the membranes
Premature labor
Meconium-stained fluid
Abnormal fetal heart tones by auscultation
Twins
Pyelonephritis

Once labor has begun, factors unique to each stage can cause one out of ten previously normal patients to be classified as being at risk. The developing intrapartum problems associated with increased risk of fetal death at birth are listed:

LABOR RISK FACTORS
Prolonged latent phase
Dysfunctional labor
Secondary arrest of cervical dilatation
Prolonged second stage
Augmentation of labor

AMNIOTIC FLUID RISK FACTORS
Meconium passage
Amnionitis

ABNORMAL FHR RISK FACTORS
Tachycardia by auscultation
Abnormal fetal heart tones (FHTs) by auscultation

PLACENTAL RISK FACTORS
Abruption
Previa
Bleeding of unknown cause

ANESTHESIA RISK FACTORS
Conduction anesthesia*
Paracervical block anesthesia

Occasionally, healthy patients with normal labor will deliver a sick infant.

TRADITIONAL MONITORING METHODS

Meconium

The appearance of meconium intrapartum has long been thought to indicate fetal distress. Thick meconium, particularly, is related to an increased neonatal death rate, low Apgar scores, and respiratory distress (meconium aspiration syndrome).

Auscultation

In 1821, auscultation of the fetal heart was suggested as a way to determine fetal distress intrapartum. Lejumeau thought that bradycardia was associated with fetal head compression.[6] In 1890, von Winckel defined the normal FHR as 120 beats to 160 beats per minute but detected no relationship between fetal distress and fetal heart rate.[7] Benson later said that "no reliable single auscultatory indicator of fetal distress exists in terms of fetal heart rate, save in the extreme degree."[8] Many studies confirm the observation that meconium and auscultation of FHR are poor indicators of intrapartum problems. Auscultation, particularly, is subject to large errors.

Potentially harmful clinical conditions were often missed when clinical teaching dictated that FHR was not to be monitored during uterine contraction and for 30 seconds thereafter. Because of this practice, based on the incorrect notion of "normal" bradycardia and on the clinical difficulty of hearing the fetal heart during contraction, data were lost and errors were made when the fetal heart was ignored during that period.

Counting errors, as shown in Figure 13-2, are particularly large at

* Under conduction anesthesia we consider caudal, epidural, and spinal. We would also include general anesthesia as a risk factor.

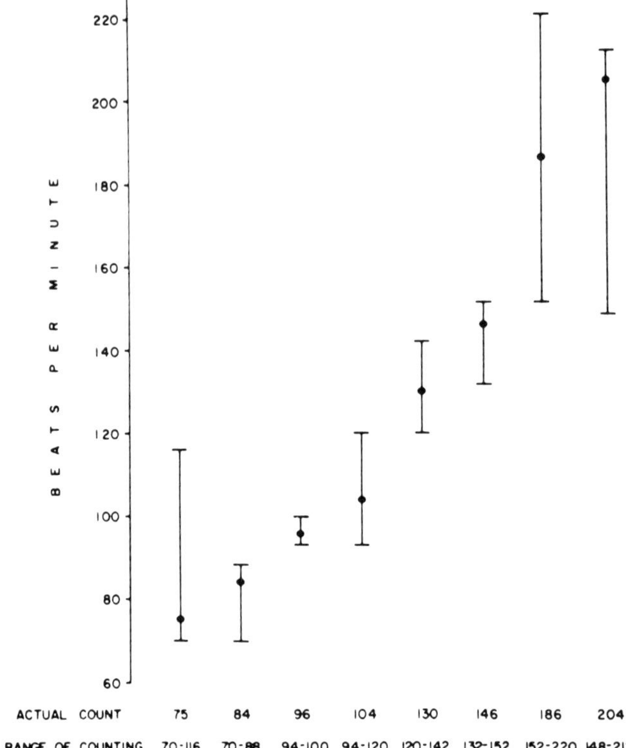

Figure 13-2. Eleven obstetricians simultaneously auscultated and recorded fetal heart rate. Compared to electronic counting, physicians made significant errors while auscultating fetuses with high and low heart rates. *Dots* = electronic counts, *lines* = the ranges of counts reported by the physicians. (Hon EH: An Introduction to Fetal Heart Rate Monitoring, 2nd ed, p 8, 1975)

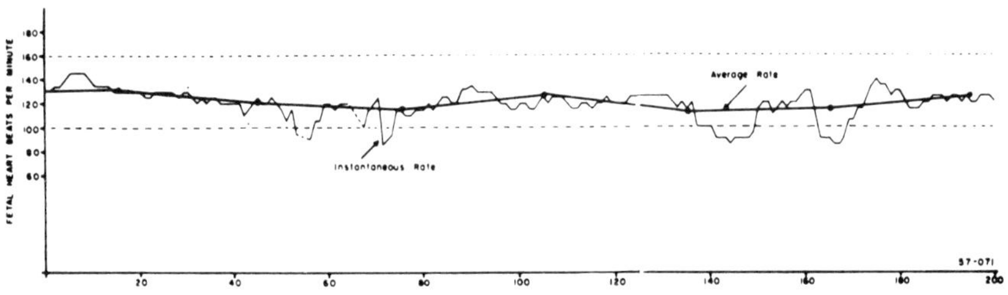

Figure 13-3. A comparison of instantaneous and average fetal heart rates is given. Significant periods of bradycardia are ignored by averaging. (Hon EH: An Introduction to Fetal Heart Rate Monitoring, 2nd ed, p 9. Los Angeles, University of Southern California School of Medicine, 1975)

Table 13-1. NORMAL FETAL HEART RATE CHARACTERISTICS

Baseline rate	120–160 beats/min
Baseline variability	>5 beats/min
Periodic pattern	Absent or early decelerations or accelerations
Fetal outcome	Vigorous; Apgar score >7

high and low heart rates. Not only is auscultation an intermittent observation, but it also requires averaging during the observation. Averaging over only 30 seconds can result in a significant error, as shown in Figure 13-3. Electronic counting remedies these weaknesses and allows continuous, beat-to-beat determination of FHR.

MONITORING FETAL HEART RATE

Fetal heart rate is assessed between contractions (*baseline FHR*) and during contractions (*periodic FHR*).[9] Normal features are summarized in Table 13-1. Normally baseline FHR varies from beat to beat, probably governed by vagal impulses, by 6 beats to 20 beats per minute. Superimposed on these rapid changes are slower shifts in baseline FHR by 6 beats to 10 beats per minute. These recur in 2 cycles to 6 cycles per minute; probably driven by fluctuations in sympathetic tone. Absence or exaggeration of these normal variabilities (rapid and slow) gives rise to concern about the fetal autonomic nervous system or the fetal heart itself. The predominant baseline FHR can be normal, fast, or slow (Table 13-2).

Since uterine contractions occur periodically, the concomitant changes in FHR are often referred to as periodic FHR patterns. These can show no change, acceleration, or deceleration relative to the preceding baseline FHR.

Hon studied FHR by using continuous electronic monitoring.[10] He defined normal FHR to be 120 beats to 160 beats per minute with a physiologic variability of over 5 beats per minute (Fig. 13-4). When the uterus

Table 13-2. BASELINE FETAL HEART RATE

	Rate (beats/min)	Duration (min)
Marked bradycardia	<100	10
Mild bradycardia	110–119	10
Normal	120–160	
Mild tachycardia	161–180	10
Marked tachycardia	>180	10

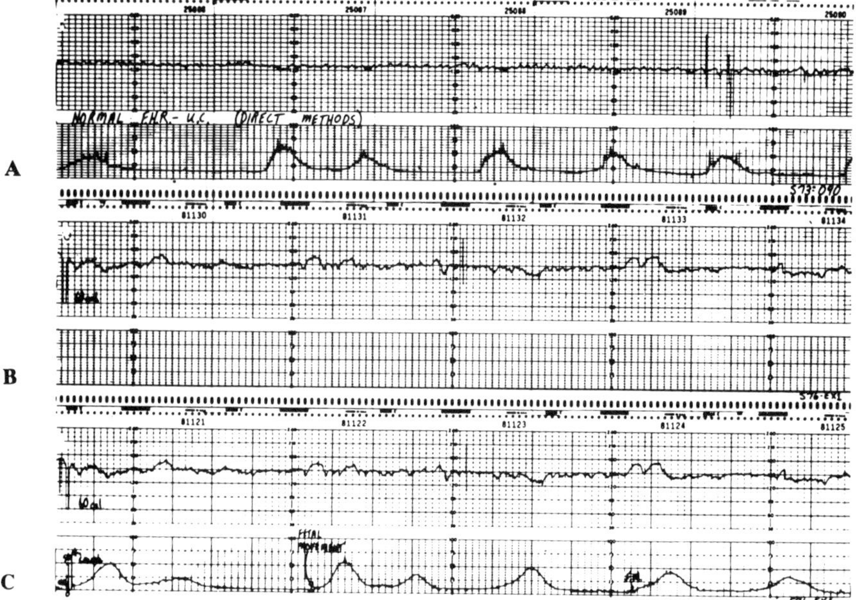

Figure 13-4. Fetal heart rate (FHR) and uterine contraction (UC). (*A*) Fetal heart rate—obtained through fetal electrocardiogram of the presenting part (scalp). Rate is calculated and plotted beat-by-beat. Beat-to-beat variability is independent of uterine contractions, which are shown on lower trace. Uterine contraction—intrauterine pressure measurement shown on lower trace. Pressure rises to 50 torr to 60 torr every 2 minutes to 3 minutes. (*B*) Fetal heart rate—Note calibration signal on the left of the record. All records should be calibrated. (*C*) Uterine contraction—the transducer has been placed at the miduterine level and opened to air, while the recording stylus has been moved to the zero position on the graph paper. It has been calibrated at 50 torr. The scale is at the left of the record. Note that variability is independent of uterine contractions. (Paul RH, Petrie RH: Fetal Intensive Care, I-1. University of Southern California, 1981. Distributed by Corometrics Medical Systems, Inc., Wallingford, Connecticut)

contracts, uterine blood flow diminishes. This alters periodic FHR 70% of the time (Fig. 13-5).

Patterns of Fetal Heart Rate

The fetal heart rate is normally variable. Spontaneous fetal movements should be associated with a change in fetal heart rate by up to 15 beats per minute. Fetal sleep and uterine contractions will also influence FHR. Thus, variability in FHR is physiologic. Indeed, lack of variability usually signals fetal distress, disease, or the effect of drugs, for instance, magnesium sulfate given to the mother.

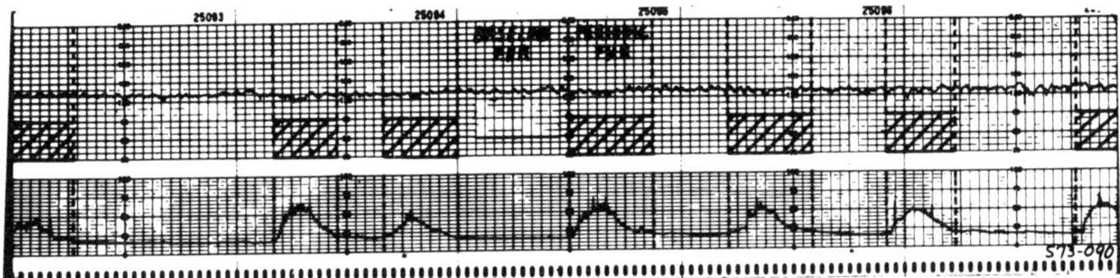

Figure 13-5. FHR and normal uterine activity are shown. The periodic fetal heart rate is measured during uterine contractions (*cross-hatched section*). The "baseline heart rate" is measured between contractions (*noncross-hatched section*). (Paul RH, Petrie RH: Fetal Intensive Care, I-10. University of Southern California, 1981. Distributed by Corometrics Medical Systems, Inc., Wallingford, Connecticut)

Periodic patterns of FHR associated with uterine contraction (Fig. 13-6) are classified under four categories: early, variable, late decelerations, and acceleration.

In *early deceleration,* FHR decreases simultaneously with the onset of uterine contraction and returns to the baseline level as the contraction ceases (Fig. 13-7). The heart rate pattern mirrors the uterine contraction pattern. This normal deceleration relates to the compression of the fetal head (the deceleration pattern can be reproduced by compressing the fetal

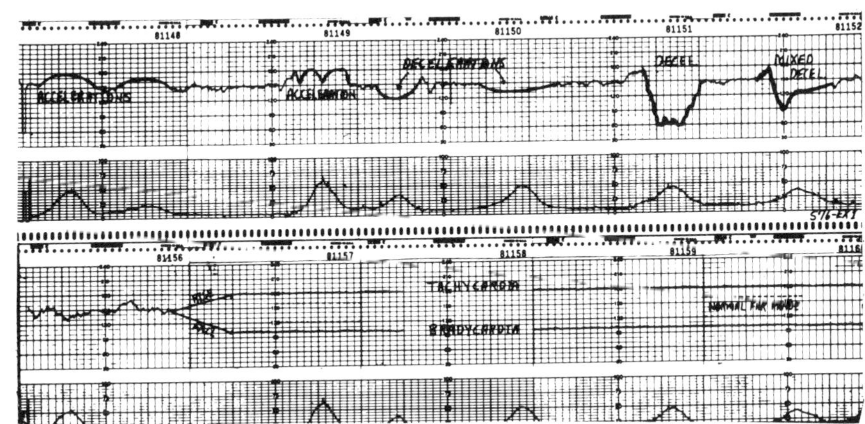

A

B

Figure 13-6. (*A*) If uterine contraction results in an FHR change, a periodic pattern emerges. Note the various shapes of acceleration (FHR increase) and deceleration traces (FHR decrease). (*B*) Tachycardia—fetal heart rate above 160 beats per minute for more than 10 minutes. Bradycardia—fetal heart rate below 120 beats per minute for more than 10 minutes. (Paul RH, Petrie RH: Fetal Intensive Care, I-10. University of Southern California, 1981. Distributed by Corometrics Medical Systems, Inc., Wallingford, Connecticut)

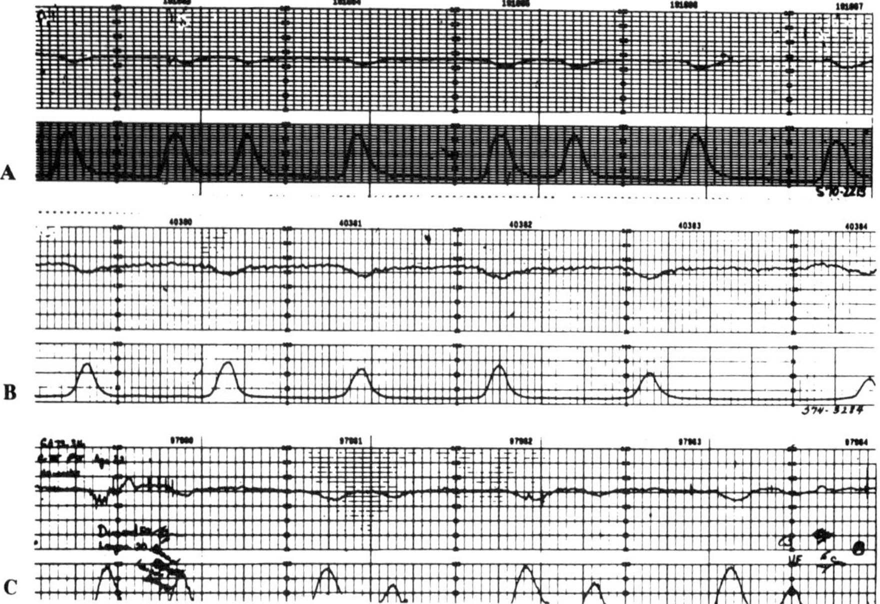

Figure 13-7. Early deceleration is shown. Slowing of fetal heart rate occurs simultaneously with onset of uterine contraction and returns to baseline at cessation of contraction. Variability is normal in *B*, much reduced in *A* and somewhat reduced in *C*. Note fetal heart rate remains above 120 beats per minute. (Paul RH, Petrie RH: Fetal Intensive Care, I-13. University of Southern California, 1981. Distributed by Corometrics Medical Systems, Inc., Wallingford, Connecticut)

head) and is mediated through a vagal reflex. It is not associated with either low Apgar scores or fetal acidosis. Early deceleration is often called *Type I deceleration.*

Variable fetal deceleration is caused by a reflex mechanism, also presumably of vagal origin, and is a result of reduced blood flow through the umbilical artery (Fig. 13-8). It is characterized by variation in onset, pattern, and form. This most common abnormal pattern is associated with acidosis and low Apgar scores. Characteristics of variable deceleration are shown in Table 13-3. If the umbilical artery is completely occluded, an acute rise in fetal aortic and left ventricular pressure results. Subsequent baroreceptor stimulation triggers a vagal response and a consequent slowing of heart rate. Alterations of blood flow in the umbilical cord can lead to changes in blood gases. The degree to which hypoxia, hypercapnia, and *p*H alterations occur determines the degree of chemoreceptor stimulation, resultant vagal stimulation, and FHR. Variable deceleration, also called *Type II decleration,* is particularly worrisome if it is associated with arrhythmias.

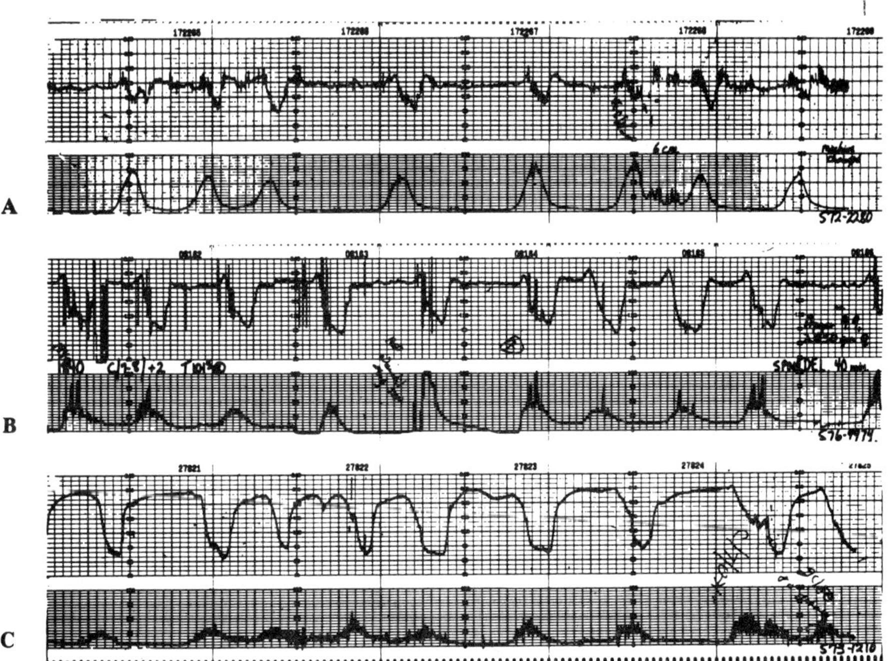

Figure 13-8. Variable deceleration is shown. Fetal heart rate traces representing mild (*A*), moderate and severe (*B*), and severe abnormalities with loss of baseline variability patterns (*C*). Onset of deceleration varies in relation to onset of uterine contraction and sometimes is followed by acceleration. (Paul RH, Petrie RH: Fetal Intensive Care, I-16. University of Southern California, 1981. Distributed by Corometrics Medical Systems, Inc., Wallingford, Connecticut)

Table 13-3. VARIABLE FETAL HEART RATE DECELERATION CHARACTERISTICS

Degree	Heart Rate (beats/min)	Duration (sec)
Mild	Any rate	<30
	70–80	<60
	>80	Any duration
Moderate	<70	>30 but <60
	70–80	>60
Severe	<70	>60

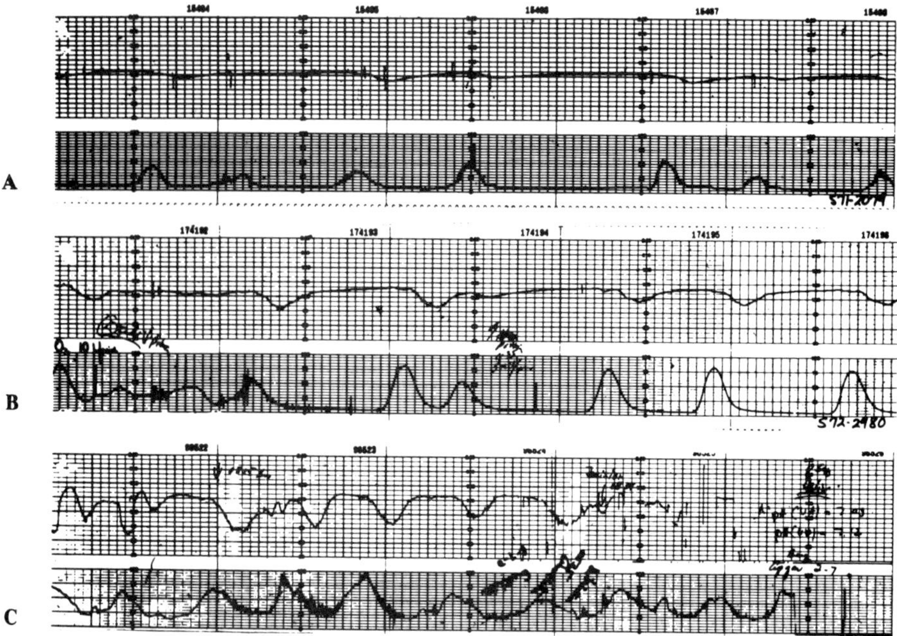

Figure 13-9. Late deceleration: *A* represents mild (<15 beats per minute) late deceleration, variability absent; *B* is moderate (15–45 beats per minute) late deceleration, with decreased variability; *C* is severe (>40 beats per minute) with absent variability. (Paul RH, Petrie RH: Fetal Intensive Care, I-14. University of Southern California, 1981. Distributed by Corometrics Medical Systems, Inc., Wallingford, Connecticut)

Instead of FHR decelerating as contraction commences, *late deceleration* begins 10 seconds to 30 seconds after a uterine contraction has started. The FHR returns to normal *after* the contraction. It is partially mediated vagally and is associated with hypoxia of the fetal myocardium secondary to insufficient uteroplacental circulation. Causes of hypoxia include hypotension, excessive uterine activity, and decreased placental exchange surface. The hypoxia may be mild, moderate, or severe (Fig. 13-9). Yet, not all babies suffering late deceleration are endangered; approximately 50% are at risk. They may be hypoxic, acidotic, or neurologically depressed. Late deceleration is also called *Type III deceleration*.

A stable FHR is abnormal (Fig. 13-9). A heart rate without variability interrupted by episodes of late deceleration is of particular concern. Kubli and colleagues graded late variable decelerations from mild to severe:[11] a slowing by 15 beats per minute is mild, 15 to 45 beats moderate, and 45 beats or more severe (Table 13-4, Figs. 13-8 and 13-9).

We ask three critical questions during severe, repetitive deceleration:[12]

Table 13-4. CLASSIFICATION OF LATE FETAL HEART RATE DECELERATION

Degree	Heart-rate Deceleration (change in beats/min)
Mild	<15
Moderate	15–45
Severe	>45

1. Can adequate oxygen–carbon dioxide exchange take place in the intervillous space between contractions?
2. To what extent is fetal blood flow to the placenta reduced, leading to deficient gaseous exchange?
3. Is cardiac output sufficient for adequate tissue perfusion?

The heart rate of the fetus may accelerate secondary to partial cord collapse (Fig. 13-6). This acceleration is brought about by uterine contraction and usually is benign.

A sinusoidal FHR pattern is seen occasionally. As shown in Figure 13-10, the frequency of variation in heart rate is much higher than the frequency of uterine contraction. It is often seen in the presence of profound anemia (isoimmunization is the most common cause), and is frequently associated with grave consequences for the fetus.[13]

Fetal *arrhythmias* are generally not associated with poor outcome, even though babies with antepartum arrhythmias are occasionally found to have congenital heart defects. The arrhythmias can be diagnosed only from a paper trace of the fetal electrocardiogram, but a suspicion of arrhythmias is raised when sharp spikes appear on the slowly moving strip chart; sharp down-spikes are indicative of missed beats (momentary arrest?), sharp up-spikes signal premature contractions (be sure to rule out

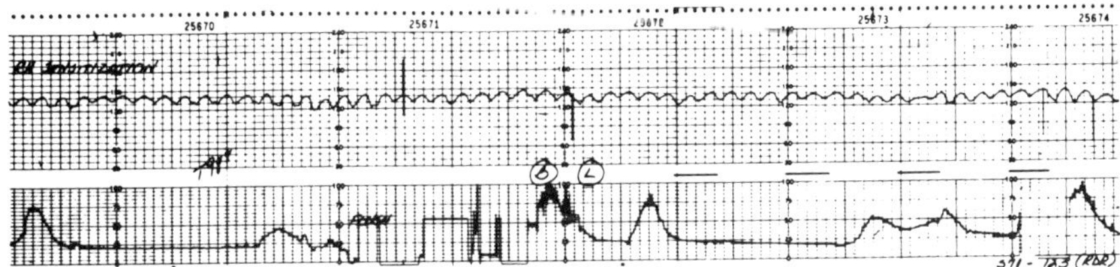

Figure 13-10. Sinusoidal fetal heart rate is shown. In this isoimmunized patient (Rh-sensitization) the cyclic, rapidly changing fetal heart rate is associated with a grave prognosis. (Paul RH, Petrie RH: Fetal Intensive Care, I-19. University of Southern California, 1981. Distributed by Corometrics Medical Systems, Inc., Wallingford, Connecticut)

artifacts!). The low voltage of the fetal electrocardiogram, interference by the maternal electrocardiogram, and background noise all contribute to difficult interpretation of the fetal ECG. If an arrhythmia is diagnosed, ultrasonic methods may be used to further define fetal cardiac status. Most arrhythmias are inconsequential and resolve within a few days after birth.[14]

The relationship of Apgar score to FHR has been much studied. A normal FHR pattern predicts, in more than 99% of the cases, a good Apgar score. Only 43% of babies with an abnormal pattern have a low Apgar score at 1 minute and 20% at 5 minutes.[15] The high false positive rate has led to additional methods of monitoring.

As a rule of thumb, slow FHR causes the obstetrical team to worry about the fetus. However, sometimes a healthy fetus maintains a relatively slow heart rate, but good variability. Before accepting this benign interpretation, confirm by auscultation and ultrasound the presence of fetal heart activity: fetal scalp electrodes can detect the *maternal* ECG with variability in maternal heart rate, while the fetus is in asystole.

FETAL SCALP *p*H

Because it is difficult to predict fetal distress from the FHR, additional data are necessary. Hypoxemia and acidosis, either limited to the fetus or suffered by the mother and then the fetus, can produce abnormal patterns of FHR. A normal pattern of FHR usually reflects a normal *p*H of fetal scalp blood. Mild tachycardia indicates mild acidosis. Variable decelerations are often associated with fetal acidosis. Late decelerations are ominous because 30% of babies will have a *p*H of less than 7.2. Fetal scalp *p*H is discussed in greater detail below (monitoring fetal scalp blood *p*H).

FETAL MONITORING TECHNIQUES

Auscultation

Auscultation of the fetal heart is best done through the back of the fetus. Move the fetal stethoscope around on the maternal abdomen until you hear the fetal heartbeat. Sometimes, it may be confused with the sound of the mother's blood flowing through the uterus. By auscultation, the types of deceleration cannot be identified because human observers cannot avoid "averaging" the pulse rate. A paper record of FHR is needed to diagnose variations.

Palpation

Palpation of the abdomen is a benign but insensitive routine to determine uterine contraction. Contractions are usually underway for approximately

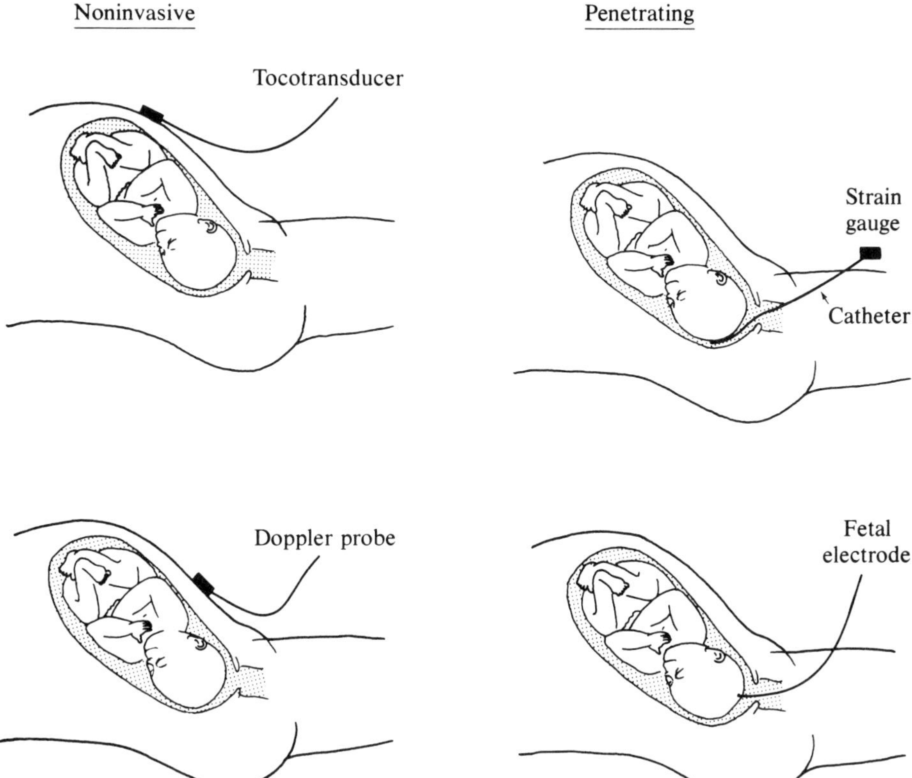

Figure 13-11. Invasive or penetrating monitoring of FHR and uterine activity is compared to noninvasive monitoring in this illustration. Note the position of the sensing device in each instance.

10 seconds before the hand can feel a change, and they persist for about 10 seconds after the palpating hand can no longer detect them.

Electronic Monitoring

Electronic monitoring of the FHR may be either invasive, meaning penetrating, or noninvasive, that is direct or indirect (Fig. 13-11). It allows instantaneous observations of heart rate.

Noninvasive

For noninvasive (external) monitoring, the sensor, placed on the mother's abdomen, transmits a signal translated into FHR. Three devices are currently in use: a phonotransducer, an ultrasound transducer, and an electrocardiogram.

The phonotransducer picks up both the first and the second heart sounds but the system transmits only the first. It is sensitive to other sounds and motion and, thus, may lead to inaccurate interpretations of heart rate. Electronic smoothing, averaging readings over several heartbeats, may reduce the influence of noise. However, unfortunately, it will also reduce our ability to detect the physiologic variability.

Ultrasound or Doppler transducers provide an alternative method for measuring FHR. Two crystals, one transmitting a wave and the other receiving the signal after it is reflected, are used. Reflection by any moving object will change the frequency of the reflected wave from the transmitted wave. The problem with the Doppler technique is that the motion of sources other than the fetal heart or heart valves, including the abdominal aorta or common iliac arteries of the maternal cardiovascular system, may be picked up. For this reason, rather precise placement of the probe over the fetal heart is important. Thus, frequent adjustment of the monitoring probe or restraint of the patient may be necessary. The Doppler system is noninvasive and relatively artifact-free. Therefore, it may be used during labor, before rupture of membranes. In clinical practice, ultrasound is the most commonly used noninvasive monitor of FHR.

The third method of measuring the FHR noninvasively uses abdominal wall electrocardiography. When the fetal electrocardiogram is obtained by placing electrodes on the maternal abdominal wall; fetal and maternal electrocardiograms are "mixed." By judicious electronic filtering, they can be separated, FHR determined, and variability calculated. Occasionally, fetal death is not recognized because the maternal electrocardiogram is mistaken for the fetal electrocardiogram. Electronic noise may be difficult to eliminate, particularly if the mother moves. Fetal age also affects electrocardiography. Gestational ages of fetuses 27 weeks to 35 weeks are associated with a smaller ECG signal than fetuses either older or younger than that.

Invasive or Penetrating

The following method is usually called invasive, but a better term is penetrating because internal electrocardiographic monitors can be used only after rupture of membranes. A sterile, spiral, metal, bipolar electrode is screwed to a depth not exceeding 2 mm into the fetal scalp. This method readily detects beat-to-beat variability and has a rather low incidence of artifacts. Noise is reduced considerably, and fetal or maternal movements have much less effect than with external methods.

Verifying FHR by auscultation is helpful at times. While auscultating what you think is the fetal heart, palpate the maternal pulse to make sure you are not listening to the maternal circulatory system. If auscultation does not work, the Doppler method may. If this does not help, ask the mother to do a Valsalva maneuver, which will slow her heart rate without affecting the FHR. Remember to disconnect the baby from the internal monitor if delivery is by cesarean section.

Uterine Activity

Noninvasive

In order to relate the FHR to the activities of the uterus, a monitor is necessary. External monitors, called *tocodynamometers,* are strapped around the abdomen (Fig. 13-11). They have transducers equipped with strain gauges. The amount of tension measured corresponds to uterine contraction. This device indicates contractions, but does not quantitate their absolute strength nor the intrauterine pressure. Fetal and maternal motions produce artifacts. Even respiration can generate artifacts and, therefore, the best placement must be found for each parturient. The system is noninvasive and may be applied before membranes rupture without risk to mother or fetus. A disadvantage is that the patient must remain relatively still or the recording will pick up artifacts.

Invasive or Penetrating

After membranes rupture, we can catheterize the uterus, monitor internally, and measure intrauterine pressures. The technique of intrauterine catheterization suggested by Miller and Paul is simple.[16]

With a rigid guide, the catheter is placed posteriorly in the interspace between the presenting fetal part and the cervix. Guide the catheter gently so that the uterus is not perforated. The intrauterine catheter can traumatize the cervix, as well as the uterus, and may become entangled in the umbilical cord. Puncture of the umbilical cord has been reported. After proper placement, remove the air bubbles from the system so that absolute pressure *in utero* can be measured directly. The flexible catheter is filled with sterile saline and one end is attached to a transducer at the height of the uterus.

The pressures generated by a uterus in labor usually have a slow crescendo followed immediately by an equally slow decrescendo (see Fig. 13-7*A*,*B*). When the mother actively bears down during a contraction, the generated pressures often exceed the range for which the recording system is calibrated; the peak pressure then cannot be read. At other times the uterine pressure curves assume a square appearance, that is, a rapid rise, a sustained peak pressure, followed by a rapid decline. Such active pushing by the patient usually indicates well-advanced labor.

Monitoring Fetal Scalp Blood *p*H

In measuring the *p*H of blood from the fetal scalp, significant progress has been made, especially considering the very small quantity of blood for analysis. A cone-shaped endoscope is inserted into the vagina and gently pressed against the fetal scalp, which smooths out the wrinkles. Now with a special, short blade a 2-mm laceration is made in the richly perfused fetal scalp. After a blood sample is obtained, maintain the cone in position, exerting gentle pressure, until bleeding has stopped.

Ideally maternal arterial blood should be collected at the same time, and fetal as well as maternal arterial *p*H, Po_2 and Pco_2 assessed simultaneously. Obviously, a fetal acidosis or hypoxemia that simply reflects maternal abnormalities will call for vigorous treatment of the mother, while abnormalities limited to the fetus direct our attention more to the fetus.

A normal fetus will show *p*H values between 7.25 and 7.35. A mild acidosis with *p*H between 7.20 and 7.24 calls at least for repeated measurements or—depending on the circumstances—for intervention. A *p*H of under 7.2 indicates distress and, in 44% of such cases, the newborn will have an Apgar score at 1 minute of 6 or less.

See Chapter 12 for details of acid–base measurements.

CRITICAL VIEWS ON FETAL MONITORING

The introduction of electronic fetal monitoring has been credited with a significant reduction in the intrapartum fetal death rate. Based upon retrospective studies, the claim has been made that roughly 2 to 3 lives per 1000 births have been saved by fetal monitoring (Table 13-5).[17–20] With

Table 13-5. ANALYTIC STUDIES OF INTRA-

Reference	No. without EFM*	No. with EFM
Chan and colleagues (1973)[17]	5427	1162
Paul and colleagues (1977)[18]	36,724 (low risk)	13,344 (high risk)
Tutera and Newman (1975)[19]	6179 (low risk)	608 (96% high risk)
Amato (1977)[20]	2981 (37% high risk)	4226 (46% high risk)

* EFM = electronic fetal monitoring.

† The numbers in parentheses are the actual numbers of intrapartum deaths.

more than 3,000,000 births per year in the United States, this translates into preventing 8000 intrapartum deaths. Prospective studies do not show comparable successes. It will take many patients to show a difference since mortality, even without monitoring, is, fortunately, low.

Respiratory distress syndrome is well recognized as a major contributor to fetal morbidity and mortality. Asphyxia in the immature baby less than 35 weeks of age may cause acidosis that, in turn, reduces production of lecithin, a surface active agent. If acidosis can be eliminated with monitoring, the incidence of respiratory distress syndrome should decrease. Neurologic damage leading to a severe neurologic deficit may also be reduced through electronic fetal monitoring. Two assumptions are made[21]: (1) that fetal monitoring could halve the prevalence of 1-minute Apgar scores under 6 and correspondingly increase the prevalence of 1-minute Apgar scores over 6, and (2) that the association between Apgar scores and neurologic outcome is causal, and a change in Apgar score would result in a change in incidence of neurologically damaged babies. These assumptions have led some to relate low Apgar scores to cerebral palsy, and express the hope that universal electronic monitoring will prevent up to one neurologic disaster per 1000 live births.

The major argument presented in opposition to electronic fetal monitoring relates to safety of fetus and parturient. Scalp abscess is the most common fetal complication of electronic monitoring. The incidence ranges from 0.3% to 5.4%. No systemic manifestations of the abscesses have been reported.[22]

Electronic fetal monitoring can also infect the mother. However, Gibbs found length of labor, number of vaginal examinations, and duration of ruptured membranes to be far more significant sources of maternal

PARTUM FETAL DEATH (IFD) RATES

IFD/1000 Births without EFM	IFD/1000 Births with EFM	Ratio	Comment
3.1 (17)†	1.7 (2)	1.8	>1500 g; congenital anomalies excluded
0.9 (34)	0.4 (6)	2.2	>1500 g; congenital anomalies and birth trauma excluded
6.0	1.6 (1)	3.7	
4.0 (12)	0.2 (1)	20.0	Congenital anomalies excluded

infection than internal monitoring.[22] With internal monitoring, injuries to uterus, intraperitoneal bleeding, and abscess formation occur, but quite rarely.

Many studies have addressed the problem of the apparent increased incidence of cesarean delivery and several have blamed the introduction of electronic fetal monitoring for this increase. A summary of these and other articles was presented at the Consensus Development Conference on Cesarean Section and are noted here:[23]

1. Fetal distress relates to many problems with potential for morbidity.
2. The diagnosis of fetal distress during the antenatal or intrapartum period is now made more frequently on the basis of new information and new technology.
3. This diagnosis is made for 1% of all births and accounts for 10% of cesarean births and 15% of the increase in the cesarean birth rates.
4. The precise diagnosis of fetal distress is still limited, despite the availability of electronic fetal monitoring and sampling of fetal scalp blood.
5. Intrapartum resuscitative intervention techniques, when successful, diminish the incidence of cesarean birth for fetal distress.
6. Intrapartum resuscitative techniques, when successful, alter the effects of fetal distress. Therefore, the infant's condition at birth may be normal despite an intrapartum diagnosis of fetal distress.

More recently, Levens and co-workers[24] showed that by using intrapartum electronic fetal monitoring only when the fetus was judged to be at high risk (including oxytocin stimulation of labor, dysfunctional labor, abnormal fetal heart rate, or meconium-stained amnistic fluid), the incidence of cesarean section increased somewhat. Also, perinatal outcome was not significantly different.

The Apgar Score

Once the baby is born, its physical status is assessed within 1 minute, and again in 5 minutes. For this, the "Apgar score" is now widely used. (For an excellent discussion of the evaluation of the neonate, see Sheila Cohen in Shnider and Levinson.[25]) The Apgar system scores are explained in Table 13-6.

Both 1-minute and 5-minute scores are important. A very low 1-minute score may presage neonatal death (up to 50%) and a 19% to 35% incidence of severe handicap for the survivors. A 5-minute score of 0 to 3 is also associated with a 59% neonatal mortality. If the newborns fail to bring their Apgar scores to normal within 20 minutes, the majority will suffer cerebral palsy.[27]

Table 13-6. THE APGAR SYSTEM[26]

Characteristic	Status	Score
Skin color	Blue, pale	0
	Body pink, extremities blue	1
	Completely pink	2
Heart rate	Absent	0
	Below 100	1
	Above 100	2
Reflex irritability	No response	0
	Grimace	1
	Cough, sneeze, or cry	2
Muscle tone	Limp	0
	Some flexion of extremities	1
	Active motion	2
Respiratory effort	Absent	0
	Slow, irregular	1
	Good, crying	2

Thus a "perfect baby" would have an Apgar score of 10, and a blue baby without heart rate, who does not respond, is limp, and makes no respiratory effort would have a 0.

While the Apgar score fails to identify many infants who have suffered intrauterine damage, a low score correlates with fetal acidemia.

REFERENCE

1. Lilien AA: Term intrapartum fetal death. Am J Obstet Gynecol 107:595, 1970
2. Antenatal Diagnosis. NIH Publication 80-1973. United States Department of Health, Education, and Welfare, III-23, 1977
3. Little WJ: On the influence of abnormal parturition, difficult labours, premature birth, and asphyxia neonatorum, on the mental and physical condition of the child, especially in relation to deformities. Trans Obstet Soc Lond 3:293, 1861
4. Aubrey R: Identification of the high-risk perinatal patient. In Aladjem S, Brown AK (eds): Perinatal Intensive Care, pp 63–94. St. Louis, CV Mosby, 1977
5. American College of Obstetricians and Gynecologists Technical Bulletin, p 44. Washington, American College of Obstetricians and Gynecologists, 1977
6. Lejumeau JA (deKergaradee): Memoire sur l'Auscultation. Applique l'Etude de la Grossesse. Paris, 1822
7. von Winckel FKLW: A Textbook of Obstetrics, Including the Pathology and Therapeutics of the Puerperal State. Philadelphia, P. Blakiston and Son Co, 1890
8. Benson RC, Shubeck F, Deutschberger J, et al: Fetal heart rate as a predictor

of fetal distress: A report from the collaborative project. Obstet Gynecol 32:259, 1968

9. Shnider SM, Levinson G: Anesthesia for Obstetrics, p 363. Baltimore, Williams & Wilkins, 1979
10. Hon EH: An Atlas of Fetal Heart Patterns. New Haven, Harty Press, 1968
11. Kubli FW, Hon EH, Khazin AF, et al: Observations on heart rate and pH in the human fetus during labor. Am J Obstet Gynecol 104:1190, 1969
12. Paul RH, Petrie RH: Fetal Intensive Care, pp 1–16. New Haven, William Mack, 1979
13. Mudler-Heubach E, Carltis SN, Edelstone DI: Sinusoidal fetal heart rate pattern following intrauterine fetal transfusion. Obstet Gynecol (Suppl) 43s:52, 1978
14. Sugarman RG, Rawlinson KF, Schifrin BS: Fetal arrhythmia. Obstet Gynecol 52:301, 1978
15. Schifrin BS, Dame L: Fetal heart patterns prediction of Apgar score. JAMA 219:1322, 1972
16. Miller FC, Paul RH: Intrapartum fetal heart rate monitoring. Clin Obstet Gynecol 21:561, 1978
17. Chan WH, Paul RH, Toews J: Intrapartum fetal monitoring maternal and fetal morbidity and perinatal mortality. Obstet Gynecol 41:7, 1973
18. Paul RH, Huey JR, Yaeger CF: Clinical fetal monitoring: Its effect on cesarean section rate and perinatal mortality: Five-year trends. Postgrad Med 61:160, 1977
19. Tutera G, Newman RL: Fetal monitoring: Its effect on the perinatal mortality and cesarean section rates and its complications. Am J Obstet Gynecol 122:750, 1975
20. Amato JC: Fetal monitoring in a community hospital: A statistical analysis. Obstet Gynecol 50:269, 1977
21. Antenatal Diagnosis. Report of a Consensus Development Conference. NIH Publication 80-1973. United States Department of Health, Education and Welfare, 1979
22. Gibbs RS, Jones PM, Wilder CJ: Internal fetal monitoring and maternal infection following cesarean section. A prospective study. Obstet Gynecol 52:193, 1978
23. Consensus Development Conference on Cesarean Childbirth, September 1980. United States Department of Health and Human Services, Public Health Service, NIH.
24. Leveno KJ, Cunningham FG, Nelson S, et al: A prospective comparison of selective and universal electronic fetal monitoring in 34,995 pregnancies. N Eng J Med 315:615:619, 1986
25. Cohen SE: Evaluation of the neonate. In Shnider SM, Levinson G (eds): Anesthesia for Obstetrics, pp 270–383. Baltimore, Williams & Wilkins, 1979
26. Apgar V: A proposal for a new method of evaluation of the newborn infant. Anesth Analg 32:260, 1953
27. The value of the Apgar score. Lancet 1:1393–1394, 1982

CHAPTER 14

Fluids and Electrolytes

Intraoperatively, we strive to balance fluids lost (hemorrhage, urine, sequestered in the blister of trauma) and infused, and to maintain (or reestablish) the normal composition of blood. Several simple and not-so-simple methods serve.

BLOOD

Volume

Blood volume ranges from about 9% of body weight in newborn infants to about 6% in women. Although blood volume can be measured with dyes and radioactively labeled proteins or cells, these measurements during surgical operations have been abandoned because the label seeps out with blood during hemorrhage, giving false readings.

Based on carefully performed studies of 150 adults, Hidalgo and co-workers have developed a formula by which to estimate blood volume from the patient's weight and height.[1] Figures 14-1 and 14-2 show nomograms that were obtained from the following formulas. For men:

$$TBV = 0.0236 \times H^{0.725} \times W^{0.425} - 1.229$$

For women:

$$TBV = 0.0248 \times H^{0.725} \times W^{0.425} - 1.954$$

TBV = total blood volume

H = height in centimeters

W = weight in kilograms

To convert pounds into kilograms, multiply the number of pounds by 0.454 and to convert inches into centimeters, multiply the number of inches by 2.54. Even though these nomograms seem scientifically respectable, the data are only rough guidelines. Edema, ascites, and differences in the body build or in the state of hydration strongly influence the relation of blood volume to height and weight.

The formula for body surface area (see Chap. 5) is similar to those for blood volume, except for the linear correction factor. It is, therefore, possible to plot blood volume against body surface area. Occasionally, we see patients in the operating room whose body surface area has already been determined, for instance in the cardiac catheterization laboratory. Figure 14-3 allows a quick estimation of blood volume when body surface area is known.

Although blood volume cannot be measured intraoperatively, a clinical impression of its adequacy can be gained by inspecting the patient. Pale mucous membrane, low arterial, central venous, and wedge pressures, and, often, but not invariably, tachycardia are important signs of a low blood volume.

Estimation of Blood Loss

The amount of blood lost during a surgical operation must be examined. A number of methods have been described; the simplest and most widely used approaches follow.

Inspection of Sponges

Have the circulating nurse display all the sponges from the operative field for inspection. Surgical sponges and laparotomy pads come in different qualities, thicknesses, and absorbencies. It is more difficult to estimate the amount of blood absorbed by the sponge if it was moist before use.

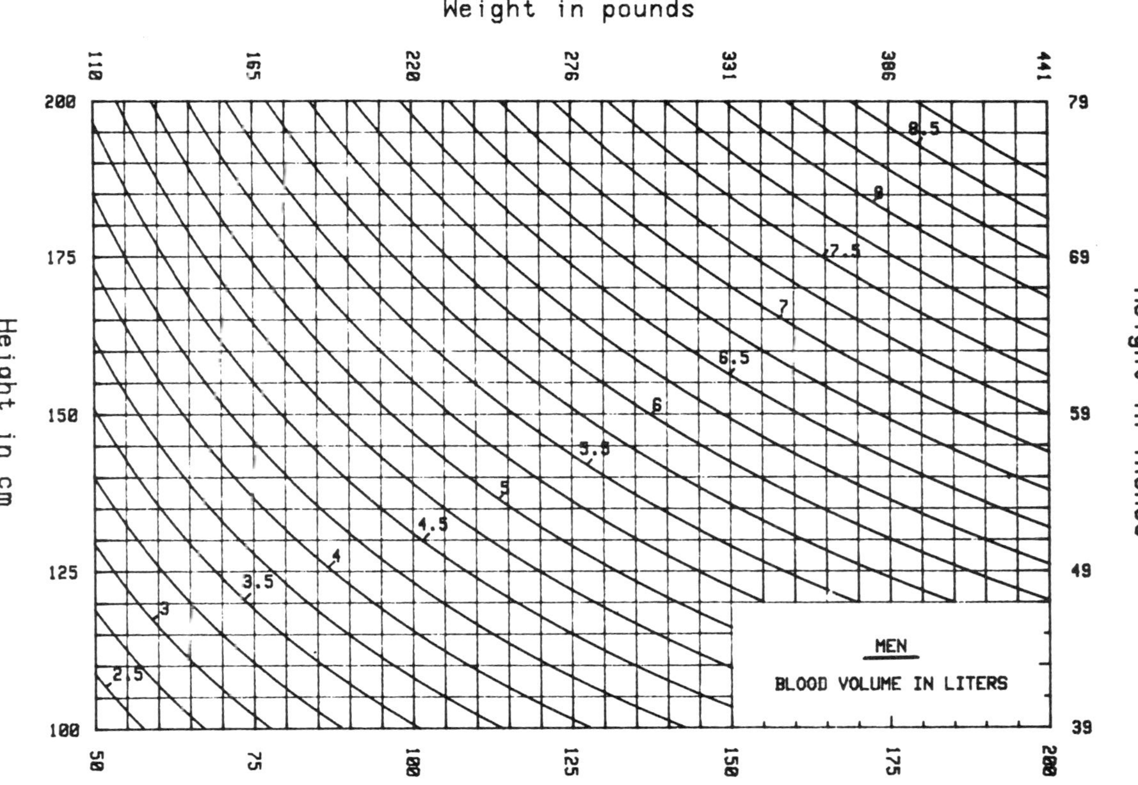

Figure 14-1. For a man, determine his height and weight and find approximate expected blood volume where the weight and height lines intersect. A 175-cm tall man weighing 75 kg has a blood volume of about 5 liters.

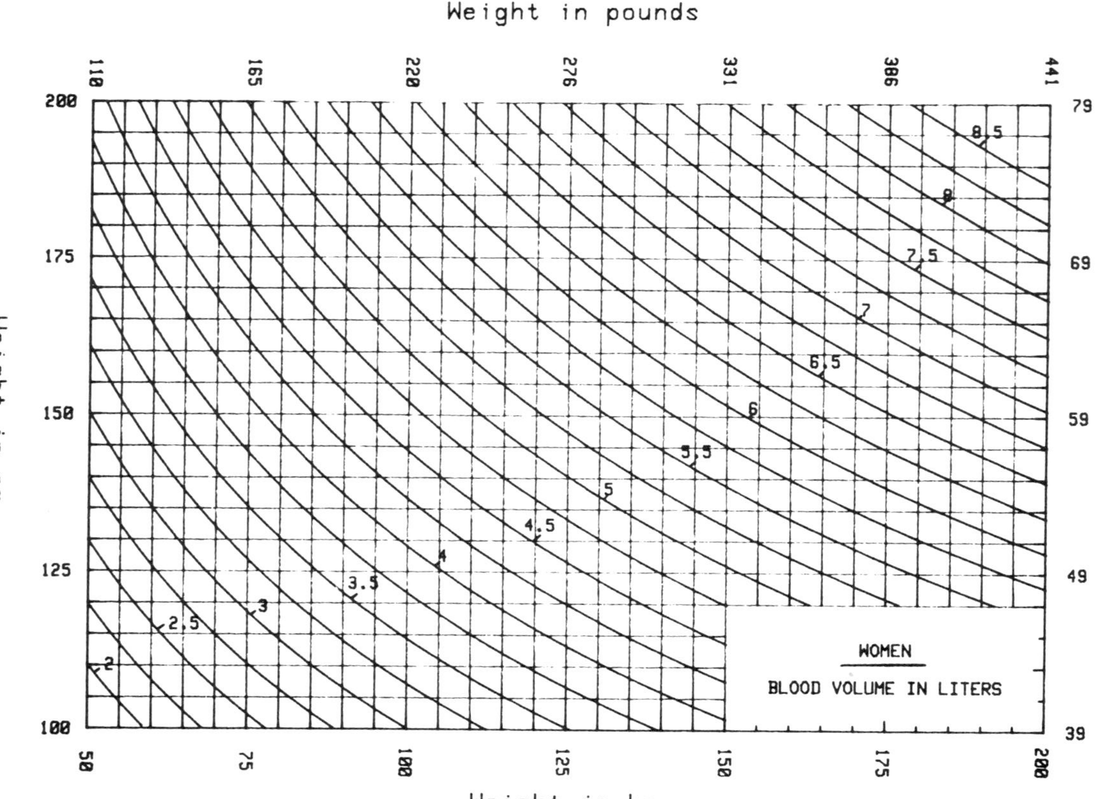

Figure 14-2. For a woman, determine her height and weight, and find the approximate expected blood volume where the weight and height lines intersect. A 160-cm tall woman weighing 75 kg has a blood volume of about 4.25 liters.

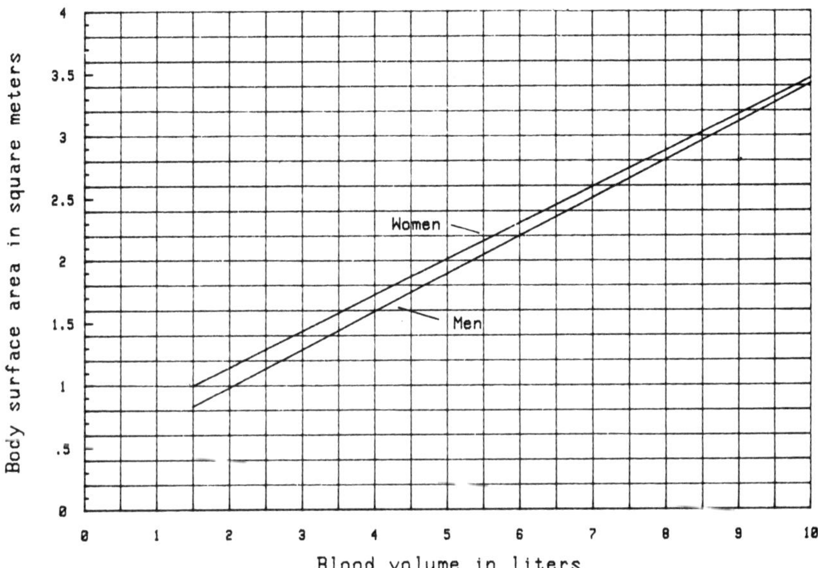

Figure 14-3. Since the formulas relating body weight and height to blood volume are similar to those relating body weight and height to cardiac index, a graph showing the estimate of blood volume as a function of surface area is shown.

Absorbent sponges may appear to be soaked with blood, yet can absorb even more blood before they begin to drip. Thus, the type of lap pads we use appear red and moist throughout after absorbing 100 ml of blood, but only after they soak up another 100 ml of blood do they begin to drip. Hanging in many operating rooms are photographs of the hospital's brand of sponges and lap pads soaked with more or less blood to help clinicians with estimation of blood loss. However, estimates by a visual inspection of sponges are subject to great error.

Weight of Sponges

Sponges and lap pads can be weighed. This method is cheap, simple, and quick. The difference in weight between dry and blood-soaked sponges can be expressed in milliliters of blood by assuming the relative density of blood to be 1. A simple kitchen scale can be used for this. Two precautions have to be taken. First, the sponges must be weighed as soon as possible because they will lose weight by evaporation. Second, premoistened sponges present a problem, but this can be overcome by measuring the solution used by the scrub nurse for wetting the sponges. A graduated vessel with sterile saline used only for wetting sponges will

Table 14-1. NORMAL BLOOD COMPONENT VALUES*

	Hematocrit	Hemoglobin
Newborn	56	18
3 months	35	11.5
1 year	36	12
6 years	40	13.5
Female adults	41	14
Male adults	44	15

* Many healthy adults have hematocrits below 40% and hemoglobin values below 14 g/dl.

serve. The amount of fluid disappearing from this container is then subtracted from the blood volume calculated by weighing the sponges.

Other Methods of Estimating Blood Loss

More complex systems have been described. These call for the extraction of hemoglobin or electrolytes from the sponges—and at the end of the operation also from drapes and gowns—by using washing machines and then measuring the color or electrical conductivity of the suspension. These expensive systems also do not account for blood sequestered in traumatized tissue and pooling on the floor or under plastic drapes.

Measuring blood collected in suction bottles is a simple matter if the blood is not diluted with irrigating solution or if the scrub nurse keeps track of how much irrigation solution has been used by the surgeon.

An old clinical rule of thumb says that one should add 25% to any estimate, whether of blood loss, or of the expected duration of the operation.

Blood Components

Hematocrit

HEMATOCRIT VALUES

Always inquire about the hemoglobin content or the hematocrit of blood before anesthesia (Table 14-1).

Several factors affect the hematocrit:

- Fluids given intravenously, depending on their composition, decrease (electrolyte solution, plasma, plasma expanders) or increase (packed red cells) the hematocrit.

- Fluids lost during the surgical procedure may consist of the patient's blood, urine, and fluids from body cavities. Some fluid is lost by evaporation.
- Fluids may shift from one compartment to another during anesthesia and operation. Procedures on the bowel often cause fluids to accumulate in the intestinal lumen, the mesentery, and the wall of the bowel. Blood and plasma may be trapped in traumatized muscle or other extravascular spaces. Edema may form in lungs or the peritoneal cavity. Interstitial fluid may move into the vascular compartment. Since these processes go on simultaneously and at different rates, it is difficult to interpret a drop or rise in hematocrit. Viscosity and oxygen-carrying capacity of a unit of blood decrease when hematocrit decreases; however, it cannot be assumed that blood volume decreases in the same proportion. It may have increased, remained the same, or decreased, depending on fluid therapy and how each of the factors mentioned contributes to the outcome.

An additional, important complexity is introduced by the relationship of intravascular to extravascular compartments. Cells, proteins, and substances such as dextran or hetastarch tend to remain within the vascular system if the surgeon does not drain them through the incision and if they do not leak out through damaged capillaries. Electrolyte and dextrose solutions freely equilibrate with the interstitial, extravascular compartment, which usually has about three times the volume of the intravascular compartment.

Hematocrit values must be interpreted in the light of other clinical evidence. For instance, an elevated hematocrit suggests that the patient may be dehydrated; conversely, a low hematocrit suggests possible overhydration. However, the high hematocrit may simply reflect an ample blood volume and a low hematocrit anemia. In infants a low tissue turgor may suggest 5% dehydration, sunken fontanels 10%, and sunken eyes 20% dehydration. Adults are suspected to be dehydrated or low in blood volume if their blood pressure falls when sitting up in bed.

No reliable, yet simple measurement is available to assess blood loss intraoperatively and, thus, fix the time when blood needs to be transfused. Some suggest giving electrolyte or colloid solution in quantities sufficient to maintain a normal cardiovascular function and to give red cells (packed cells or whole blood) when the hematocrit falls below 30%. Others recommend the use of formulas, such as the one published by Gross.[2] This formula equates the allowable blood loss (V_L) to the estimated blood volume (EBV) of the patient multiplied by a ratio of the permissible *de-*

crease of hematocrit to the *average* between the initial and the minimal allowable hematocrit. The formula is

$$\text{EBV} \times \frac{H_0 - H_f}{H_{av}} = V_L$$

where

V_L = allowable blood loss

EBV = patient's estimated blood volume (see Figs 15.1 and 15.2)

H_0 = patient's initial hematocrit concentration

H_f = patient's minimal allowable hematocrit concentration

$H_{av} = (H_0 + H_f)/2$

Assume a patient with an estimated blood volume of 5 liters and set a minimal allowable hematocrit of, for instance, 28%. Let the patient's initial hematocrit be 39%. The allowable blood loss could then be calculated as follows:

$$5 \times \frac{39 - 28}{\left(\frac{39 + 28}{2}\right)} = 1.6$$

With another calculation one can approach the question from the other end, namely how much whole blood or packed cells must be administered to change the hematocrit by a desired amount?[3]

ml transfusion required = desired change in hematocrit × kg × factor

where kg is the weight of the patient.

The factor varies with the volume of blood per body weight. For a rough estimate, the following figures (assuming 100 ml blood/kg for infants and 70 ml blood/kg for adults) can be used:

	Packed cells	**Whole blood**
	(Hct 70%)	(Hct 40%)
Children under two	1.5	2.5
Children over two and adults	1.0	1.75

Thus, for an adult with a hematocrit of 28% and weighing 70 kg, how much whole blood would be required to bring the hematocrit to 35%? Given the desired change of 7% in the hematocrit:

$$7 \times 70 \times 1.75 = 858 \text{ ml}$$

Clearly, these estimates provide only guidelines, but they are useful in gaining an idea of the approximate magnitude of transfusions required to approach a desired goal.

HEMATOCRIT DETERMINATIONS

Arterial, venous, or capillary blood may be used for hematocrit determinations. A standard method is now the *microhematocrit*, which employs a capillary tube treated with heparin. When blood is drawn from the artery or vein, but spinning is delayed, an anticoagulant has to be used. This should be EDTA or balanced oxalate, because other anticoagulants affect cell volume. When drawing blood from an arterial catheter, be sure that the first sample withdrawn, still containing some of the flushing solution, is not analyzed. Venous blood should not be drawn from a site proximal to an IV catheter through which blood or other fluids are being administered. This is an obvious precaution, yet we tend to forget about it. Capillary sticks are used, particularly, in infants. After lancing a heel or finger, wipe off the first drop of blood and allow spontaneous bleeding. Keep in mind that squeezing the tissue dilutes the blood, reducing hematocrit. Capillary blood already has a slightly lower hematocrit than venous or arterial blood.

Do not stick earlobes. Hemostasis is sometimes difficult in this area. When using the finger, do not stick the center of the finger pad. It is more sensitive than the side. Bring the unmarked end of the microhematocrit capillary into contact with blood and let capillary action perform its feat of sucking blood up. Fill the capillary to roughly two-thirds and seal the end of the tube with a dab of clay. Leave the other end open. Put the capillary into a centrifuge, the closed end firmly seated against a rubber stopper, the open end facing inward. Spin the sample as long as is recommended, usually 3 minutes to 5 minutes. Centrifuges differ in their force; therefore, it is important to follow the instructions that come with the instrument. After spinning, the hematocrit is read on an appropriate reader supplied by different manufacturers. The hematocrit is expressed in terms of the red cell volume as a percentage of the total sample volume.

An interesting relationship between hematocrit and bleeding time must be remembered. The increased bleeding time observed in anemic patients can be shortened by nothing more than elevating the hematocrit with the help of washed red cells. Conversely, a high hematocrit may predispose to clotting—even intravascularly. Thus, monitoring the hematocrit perioperatively and keeping it within a normal range may help in the management of clotting disorders.[4]

Bleeding and Clotting: Testing During Anesthesia

During anesthesia, unusual oozing and bleeding sometimes arise in patients who gave no history of bleeding or clotting disturbances, and in whom there was no reason for detailed preoperative studies. When this happens, draw blood from a fresh vein. Once again, do not draw blood from a vein proximal to an intravenous infusion site. Order the necessary tests from the hematologic laboratory. These will include prothrombin time (PT) and a partial thromboplastin time (PTT) to screen for deficiencies in the coagulation factors. The platelet count should be over 100,000 platelets/mm^3. When indicated, plasma fibrinogen levels should be determined.

While the aforementioned tests are underway, you can concurrently perform several simple tests during anesthesia:

Capillary Fragility

On the arm not being used for intravenous therapy or invasive monitoring, mark all nevi and petechiae with a pen. Then, inflate a blood pressure cuff to mean blood pressure or to about 90 torr, whichever is lower, and keep it there for 5 minutes. Then, count the new, unmarked petechiae. In 5 minutes, recount them. Up to 20 new petechiae are normal. Petechiae developing under the cuff are discounted. This is called the *Rumpel–Leede test*, during which many petechiae develop in patients with vasculitis, connective tissue disease, and some platelet abnormalities.

Bleeding Time

Apply a blood pressure cuff to the arm not used for intravenous therapy or invasive monitoring and inflate the cuff to 40 torr. Prepare the skin with alcohol as for an IV puncture and let it dry. Then make two punctures about 2 cm apart, each about 3 mm long and 2 mm deep, but not over a vein. Touch the blood, but not the wound, with filter paper every 30 seconds so that the blood is absorbed. Bleeding should cease in about 5 minutes. Bleeding for 8 minutes or more is abnormal. This is known as *Ivy bleeding time*, which is prolonged in patients who have taken aspirin, who are thrombocytopenic, or who are under the influence of anticoagulants.

Clotting Time

Obtain 3 ml of blood without tissue trauma, meaning from an established arterial catheter or, if a new vessel is punctured, from the second rather than the first syringe. Place 1 ml each into three clean, dry, test tubes kept at 37°C in a water bath. Tilt the first tube every 30 seconds until the blood no longer flows. Do the same to the second, and finally, to the third. Record the time before the blood in each tube clotted. Normally the time for this *Lee–White test* lies between 9 minutes to 14 minutes. Clotting time is prolonged when anticoagulants are used or when a severe deficiency in clotting factor exists.

A simple version of this test is often used and is known as the "*tube-on-the-wall*" *test*. For this, 5 ml of blood are placed in a dry tube taped to the wall so that the tube is not shaken and is kept at room temperature. If no clot forms in 10 minutes, anticoagulants are present, or fibrin or clotting factors absent. A clot should retract within 2 hours. If it fails to do this, severe thrombocytopenia may exist. If the clot forms and then dissolves, fibrinolysins may be at work or fibrinogen may be very deficient. This test is recommended as a rough screen for patients suspected of having disseminated intravascular coagulopathy (DIC) or in whom it might develop. If the supernatant serum is pink or red, hemolysis is present, check for compatibility of transfused blood and other factors leading to red cell destruction.

The Activated Coagulation Time Test

When heparin is used for cardiovascular operations, the adequacy of anticoagulation and, subsequently, of the degree of heparin reversal needs to be monitored. The activated coagulation time (ACT) can be measured in the operating room and is helpful even though, in hypothermia and hemodilution, it becomes inaccurate.[5] Commercially available analyzers make the test quite simple, and the ACT reflects the overall status of coagulation.

The presence of other factors influencing the coagulation time is also reflected in the ACT; thus, platelet activity affects ACT.[6] This is clinically desirable as it leads the clinician to adjust heparin and protamine therapy to the needs of the patient. With heparin therapy, a dose-dependent lengthening of coagulation time is observed. For bypass we maintain the ACT at or near 400 seconds. Remember that it takes at least 20 minutes before an agent injected intravenously is completely mixed with the entire blood volume. For patients with low cardiac output, it can take much longer.

Heparin Biotitration

The amount of heparin in a given sample of blood can be determined by an automated titration system, for instance the Heparin Analyzer.* The manufacturer makes available test cartridges that contain the reagents necessary for testing; that is, protamine solutions in different concentrations are shown on the cartridge label. Typically, a cartridge consists of

* HemoTec, Inc., Englewood, Colorado

four chambers into each of which 1.5 ml of whole blood is injected. The automated analyzer then bubbles air through all chambers, mixing the protamine solutions with the blood sample and enhancing the formation of a clot. The system then uses a photo-cell assembly to detect the chamber in which the first clot has formed. The ratio of protamine to heparin in this chamber is assumed to be nearest to the neutralization point. With a bit of microprocessor wizardry the unit then displays the clotting time in minutes and seconds and, if desired, other data. For instance, the analyzer contains formulas for blood volumes in men and women. The height and weight of the patient can be entered, and the system will present an estimated blood volume as well as the amount (in milligrams) of protamine needed to complete the neutralization of heparin or, conversely, the dosage of heparin needed to reestablish a desired level of heparinization.

Dextrans and other surfactants in blood may interfere with the assay. The resolution capability of the assay cartridges ranges from 30 units to 50 units of heparin per kilogram of body weight, depending on the selected cartridge. Cartridges come in different strengths. Unfortunately, they have a limited shelf life of 60 days when maintained under refrigeration.

Thromboelastogram

It is also possible to assess the fibrin clot in blood or plasma. Since the formation of the clot depends on the balance of a number of cellular components and clotting factors, the definition of the clot's formation, strength, and persistence describes the entire clotting system and thus allows clinical conclusions about the adequacy of the clotting mechanism or the success of anticoagulation (or its reversal). A commercially available unit, the Thrombelastograph,* makes these measurements available to clinicians in the intensive care unit or the operating room.

The unit's operation relies on the principle that a pin inserted into a cup filled with plasma or blood will not be influenced by any motion of the cup as long as nothing but liquid blood or plasma links cup with pin. Once fibrin strands form between pin and cup, oscillations of the cup are transmitted to the pin. These forces acting on the pin are then recorded and form a so-called thromboelastogram. In Figure 14-4 we see the straight line drawn by the recording system as long as no fibrin strand is sensed. As strands form, the cup's oscillations are transmitted to the pin and the recording assumes the outline of a suppository. The bulge of this suppository reflects the time of strongest fibrin development, and much later its narrower tail end reflects the dissolving of the clot. In case of early narrowing, fibrinolysis must be suspected. Delayed formation of the sup-

* Litton Datamedix, Sharon, Massachusetts

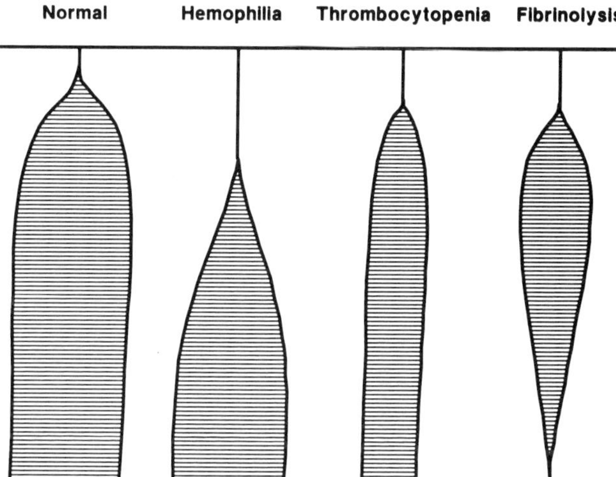

Figure 14-4. Thromboelastograms. A sensitive pin is positioned in an oscillating cup filled with the blood or plasma. When fibrin strands begin to tug on the pin, a record is generated. The time axis runs from top to bottom, therefore examine first the point (top) of the thromboelastogram before the pin is hindered by fibrin. As more fibrin gradually forms, the thromboelastogram grows fatter. The forms show the typical changes with the indicated conditions.

pository's shape suggests a clotting disorder such as hemophilia; a narrow one, thrombocytopenia; a fat one, hypercoagulability. The system has been praised by some as being clinically useful (*e.g.*, in patients undergoing liver transplants, where major shifts in fibrinogen–fibrin homeostasis and clotting disorders are common) and criticized by others as being too nonspecific as it fails to identify the specific factors that can lead to an abnormal thromboelastogram.

Osmometry

The particles in solution in blood and urine that contribute to their osmotic pressure may undergo significant shifts during anesthesia, for instance, when the concentration of glucose or ketones rises in a diabetic patient.

The osmotic pressure is measured in milliosmols (mOsm). An *osmolar* solution contains 1 osmol per liter of solution. An *osmolal* solution contains 1 osmol per kilogram of solution.

The osmolality is best measured by freezing point depression—a laboratory procedure. Each particle in a solution contributes to its molality, and thus to its osmolality. For salts that dissociate, each mole of, for instance, NaCl, contributes 2 osmols. In the body, NaCl is only about

93% dissociated. The osmolality of sodium chloride is therefore equal to 1.86 times the molality.[8]

The osmolality of blood becomes important when gradients are generated that cause fluids to shift from a compartment of low osmolality to one of high osmolality. In clinical practice this is seen when mannitol or hypertonic saline is administered; the intravascular osmolality is raised above that of the intracellular compartment; that is, the tonicity of the two compartments is not equal, one being hypertonic to the other. In another common example, the osmolality of blood may be raised by the ingestion of alcohol; however, the intravascular compartment may remain isotonic to the intracellular compartment as alcohol freely crosses the cell membranes. An assessment of osmolality gives no clue to the relative tonicity of the solution.

The most important solutes contributing to osmolality are sodium and its anions, glucose, and urea. Since these can be measured chemically by direct means, a freezing point determination may seem superfluous. However, when the calculated osmolality does not agree reasonably well with the measured osmolality, one must suspect the presence of substances not measured in blood. These may be ethyl alcohol, mannitol, methanol, ethylene glycol, or other substances of low molecular weight. Another possibility is that the serum water is unusually low, as for instance in the presence of substances replacing water, such as with hyperlipidemia or hyperproteinemia. Thus, whenever there is an indication to order a freezing point depression, it is desirable to calculate the approximate osmolality of blood. This is done as follows:

glucose: take mg per 100 ml × 10/180 = mmol/l

blood urea: take mg per 100 ml × 10/28 = mmol/l

sodium: mEq/l × 2 = electrolytes in mmol/l

(The sodium salts are assumed to be only 93% ionized, but serum contains only about 93% water. These factors cancel, on the average, and one can therefore simply use the absolute values in milliequivalents per liter for the sodium salts.)

For normal blood containing Na 140 mEq/l (together with its anions representing 280 mOsm), glucose 90 mg/dl (5 mOsm), and blood urea nitrogen 14 mg/dl (5 mOsm), the osmolality is calculated as 290 mOsm. Whenever the discrepancy between the value thus calculated and the one measured by freezing point depression exceeds 10 mOsm, a laboratory error or the presence of factors not assessed (such as alcohol or mannitol) must be suspected.

These considerations pay dividends in the emergency room, when a patient in coma is admitted who may have ingested, for instance, ethylene glycol or methanol. The freezing point may then be more than 10 mOsm higher than values calculated from sodium, urea, or glucose. In the operating room during transurethral prostatectomy, the sodium values may fall acutely as sodium-free water enters the vascular system. If glycine is used, once again there may be a discrepancy between freezing point depression and calculated osmolality. In diabetics with hyperglycemia, the calculated and freezing point osmolalities may be in good agreement and, depending on the levels of sodium and urea, may show elevated levels.

Finally, it must be mentioned that sodium and glucose do not cross the cell membranes as readily as is true for urea and some other substances that exert osmotic pressures (such as alcohol). Thus, it is possible to have an osmotic gradient across the cell membrane, leading to shifts in water across the cell membranes even though the total osmotic pressure in serum may be normal. It is therefore useful to recalculate the osmolality of serum, reckoning only sodium and glucose. A patient in renal failure may have a normal total osmolality of 290 mOsm/kg (Na 124 mmol/l, blood urea nitrogen 98 mg/dl, glucose 90 mg/dl) but a reduced effective osmolality, which becomes apparent when the urea is omitted from the calculation, revealing an effective osmolality of only 255 mOsm/kg. This shows the excess of water present in this patient and the relative hypotonicity of his serum.

A poor man's substitute is the simple measurement of the total solids in plasma or urine by using a small, hand-held refractometer (T-S Meter*). This optical instrument is scaled to allow a direct reading of urine, relative density, or light refraction of serum or plasma.

Tables permit a conversion of the refraction index into, for example, percentage of total solids. The total solids are made up of salts, proteins, glucose, and lipids. Thus, while there does not have to be a direct, linear relationship to osmolality, in many clinical situations the solids and osmolality are parallel. When, during infusion therapy, the percentage of total solids in plasma changes, further investigations are in order. Relative density of urine is usually not monitored during anesthesia. Should the need arise, this handy instrument will serve for a quick, on-the-spot analysis.

Electrolytes

It has become feasible, intraoperatively, to measure some electrolytes repeatedly. This is often practiced during transurethral resection of the prostate, during which large volumes of electrolyte-free solution may gain access to the patient's circulation through open venous channels in the

* American Optical, Buffalo, New York

prostatic bed.* The irrigation solution used by the urologist is either distilled water or a 1.2% to 2.5% glycine solution. Any of these solutions dilute the electrolyte components of blood. Distilled water and 1.2% glycine are hypotonic and, therefore, also produce shifts of extracellular water into the intracellular space. Two and one-half percent glycine is approximately isotonic and, therefore, not associated with fluid shifts, but acts as a simple diluent.

Because acutely induced hyponatremia and hypokalemia may disturb the cardiovascular and central nervous systems profoundly, monitoring sodium and potassium concentrations in blood during these operations is recommended.

Sodium

Sodium levels in normal serum are between 135 mEq/l and 148 mEq/l. During transurethral prostatic resections and percutaneous nephrolithotomy or nephrolithotripsy, these levels may fall to 115 mEq/l, sometimes even within 15 minutes. The patient may be confused, complain of chest pain, and show wide QRS complexes and elevated ST segments on the ECG. With even lower levels, near 100 mEq/l, seizures may occur. Ventricular tachycardia or fibrillation may supervene when the sodium falls below 100 mEq/l.

Potassium

Potassium levels are often monitored during cardiopulmonary bypass. Changes in *p*H may be associated with shifts in potassium, an alkalosis resulting in hypokalemia or an acidosis in hyperkalemia. These shifts amount to roughly 0.3 mEq/l to 0.6 mEq/l of potassium per 0.1 *p*H unit. Patients with normal potassium concentrations usually tolerate such shifts in *p*H well. For patients who are digitalized or who initially have borderline values of potassium, in other words, values outside the normal range of 3.5 mEq/l to 5.3 mEq/l, the shifts in *p*H may be more dangerous. Hyperventilation, with resultant respiratory alkalosis, can lead to cardiac arrest in hypokalemic patients. Chronic hypokalemia (as induced by diuretic medication, for example) may also render resuscitation more difficult, or impossible, in cases of hypoxia.[9]

A careful method of collecting blood for potassium analysis is particularly important because hemolysis of only 0.5% of red cells can increase serum potassium by 0.5 mEq/l. Rapid withdrawal of blood through

* Large volumes of irrigation fluid may also gain access to the patient's vascular system during transcutaneous nephrolithotomy. This may lead to cardiovascular changes, but—as long as physiologic solutions are used—not to shifts in electrolytes.

a small needle causes hemolysis. Muscular exercise may also elevate the potassium concentration. It is, therefore, not advisable to have a patient "pump his hand" in order to make the veins stand out before drawing blood. This exercise of the arm with a venous tourniquet may increase potassium in the plasma by roughly 10%.

Hill and colleagues found that the presence of heparin in the sample can reduce the potassium concentration by dilution if too much heparin has been used, and also by a specific and unexplained heparin effect.[10] In order to minimize this problem, sampling syringes should be wetted with heparin and all excess heparin ejected before aspirating blood from veins or arteries. Platelets are rich in potassium. During clotting platelets release potassium. Serum may therefore contain 0.1 mEq/l to 0.7 mEq/l more potassium that plasma or whole blood with intact red cells.

Calcium

Calcium occurs both in a bound and an unbound form; the latter is frequently referred to as *ionized calcium*. Since the ionized calcium is believed to be responsible for the physiologic effectiveness of calcium, this fraction is of greater interest to the clinician than the total serum calcium. The amount of calcium available in the free, ionized form depends on the *p*H and on the amount of protein available to which calcium can bind. Normal values of ionized calcium are 2.1 mmol/l to 2.6 mmol/l. Since *p*H so powerfully affects the degree of ionized calcium, care must be taken not to alter the *p*H of blood to be analyzed for calcium. Blood drawn for measurements of ionized calcium is, therefore, best handled with the same anaerobic technique as for measurements of *p*H.

Methods of Measurement

Clinical laboratories usually measure electrolytes in serum. Blood is allowed to clot, and the remaining serum is analyzed. *Plasma* is the cell-free liquid that contains the clotting factors. When time permits, let the laboratory do the analyses. No operating room can afford to duplicate the facilities of a clinical laboratory, or attempt to exercise the quality control of a trained staff of experts in different fields.

Many intensive care units and operating rooms have their own automated analyzers for electrolyte determinations. These devices calibrate and clean themselves, are rapid, and are quite precise. They can use whole blood plasma or serum.

Automated analyzers use a potentiometer and ion-selective electrodes (ISEs), resembling little batteries, that develop a voltage when the concentration of the electrolytes in the sensing electrode increases. The principle is similar to that of the *p*H electrode (see "Measurement of *p*H";

Chap. 12). In order to make each electrode specific to one species of ion, special membranes are used that permit only one species to migrate across the membrane to the electrode. For sodium analysis, for instance, a sodium-selective glass is employed.

Recently, small analyzers have become available that are light in weight and use disposable test cards that make analysis for *p*H, K^+, and Na^+ even simpler and quite rapid.* The system also uses ISEs.

ISEs have the advantage over flame photometers in cases of hyperlipidemia or hyperproteinemia, conditions in which some of the plasma water has been displaced by other components. Flame photometers measure the concentration of ions in a volume of plasma, whereas ISEs report the activity of the electrolytes in the plasma water proper.

The serum samples should not be left exposed to air because after 2 hours the evaporation of serum water will cause sodium and potassium to read 6.9 and 0.23 mEq/l higher, respectively, than in an immediately analyzed sample, while bicarbonate falls in that time span by about 3.5 mmol/l. This divergent shift of electrolytes versus bicarbonate exaggerates the effect of dehydration on the anion gap, which may increase by 6.5 mmol/l in 2 hours.[11]

The Anion Gap

The anion gap is often calculated from the serum values for sodium, potassium, chloride, and bicarbonate. Under normal circumstances the sum of the concentrations of the two principal cations, namely sodium (140 mEq/l) and potassium (5 mEq/l), equals the concentration of the measured anion, namely chloride (100 mEq/l), plus the calculated bicarbonate (25 mEq/l), plus the estimated anions contributed by proteins, sulfates, and phosphates. On the one hand, a normal anion gap can be expressed as zero, when the *estimated* anions are *in*cluded in the reckoning; on the other hand, a normal anion gap would be about 25 mE/l when the *estimated* anions are *ex*cluded. When the sum of the cation concentrations exceeds that of the anions so calculated, one must assume that a new species of anion (*e.g.*, lactate) has been added. Thus, an anion gap usually bespeaks the presence of organic acids normally not present. The calculation of the anion gap is an easy bedside exercise that can help the clinician to monitor the patient's metabolic progress. However, one must be aware that a shift in acid–base status may affect the anion gap even in the absence of unexpected organic acids. The presence of acidemia will cause the anion gap to appear smaller than it really is, while alkalemia does the opposite.[12]

* Sentech, Arden Hills, Minnesota

Glucose

Normal values for glucose range from 70 mg/dl to 105 mg/dl of plasma. Arterial and capillary concentrations of glucose may be 5 mg/dl higher in the fasting state than is true for venous blood glucose. Blood glucose is about 5 mg/dl lower than plasma glucose.

Glucose in fasting patients is sometimes low. Hypoglycemia during the induction of anesthesia is of sufficient concern that many anesthesiologists use a glucose-containing solution intravenously for the initial fluid therapy. With rapid infusion of a liter of solution containing 5% glucose (50 g), blood glucose may rise to 250 mg/dl or more. In patients with diabetes, much higher levels can occur if insulin is insufficient.

Chemical laboratories have a number of good methods of measuring blood glucose. In the operating room, test strips (Dextrostix, Chemstrip, and others) are widely used and quite helpful. The strips are treated with enzymes that convert glucose and produce a color change. These tests provide a useful way to estimate ranges of glucose. It is important to adhere to the manufacturer's recommendations for best results. Capillary, venous, or arterial blood, rather than serum or plasma, can be used, but should not contain anticoagulants with fluoride; this interferes with the reaction. The blood should be at room temperature.

Instead of assessing the color change visually, several instruments can measure the color change by reflectant colorimetry. The instruments are small, electrically powered, portable units that cover a range from 10 mg/dl to approximately 400 mg/dl, and have an accuracy of approximately 5% to 10% better than that of the visual method within that concentration range. The manufacturers supply calibration methods. For intraoperative checking of blood glucose, these little instruments are sufficiently accurate, very convenient, and quite inexpensive. Determinations of blood glucose can be made within a few minutes.

URINE

Volume and Relative Density

Catheterization of the bladder is not without complications. Infection from an indwelling catheter can lead to a chronic, smoldering urinary tract infection that, after years, may lead to an ascending pyelonephritis. Nevertheless, in major surgical procedures when monitoring renal function is essential or when large volumes of fluid are given intravenously, the bladder must be catheterized. The common method is to insert a soft, rubber, Foley catheter, taking appropriate surgical precautions for sterility. The catheter is connected to a closed, sterile, disposable collection system placed so that the anesthesiologist can watch the volume of the urine accumulating during the operation. Since contamination is possible, good practice calls for a precaution: keep the collecting bag and the collecting tubes of the catheter system below the level of the bladder so that no urine can flow back into the bladder. Reflux occurs when no one watches for it, for example, during positioning or transferring the patient from a table to a stretcher.

An alternative method deserves attention. Instead of inserting a catheter through the urethra, it is possible to insert a plastic catheter through a large-bore needle placed into the full bladder suprapubically, after surgical preparation of the skin. A plastic catheter is advanced through the needle into the bladder and the needle is withdrawn. The urethral mucosa is not traumatized and no nidus for infection in the urethra is produced. The catheter can be left in place postoperatively for hours or days, and the patient can begin to void before the catheter is removed. The incidence of infection with this method is said to be lower than that with transurethral indwelling catheters.[13]

Intraoperative urine volumes are frequently kept at 1 ml/kg/hr. These volumes indicate a urine production greater than that in healthy people who regulate their own fluid intake. While a volume of 1 ml/kg/hr appears to be well tolerated and certainly demonstrates brisk renal function, lower volumes are acceptable. The average adult excretes approximately 1200 ml of water a day in urine, but not less than 500 ml. An entirely normal urine production, therefore, could be 50 ml/hr. Even 30 ml/hr is well within physiologic ranges for a healthy adult weighing 70 kg. Without a good indication (*e.g.*, malignant hyperpyrexia or barbiturate poisoning), there is no benefit in pushing urine production intraoperatively to more than 1 ml/kg/hr. When large volumes of fluids are given intraoperatively and when the bladder cannot empty itself, cardiovascular symptoms may appear in lightly anesthetized patients. Hypertension produced by an overdistended bladder is sometimes seen during light anesthesia or early after the operation. The arterial pressure quickly returns to normal when the urine is drained by means of a catheter.

Urine volume must be assessed in the light of urine relative density, which is easily determined with a gravimometer, a small float that will swim more or less immersed in urine, depending on its relative density. Assuming normal kidney function—not always a safe assumption in patients in the intensive care unit or the operating room—a dilute urine with relative density under 1.007 coupled with a brisk diuresis suggests overhydration, whereas scant urine and a relative density at or above 1.025 suggest dehydration. A relative density of between 1.014 and 1.018 is desirable as it suggests that the kidneys are functioning adequately and that hydration lies in a normal range.

In both the intensive care unit and the operating room we encounter patients with renal disease. Urine volume, relative density, and glucose content may then no longer reflect prerenal conditions, but may be affected by the kidney's inability to fulfill its normal role. In the acute monitoring phase under discussion in this text, information about urinary electrolytes assists in making the diagnosis of renal failure, particularly acute tubular necrosis, a condition of special concern in the intensive care unit and the operating room. In the urine of patients with normal renal function and normal electrolyte intake, we should find 75 mEq/l to 100 mEq/l of sodium and an equal amount of chloride as well as 20 mEq/l to 30 mEq/l of potassium. The term F_{ENa} stands for the fractional excretion of filtered sodium and allows us to differentiate between prerenal azotemia (F_{ENa} is smaller than 1) and acute renal failure (F_{ENa} is larger than 5). The term gives the value of the ratio of urinary (U_{Na}) to plasma sodium (P_{Na}) in percent multiplied by the ratio of plasma creatinine (P_{Creat}) to urinary creatinine (U_{Creat}) according to the formula

$$F_{ENa} = \frac{(U_{Na}) \times (P_{Creat})}{(P_{Na}) \times (U_{Creat})}$$

In patients with healthy kidneys who take no added salt in their diet the percentage should be close to 1.

The excreted fraction of filtered sodium (F_{ENa}) is informative only in patients who already have a lowered rate of urine production. Shin and co-workers report that renal dysfunction and perhaps even acute renal failure must be anticipated in patients who have a normal rate of urine production but whose creatinine clearance falls to less than 25 ml/min within 6 hours after trauma, anesthesia, and operation.[14]

Glucose in Urine

In addition to measuring the volume of urine, sometimes it is necessary to check the concentration of glucose. In the operating room, an easy and quick test is the Clinitest. For this, five drops of fresh urine are placed by a medicine dropper into a dry test tube. The dropper is then rinsed with water and ten drops of water are added to the test tube. Next, one Clinitest tablet (Ames) is dropped into the test tube. A chemical reaction results. Allow this to proceed without shaking the tube and wait for 15 seconds after it has stopped. Shake the tube gently and compare the color of the urine sample with the color chart provided by the company. Remember that many patients who are not diabetic can spill sugar in their urine. The renal threshold for glucose in otherwise healthy patients is around 180 mg/dl. With the rapid intravenous infusion of glucose-containing solutions, these values can easily be exceeded. It is, therefore, not advisable to put a patient receiving intravenous glucose on the "sliding scale," which calls for the administration of insulin, depending on the amount of glucose detected in urine.

MONITORING APPROACHES IN THE INTENSIVE CARE UNIT

The monitoring principles outlined throughout this book also apply to patients in the intensive care unit. This includes, specifically, respiratory and cardiovascular monitoring and the repeated assessment of renal function. However, because the vital functions of these patients have to be watched and deviations treated over the course of days rather than just hours, concerns arise about metabolic functions in addition to electrolyte and acid–base disturbances. Hence, the monitoring of patients in the intensive care unit includes repeated measurements of several variables that reflect metabolic and hepatic activities. These may become deranged simply because the patient starves or is stressed from infection or extensive trauma, or because the patient suffers from a combination of these adversities and an underlying disease. We give here a brief review of some of the general points that require attention, but we omit reference to problems that relate to specific organs such as hepatic, pancreatic, or thyroid diseases.

Physical Examination

The general assessment includes inspection of skin turgor and body weight, largely indices of total body water. In infants these can change rapidly enough to warrant daily assessment. Even in adults with diarrhea (or overhydration), turgor and weight can change markedly within a day.

Bowel sounds are an important indicator of intestinal activity. Early, postoperatively, they are often absent, either because the abdominal cavity was entered by the surgeon (such mechanical irritation can arrest bowel activity) or because one of the major inhalation anesthetics had been given. Under deep anesthesia they arrest bowel activity. If nothing but anesthesia was the cause for the ileus, bowel sounds should return in a matter of hours. With surgical manipulation of the abdominal cavity or resection of bowel, the ileus may not resolve for 1 day to 3 days, depending on the operation and the patient's general status. With infection, of course, ileus may persist longer.

Laboratory Studies

General

In addition to monitoring the vital signs during the early and acute phases of a patient's stay in the intensive care unit, many intensive care specialists obtain values of the following variables several times daily: urine glucose, urine specific gravity, and acid–base parameters. Once daily the following variables are commonly monitored: electrolytes (Na^+, Cl^-,

K^+, Ca^{2+}, PO_4^{2+}), liver enzymes, bilirubin, plasma osmolarity, blood glucose, and fluid input and output.

Nitrogen Balance

Patients in the intensive care unit tend to destroy their muscle mass, and thus lose nitrogen, while they find it difficult to take up enough nitrogen to keep the balance in equilibrium. To determine the daily nitrogen balance, estimate the 24-hour nitrogen output and subtract it from the estimated nitrogen intake. Such estimates are clinically useful (accurate determinations are research procedures). They are performed as follows:

$$N_{out} = UUN \times \text{urine volume} + .2 \times UUN + 2 \text{ g/day}$$

where

$$N_{out} = \text{the nitrogen loss in grams per day}$$

$$UUN = \text{urine urea nitrogen in grams per liter}$$

$$(\text{Urine volume} = \text{measured in liters per day.})$$

Twenty percent of UUN is added in order to compensate for the fact that urea contains only about 80% of the nitrogen excreted in the urine; 2 g/day are added to account for other, unmeasured nitrogen losses.

$$N_{in} = N_{intake\ oral}(\text{in grams protein/6.25}) + \text{gram nitrogen given IV}$$

(the protein is divided by 6.25 to arrive at an approximation of nitrogen in protein).

Immune Status

To monitor the susceptibility to infection so important in patients with malnutrition resulting from disease or surgical intervention, the total lymphocyte count is helpful:[14]

$$\text{total lymphocyte count} = \frac{\%\ \text{lymphocytes}}{100} \times \text{total white blood cells}$$

The total lymphocyte count so determined should be above 1200 lymphocytes/mm^3. Counts between 800 and 1200 lymphocytes/mm^3 indicate moderate depletion; those below 800 lymphocytes/mm^3 indicate severe depletion.

Proteins

Deficiency of albumin has long been recognized to reflect or presage the arrival of protein calorie malnutrition. In general, albumin levels of 3 g/

dl to 3.5 g/dl suggest a mild, those of 2.4 g/dl to 3 g/dl a moderate, and those below 2.4 g/dl a severe malnutrition. More detailed studies of individual amino acids have been reported, but these require special facilities and interests.[15]

Data Acquisition and Display

In contradistinction to the operating room, data in the intensive care unit serve a multitude of users. This is true because multiple organs may be affected and multiple teams of experts may participate in the care of the patient. Data of interest to the nephrologist do not overlap with those of concern to physical therapists; many data used by the hyperalimentation

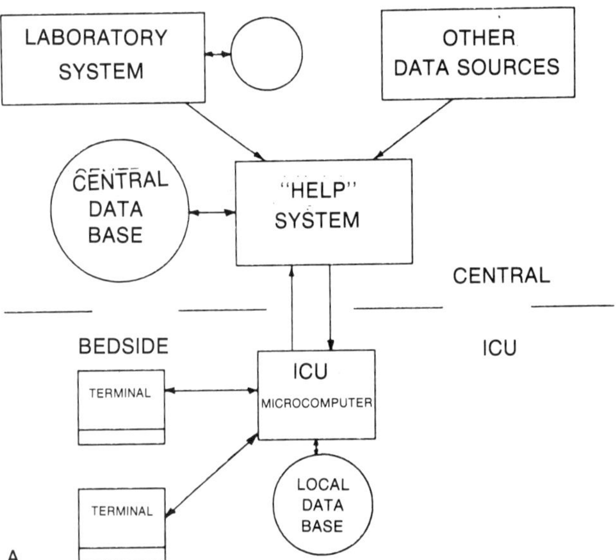

Figure 14-5. (*A*) Block diagram of the network and distributed data base for the Latter Day Saints' Hospital "HELP" system for data management. (*B*) Intensive care unit rounds report: an organ system-oriented computer report that is used during rounds. Space is provided for information not contained in the computer report. (*C*) Infection control report with an alert. (*A*: Gardner RM, West BJ, Pryor TA: Distributed data base and network for ICU monitoring. In Computers in Cardiology, p 307. Salt Lake City, IEEE Computer Society, 1984. Copyright © 1984 IEEE. (*B*: Bradshaw KE, Gardner RM, Clemmer TP, et al: Physician decision-making—evaluation of data used in a computerized ICU. Int J Clin Monit 1:81–91, 1984. *C*: Evans RS, Gardner RM, Bush AR, et al: Development of a computerized infectious disease monitor [CIDM]. Comput Biomed Res 18:103–113, 1985)

B

```
                      L D S   H O S P I T A L   I C U   R O U N D S   R E P O R T
                                        DATA WITHIN LAST 24 HOURS

NAME:                                        NO.                ROOM: 4S30                                  DATE: OCT 31 07:00
DR. BOX, TERRY D.                 SEX: M     AGE:  74   HEIGHT: 176   WEIGHT:  72.50   BSA:  1.88   BEE:  1436    MOF:    7
==========================================================================================================================
CARDIOVASCULAR: 0                                                          EXAM: _____________________________________
   -- NO CARDIAC OUTPUT DATA AVAILABLE                                           _____________________________________
                   SP    DP    MP   HR  : LACT          CPK          CPK-MB        LDH-1        LDH-2
 LAST VALUES      142    72    96  130  :
 MAXIMUM          161   128   134  136  : 2.1 (04:30)     (     )     (     )     (     )     (     )
 MINIMUM           91    47    69   70  :
 HEART RATE =        QRS =        PR =        QRS AXIS =
 -- NO ECG DECISIONS AVAILABLE --
==========================================================================================================================
RESPIRATORY: 3
OCT 31 83     pH     PCO2    HCO3   BE   HB    CO/MT   PO2   SO2   O2CT   %O2  AVO2  VO2   C.O.  A-a  Qs/Qt  PK/ PL/PP  MR/SR
31 05:20 A   7.51    48.2    38.4  14.6 11.8   2/ 1     56    89   14.7    5
         SAMPLE # 15, TEMP 38.0, BREATHING STATUS : NASAL CANNULA
         MODERATE METABOLIC ALKALOSIS
         HYPOVENTILATION MARKEDLY IMPROVED
         MODERATE HYPOXEMIA
        RATE   VT    VE    VC    MIF    COMP    VD/VT    VCO2   EXAM:                                X-RAY:

    ON  ------ ----- ----- ------ ------- -------- -------- --------  :                                 :
    OFF ------ ----- -----                                            :                                 :
==========================================================================================================================
NEURO AND PSYCH: 0
    GLASGOW 15 (00:15) VERBAL ________   EYELIDS ________   MOTOR __________   PUPILS ________     SENSORY _______

    DTR ___________   BABIN. _________   ICP ____________   PSYCH __________
==========================================================================================================================
COAGULATION: 0
    PT:          (     ) PTT:        (     ) PLATELETS:  268 (05:20)   FIBRINOGEN:      (     ) EXAM: ______________________
    FSP-CON:     (     ) FSP-FT:     (     ) 3P:     (     )                                        ______________________
==========================================================================================================================
RENAL, FLUIDS, LYTES: 2
    IN   6082 CRYST   3168  COLLOID            BLOOD        NG/PO    1865 : NA    143 (05:20) K      4.5 (05:20)  CL   101   (05:20)
    OUT  4729 URINE   1610  NGOUT              DRAINS 1000 OTHER    2119 : CO2    34 (05:20) BUN 49   (05:20)  CRE   4.6 (05:20)
    NET  1354 WT     72.50  WT-CHG     0.00 S.G.   1.018                 : AGAP  15.4        UOSM                UNA       CRCL
==========================================================================================================================
METABOLIC --- NUTRITION: 0
    KCAL      2427  GLU  226   (05:20)   ALB    2.1 (04:30)  :  CA    7.7 (04:30)   FE        (     )  TIBC        (     )
    KCAL/N2    596  UUN        (     )   N-BAL               :  PO4   4.3 (04:30)   MG        (     )  CHOL   148 (04:30)
==========================================================================================================================
GI, LIVER, AND PANCREAS: 1                                                                                     EXAM:
    HCT      36.4 (05:20)  TOTAL BILI    4.8 (04:30)  SGOT   84 (04:30)  ALKPO4  281 (04:30)  GGT      131 (04:30) __________
    GUAIAC 1+     (00:00)  DIRECT BILI   3.4 (04:30)  SGPT   81 (04:30)  LDH     327 (04:30)  AMYLASE  (     )     __________
==========================================================================================================================
INFECTION: 1
    WBC  9.0 (05:20) TEMP  38.2 (02:00) DIFF  17B, 48P, 23L, 11M,  1E (05:20) GRAM STAIN: SPUTUM ___________ OTHER __________
CULTURES:
    BLOOD _______  SPUTUM ________  URINE __________  CSF ________  CATH ________  WOUND _________  OTHER ______________
==========================================================================================================================
SKIN AND EXTREMITIES:
    PULSES ________  RASH ________  DECUBITI ____________
==========================================================================================================================
TUBES:
    VEN ________  ART ________  SG ________  NG ________  FOLEY ________  ET ________  TRACH ________  DRAIN______

    CHEST _____________  RECTAL ______  JEJUNAL ________  DIALYSIS ________  OTHER ______________________________________
==========================================================================================================================
MEDICATIONS:

MEPERIDINE (DEMEROL), INJ               MGM   IM      50.0   METAPROTERENOL (ALUPENT), SOLUTION       MGM   INHAL    50.0
AMPICILLIN, INJ                         MGM   IV      6000   RIOPAN, LIQUID                           ML    ORAL      300
NYSTATIN, SUSPENSION                    ML    ORAL    15.0   AMPHOJEL, LIQUID                         ML    ORAL       60
CLINDAMYCIN (CLEOCIN), INJ              MGM   IV      1200   PROMETHAZINE (PHENERGAN), INJ            MGM   IM       25.0
CEFOXITIN (MEFOXIN), INJ                MGM   IV      2000   INSULIN REGULAR, INJ                     UNITS IV        200
```

Figure 14-5. *(continued)*

team are not consulted by the respiratory therapists. Thus, all teams need specific data and all generate data in the course of their work. To present all the data to all the teams all the time would make it more difficult for individual specialists. Reed Gardner from the Latter Day Saints' Hospital in Salt Lake City has therefore presented an interesting solution to the problem, exploiting the power of computers. In his hospital each team can request data that are limited to information of special concern to the team or specialist.[16–18] Figure 14-5*A*, *B*, and *C* shows examples.

C

```
          INFECTIOUS DISEASE MONITOR REPORT FOR 01 APR 1984
                        FOR LAST 24 HOURS
                     PRINT TIME:   4/1/84.12:30

***** PATIENT WITH POSSIBLE NOSOCOMIAL WOUND *****
***** PATIENT NOT ON APPROPRIATE ANTIBIOTIC *****
***** AMPICILLIN WOULD BE THE LEAST EXPENSIVE ANTIBIOTIC *****
@PAT: 6001200 SMITH, JOHN NMI              66    M     6N92   MR#: 407712
 DOC: 999 DOE, RALPH JR.         SERVICE: ________     R-FACTOR: 1 2 3 4 5
 ADMITTED: 03/29/84.14:32       ADMIT DIAG: ABDOMINAL ABSCESS
 PREV. ADMIT 02/29/84       PREV. DSCH  03/06/84
 SURGERY:      clean               SURGEON: 999
  03/01/84.7:30  APPENDECTOMY
 PAT. IS ALLERGIC TO SULFONIMIDES
 CURRENT ANTIBIOTICS
  03/29/84.19:14 CEFAZOLIN (ANCEF)   1000 MGM, INJ              Q  6 HRS
 CULTURE RESULTS          -PRELIMINARY REPORT-               ANAER CULT
  SOURCE: WOUND                               COLLECTED: 03/29/84.17:45
  STAIN: NUMEROUS WBCS
         NUMEROUS GRAM POSITIVE COCCI IN GROUPS
         FEW GRAM NEGATIVE BACILLI
         FEW GRAM POSITIVE BACILLI
  RESULT: NO ANAEROBES ISOLATED
 CULTURE RESULTS           -FINAL REPORT-                    ROUTINE CULT
  STAIN: NUMEROUS WBCS
         FEW GRAM POSITIVE COCCI IN GROUPS
         FEW GRAM NEGATIVE BACILLI
         FEW GRAM POSITIVE BACILLI
  RESULT: ESCHERICHIA COLI    MODERATE GROWTH
   SENSITIVE TO: Ampicillin,Carbenicillin,Cephalosporin,Chloramphenicol
                 Gentamicin,Cefoperazone,Trimethoprim-sulfamethoxazole
                 Tobramycin,Amikcin,Cefamandole,Cefoxitin,
   INTERMED TO:  Moxalactam,Cefotaxime,Piperacillin,
   RESISTANT TO: Tetracycline
  RESULT: ENTEROCOCCUS    HEAVY GROWTH
   SENSITIVE TO: Ampicillin, Chloramphenicol,Vancomycin,
   INTERMED. TO: Erythromycin
   RESISTANT TO: Cephalosporin,Clindamycin,Penicillin-G,Tetracycline
```

Figure 14-5. *(continued)*

REFERENCES

1. Hidalgo JU, Nadler SB, Bloch T: The use of the electronic digital computer to determine best fit of blood volume formulas. J Nucl Med 3:94, 1962
2. Gross JB: Estimating allowable blood loss: Corrected for dilution. Anesthesiology 58:277–280, 1983
3. Cassady JF, Patel RL, Epstein BS: Calculations for predicting blood transfusion needs (letter to the editor). Anesthesiology 59:491, 1983
4. The bleeding-time and the haematocrit. *Lancet* i:997–998, 1984
5. Culliford AT, Gitel SN, Starr N, et al: Lack of correlation between activated

clotting time and plasma heparin during cardiopulmonary bypass. Ann Surg 193:105, 1981

6. Moorehead MT, Westengard JC, Bull BS: Platelet involvement in the activated coagulation time of heparinized blood. Anesth Analg 63:394–398, 1984
7. Kang YG, Martin DJ, Marquez J, et al: Intraoperative changes in blood coagulation and thromboelastographic monitoring in liver transplantation. Anesth Analg 64:888–896, 1985
8. Gennari FG: Serum osmolality. New Engl J Med 310:102–105, 1984
9. Wong KC, Port JD, Steffins J: Cardiovascular response to asphyxial challenge in chronically hypokalemic dogs. Anesth Analg 62:991–994, 1983
10. Hill AB, Nahrwold ML, Noonan D, et al: A comparison of methods of blood withdrawal and sample preparation for potassium measurements. Anesthesiology 53:60, 1980
11. Nanji AA, Blank D: Spurious increase in the anion gap due to exposure of serum to air (letter to the editor). New Engl J Med 307:190–191, 1982
12. Madias NE, Ayus JC, Adrogue HJ: Increased anion gap in metabolic alkalosis: The role of plasma–protein equivalency. New Engl J Med 300:1421–1423, 1979
13. Fram BA, Rossier AB, Blunt K, et al: Experience in the urologic management in 120 early spinal cord injury patients. J Urol 119:485, 1978
14. Shin B, MacKenzie CF, Helrich M: Creatine clearance for early detection of posttraumatic renal dysfunction. Anesthesiology 64:605–609, 1986
15. Siegel JH: Integrated approaches to physiologic monitoring of the critically ill. In Gravenstein JS, Newbower RS, Ream AK, et al (eds): An Integrated Approach to Monitoring, pp 41–57. Boston, Butterworths, 1983
16. Lakshman K, Blackburn GL: Monitoring nutritional status in the adult critically ill. J Clin Monit 2:114–120, 1986
17. Gardner RM, West BJ, Pryor TA: Distributed data base and network for ICU monitoring. In Computers in Cardiology, p 307. Salt Lake City, Utah, IEEE Computer Society, 1984
18. Bradshaw KE, Gardner RM, Clemmer TP, et al: Physician decision-making—evaluation of data used in a computerized ICU. Int J Clin Monit 1:81–91, 1984
19. Evans RS, Gardner RM, Bush AR, et al: Development of a computerized infectious disease monitor (CIDM). Comput Biomed Res 18:103–113, 1985

CHAPTER 15

The Anesthesia Record

In the early days of ether and chloroform, anesthesia was much more an art than a science. Few measurements were possible, fewer were made, and none were recorded. An important change came about in 1894 when Codman and Cushing first plotted intraoperative vital signs on a record.[1] Today's anesthesia records clearly show their ancestry when we compare them to the first record, but today's record has grown in complexity just as much as is true for anesthesia in general. As we shall see, certain aspects of record keeping in the operating room are essential for monitoring. What is being said for the anesthesia record is equally valid for the records in the intensive care unit.

Today we are bound to keep an anesthesia record, even though any experienced anesthesiologist can remember numerous instances when the anesthesia record played no part at all in the welfare of the patient and was kept only because not doing so would have challenged established custom and requirements of the Joint Commission on Accreditation of

Hospitals (JCAH). By the same token, who cannot recall cases where information on the record made a significant difference to the patient or, at times, to an anesthesiologist in court defending himself against a malpractice claim? Unfortunately, no one can predict in which case the record will prove to be helpful or vital. Therefore, we need to write one for every patient and we need to write it well.

In the following pages we will discuss four aspects of the record: the record as log book, as clinical management tool, as trend and pattern plotter, and finally, as medico-legal document.[2] Even though these categories overlap, they focus attention on the cardinal features of the anesthesia record.

THE RECORD AS LOG BOOK

Preoperative Evaluation Form

Demographic and historical data fall into this category. These data are often so voluminous that many anesthesiologists now use separate preoperative evaluation forms (Fig. 15-1) on which to record facts of the patient's medical and drug history, family history as far as it is of interest to the anesthesiologist (*e.g.*, familial malignant hyperthermia), relevant laboratory data (*e.g.*, hemoglobin or hematocrit, electrolytes, urine values), ECG and radiologic findings, data from liver or lung function studies, allergies, and anatomic details such as dental status, likelihood of difficult intubation or venous access. Results from an Allen's test, as well as a description of the physical examination (including weight, height and the ASA physical status) all fit on the preoperative evaluation form.

The ASA physical status system, introduced and revised by the American Society of Anesthesiologists, has become an integral, if often misunderstood—part of the anesthesia record.[3] It is misunderstood because it is *not*, as believed by many, an assessment of risk; it is an assessment of the patient's preoperative condition. Many factors unrelated to the patient's physical status affect the anesthetic and the operative risks. The ASA classification, as revised in 1974, consists of the following categories:

1. A normally healthy patient
2. A patient with mild systemic disease
3. A patient with severe systemic disease that is not incapacitating
4. A patient with an incapacitating systemic disease that is a constant threat to life
5. A moribund patient who is not expected to survive 24 hours with or without the operation

Some have added a sixth category for organ donors whose circulation and ventilation is maintained until the organs in question have been removed.

SURGERY DATE ________________

PATIENT NAME

PREOPERATIVE EVALUATION FOR ANESTHESIA

OP PROPOSED:

DATE: | SURGEON:

PROBLEMS RELATED TO ANESTHESIA:

WT.

HT.

Pulse

BP

HCT HGB

WBC PLTS

ALLERGIES: HABITS: Smoking–
ETOH–

Urine:
SG
Protein
Glucose
HGB
Other

CURRENT MEDS:

ILLNESS:

OPERATIONS:

ANESTHETICS:

LYTES

BUN CR.

CNS– GI–

CV– GU–

Glucose

PUL.– OTHER–

COAG

PHYSICAL EXAM:

Misc. Lab Studies

TEETH– AIRWAY–

LUNGS–

ECG

HEART–

CXR

OTHER–

ANESTHESIA PLAN:

ASA:

PreOp Medication as written in the Physicians' orders.

1. ________ NPO @: ________

2. ________ Meds to be given @ ________

3. ________ Signed: ________ M.D.

Figure 15-1. Preoperative evaluation form used at Shands Hospital at the University of Florida.

In an emergency, the number of the relevant category should be preceded by an E. Note that the patient's age is not a classifying factor. Conscientiously adhering to these straightforward, but general, classifications of physical status has much merit and may prevent varied interpretations.[4]

Many anesthesiologists follow the ASA recommendation to assess the patient's condition again after anesthesia. It is not customary to repeat the ASA classification, but it is necessary to judge the patient's condition as influenced by the anesthetic and the operative procedures. Unfortunately, no generally accepted guidelines or definitions for postoperative evaluation exist. A postoperative score proposed by Aldrete and Kroulik for the recovery room has been adopted by some anesthesiologists.[5] Activity, respiration, circulation, consciousness, and color are repeatedly graded on a scale of 0 to 2 to gauge the recovery from anesthesia rather than to assess overall physical status. Collins has proposed a more elaborate system that is also used repeatedly to monitor the patient's recovery or deterioration.[6] Neither system considers the patient's preoperative physical status, as assessed by the ASA classification, or the patient's physical status as influenced by the surgical procedure. Also, neither system is a risk classification. We hope that one of the current systems or perhaps a new classification will someday be universally adopted, so that the assessment of the patient as he leaves the operating room can become better defined and standardized.

Informed Consent

The patient must be informed well before the operation about the details of the anesthetic, its hazards, and other available anesthetic options. The physician should leave no doubt about the anesthetic option he deems best; it is unfair to confront the patient with options from which he cannot select the safest because he is not an expert in anesthesia. Usually there will be a separate "informed consent form" especially spelling out the circumstances and risks of anesthesia. These forms are of legal concern to attorneys and are often drafted with their help, as was true for the sample shown in Figure 15-2.

The Anesthesia Record

The logbook functions of the anesthesia record proper include the *who*, *when*, *what*, *where*, and *how* questions.

Who

The name and hospital number of the patient, the fact that the patient was properly identified (patients with common names have been given

SHANDS HOSPITAL AND CLINICS, INC.

CONSENT TO ANESTHESIA

I understand that any type of anesthesia sometimes results in minor complications.

I also understand that any type of anesthesia is associated with substantial risks and hazards. These risks and hazards include long lasting or possibly permanent damage to my brain, heart, nerves, liver, kidneys, lungs, and other organs and body structures. Even paralysis and death may result from anesthesia. These substantial risks and hazards are fortunately very rare.

Dr. ________________ has explained the nature and alternative choices of anesthesia to me and has given me an adequate opportunity to discuss the associated risks and hazards. I consent to local, regional, or general anesthesia to be administered by a member of the Department of Anesthesiology. I consent only to the administration of local, regional, general (strike out whatever is not desired) by a member of the Department of Anesthesiology.

(Patient's Signature)

(Witness) (Date) (Time)

The patient is unable to consent because:

I thereby consent for the patient.

(Relationship to Patient) (Signature)

(Witness) (Date) (Time)

6/82: Consents

Figure 15-2. Informed consent form used at Shands Hospital at the University of Florida.

wrong drugs or even a wrong operation), and the personnel (from surgeons to scrub nurses and circulators to anesthesiologists) need to be listed. In one law suit the anesthesiologist could not recall the name of the circulating nurse in the operating room, whose testimony might have helped him in his case.

When

The date of the anesthetic and the times of starting and ending anesthesia and operation or applying and removing a tourniquet are important items. The times of administering drugs or initiating resuscitation are of equal significance. The time span during which a relief anesthetist took over the care of the patient has been the subject of intense scrutiny in some law suits.

What

The drugs given preoperatively, the number of the anesthesia machine (in case of difficulties with it), the pre- and postoperative diagnosis, the operation performed, as dictated by the surgeon, and the monitors in use should all be recorded. (In one law suit the anesthesiologist was challenged by the plaintiff's attorney to prove that an electrocardiograph had been used in the case. To his dismay no one in the operating room could remember whether the monitor had been turned on, and he had failed to record information about its use.) One should also record not only the drug and dose of a spinal or epidural anesthetic but brand and lot number of the drug as well. Should the patient develop a complication such as meningitis, this information will be needed. In several law suits the details of cannulation of a vein or artery became subjects for questioning. Some attorneys now advise that we also record the setting of the alarm limits and the fact that the alarms were armed (or disarmed).

Where

Include on the record such mundane items as the identification of the operating (or diagnostic or other treatment) room (in case of a problem with the room or its supplies, including gas supply).

How

The type of anesthesia system and difficulties encountered, for instance, with intubation, and how they were overcome belong in the anesthetic record so that in the future patients are not exposed to the same problems and risks.

The patient's position must be described. Many like to use simple diagrams with stick people. In addition to this, special precautions taken with "donuts" under the head, or padding under the heels or elsewhere, should be recorded. Pressure injuries to the nerves and skin are not uncommon and it is prudent to record what steps were taken to prevent them.

THE RECORD AS A CLINICAL MANAGEMENT TOOL

A good record helps the clinician to adjust the administration of drugs and fluids and the settings of a ventilator. For instance, without recording (or remembering—which is not easy and may lead to gross mistakes) the dose and time of the injection of, for instance, a narcotic, it will be difficult to estimate when to reinject or how much of an antagonist to give. Several monitored variables assist in this process of making a decision, but a good record will render valuable guidance to the clinician. By the same token it is mandatory to record the values of arterial oxygen tension when one tries to gauge the success of changing inspired oxygen concentration or the addition of positive end-expiratory pressure. The same can be said for fluid management; only a good record will allow the construction of a running balance of loss versus input. Without a reliable anesthesia record, clinical management of complex anesthetic cases becomes haphazard.

THE RECORD AS A TREND AND PATTERN PLOTTER

Sampling Rate

The rate at which variables should be recorded must be adjusted to the individual variable and clinical circumstances. For uneventful, routine cases, an entry every 5 minutes is traditional and apparently sufficient. In critical emergencies, nothing but continuous monitoring of cardiovascular variables is acceptable.

Another perspective on the frequency with which measurements are needed is offered by the observation that humans can usually survive for 3 minutes without circulation before suffering permanent brain damage. This 3-minute figure is often quoted, yet it is a very rough estimate. Without perfusion of the brain, a feverish, hypoxic old man will suffer permanent damage in far less than 3 minutes and a hypothermic child in barbiturate coma will survive much longer without brain damage. Nevertheless, the 3-minute limit is widely accepted. A useful rule of thumb is that data should be recorded at twice the rate at which they significantly change. If the "3 minutes to disaster" rule is accepted, the patient should be monitored every 1.5 minutes (half of 3 minutes). This is done with heart rate and ECG, but, at least currently, not with blood pressure, even though it can change markedly in about 15 seconds.

The Trend Plot

Trend plots are generated when we record over time the repeated measurements of arterial pressure, heart rate, respiratory rate, inspired and expired oxygen, inspired and expired CO_2 concentrations, temperature, and the saturation of hemoglobin with oxygen.

Trend plots allow for extrapolation; lines are drawn to the plotted values and it becomes clear where they would lead if the trend were to continue. Graphs of vital values are as important to anesthesia as the compass is to navigation: a little deviation can be tolerated for a short time, but corrections must soon be made to avoid missing the destination by a wide margin.

A trend in vital signs can develop, and often reverse, within seconds. For instance, with sustained positive pressure in the airway, arterial blood pressure can fall precipitously, and within 15 seconds it may not be measurable. During intubation of the trachea, arterial pressure and heart rate may double within 15 seconds.

With brisk, but not catastrophic hemorrhage, or with a slowly evolving overdose of an inhalational anesthetic, heart rate and arterial pressure first change gradually but then fall below critical levels in a matter of minutes. Because such gradual changes are far more common than the catastrophic changes that occur with massive hemorrhage, ventricular fibrillation, or excessive pressure in the airway, the graph is customarily updated manually every 5 minutes. Automated noninvasive blood pressure recording devices can update the data more often, or even continuously.

Arterial oxygen can change drastically within less than a minute. For instance, arterial Po_2 may drop from 100 torr to 30 torr in less than a minute when the lungs are ventilated with an oxygen-free gas mixture. This can be well monitored with a pulse oximeter. In routine care, the trends in oxygen tension proceed much more slowly. Arterial CO_2 changes quite gradually, for example, by about 3 torr to 5 torr per minute, even when the lungs are not ventilated.

Similarly, temperatures also tend to change gradually. In most instances, recording temperature every 10 minutes will suffice to detect the slow trends of cooling or heating. Even in malignant hyperthermia, when temperature may rise relatively quickly, minutes rather than seconds are required for the trend to be established.

The Pattern Plot

Our eyes can easily discern trends when a variable is plotted on a graph rather than numerically jotted down one number under the other. When more than one trend is graphically displayed, the eye begins to recognize patterns that may have great clinical significance. For instance, a simultaneously falling arterial blood pressure and rising heart rate raise concern about hypovolemia. When the central venous pressure falls and the capnogram simultaneously shows less CO_2 in the end-expired breath, hypovolemia, and a reduced pulmonary blood flow (less CO_2 being delivered to the lungs) secondary to hypovolemia, become almost a certainty. Light anesthesia is frequently betrayed by a rising heart rate and blood pressure, while increased CO_2 in the expired air, tachycardia, and, initially at least, hypertension, signify hyperthermia, which is readily confirmed with a thermometer. One of the most ominous patterns is falling blood pressure and slowing heart rate in the face of low oxygen saturation, the harbinger of cardiac arrest and brain damage.

THE RECORD AS A MEDICO-LEGAL DOCUMENT

One of the most telling images of the anesthesia record as a medico-legal document is the picture of a record enlarged ten times and mounted on a board, where it can be viewed by all members of the jury, the judge, and the defendant anesthetist, while the plaintiff's attorney with excruciating care goes over every ambiguity, contradiction, omission, and error of the record. Illegible entries will be made to appear the work of a sloppy clinician. The only thing that could make matters worse would be the demonstration that the anesthesia record was improperly altered.

No malpractice case will come to settlement or trial without a detailed analysis of the record. A well-kept record will cast a positive light on the clinician, a carelessly finished one the opposite. A good record will show that attention had been paid to the record as a log book, as a clinical management tool, and as a trend and pattern plotter. Be sure that the record does not contradict other medical documents, such as the notes written by operating or recovery room personnel. In emergencies, where keeping time may become impossible and remembering details about events and treatment may be difficult, consult with other personnel in the unit to arrive at a common estimate of the times and events that took place. Errors will occur and corrections will be necessary in the anesthesia record. A good way to execute such correction is to cross out the error with a single line so that the erroneous value can still be read. Then write the correct value in, give the time and date of the correction, and initial the correction so that the author of the correction can be identified.

We know of no anesthesiologist, nurse anesthetist, or intensive care specialist with a permanent halo; we assume therefore that everyone will make mistakes. Honest records will show these mistakes. There is a powerful temptation to obscure mistakes because they are embarrassing and may be costly. Experts in the field of malpractice insurance, however, urge us to let the record show all mistakes. It is far better to know at the outset that a mistake has been made and that, should the patient have been harmed, actions will be taken to reach a settlement with the patient or his relatives. Such settlements allow a timely payment to the plaintiff and avoid costly litigation, which is in the interest of everyone. The patient will avoid the great costs and often years of delay entailed in a lawsuit and will be assured of payment. If a suit comes to court, the patient still runs the risk of losing. Honest records are best!

The JCAH Requirements

The JCAH is concerned with the establishment and maintenance of adequate standards of anesthesia services and has repeatedly stated that written records must be kept.[7] The JCAH does not provide a sample of such records, but does enumerate what is expected of an acceptable anesthesia service.* This includes the key factor that the anesthesia services must be directed by a physician member of the medical staff and that it is his or her responsibility to assure "that the quality and appropriateness of anesthesia care are monitored and evaluated and that appropriate actions based on findings are taken." The quality and appropriateness of anesthesia care are impossible to assess without the help of carefully kept records detailing the steps and procedures employed in the anesthetic care of the patient. The JCAH also requires that written policies relating to the delivery of anesthesia care be kept. This includes the policy that provides for "the preanesthesia evaluation of the patient by a physician—with appropriate documentation in the patient's medical record of pertinent information relative to the choice of anesthesia and the surgical or obstetrical procedure anticipated," and that "the preanesthesia medical record entry refers to the use of general, spinal, or other regional anesthesia." The policies also prescribe that "the preanesthesia record entry includes the patient's previous drug history, other anesthetic experiences, and any potential anesthetic problems," as well as "the review of the patient's condition immediately prior to the induction of anesthesia." Written policies are to define the steps that assure "the safety of the patient during the anesthetic period." The JCAH also requires "the recording of all pertinent events that take place during the induction of, maintenance of, and emergence from anesthesia, including the dosage and duration of all anesthetic agents, other drugs, intravenous fluids, and blood or blood components." Finally, the JCAH calls for pertinent postanesthesia entries in the medical record of patients who have been given anesthesia. These notes should show date and time when they were written and should be prepared by the person who administered the anesthetic. These requirements clearly show how much importance is attached to the records that describe the patient's sojourn through the pre-, intra-, and postoperative phases of the surgical or diagnostic procedures requiring anesthesia.

* Joint Commission on Accreditation of Hospitals: Accreditation Manual for Hospitals. Chicago, JCAH, 1987

TYPES OF RECORDS

The Anesthesia Record

The Hand-Written Record

Many anesthesia services have their own records, for example, the records from the University of Florida (Fig. 15-3) and the VA hospital system (Fig. 15-4) and a recovery room record (Fig. 15-5). Two principal difficulties arise with the manual completion of the anesthesia record:

1. During induction of anesthesia and critical phases of an operation or anesthesia administration, the clinician may need to concentrate all of his attention on the patient and use both of his hands for clinical tasks unrelated to record keeping. This means that, during many anesthetic procedures, no data are recorded manually for minutes on end. Once the critical phase has passed, the clinician reconstructs from memory what happened and what was observed. Often human memory is called on to recover such information for 20 minutes or more. That this leads to many entries giving wrong times of events, false doses of drugs, and incorrect values of monitored physiologic variables goes without saying.[8–10]
2. The variables recorded during the early days of record keeping included heart rate, blood pressure, and respiratory rate. A few notations commented on the patient's appearance (*e.g.*, "cool and sweaty") and the times when ether was administered. To this skeleton of information we have added for even the routine cases, in the intervening 80 years, information on the flow of oxygen, nitrous oxide, and anesthetic vapor, the injection of barbiturates, narcotics, muscle relaxant drugs, and antagonists, the infusion of fluids and blood, the pressures and tidal volumes generated by the ventilator, the concentrations of inspired oxygen and end-expired CO_2, the patient's temperature, and whether or not a sinus rhythm was observed in the ECG! Small wonder that hand-written records contain many subtle as well as gross mistakes. Indeed, one could ask whether, in fairness to the patient, the anesthesiologist should be permitted to keep anything but a rudimentary record; in many cases a complete record will demand too much attention that is withheld from the patient!

The Automated Record

In response to the problems besetting manual record keeping, a number of investigators have presented automated record-keeping systems.[11] Industry, too, has recognized the need and has made available systems that chart vital signs and other variables automatically. The Datatrac* prints

* Datascope Corp., Paramus, New Jersey

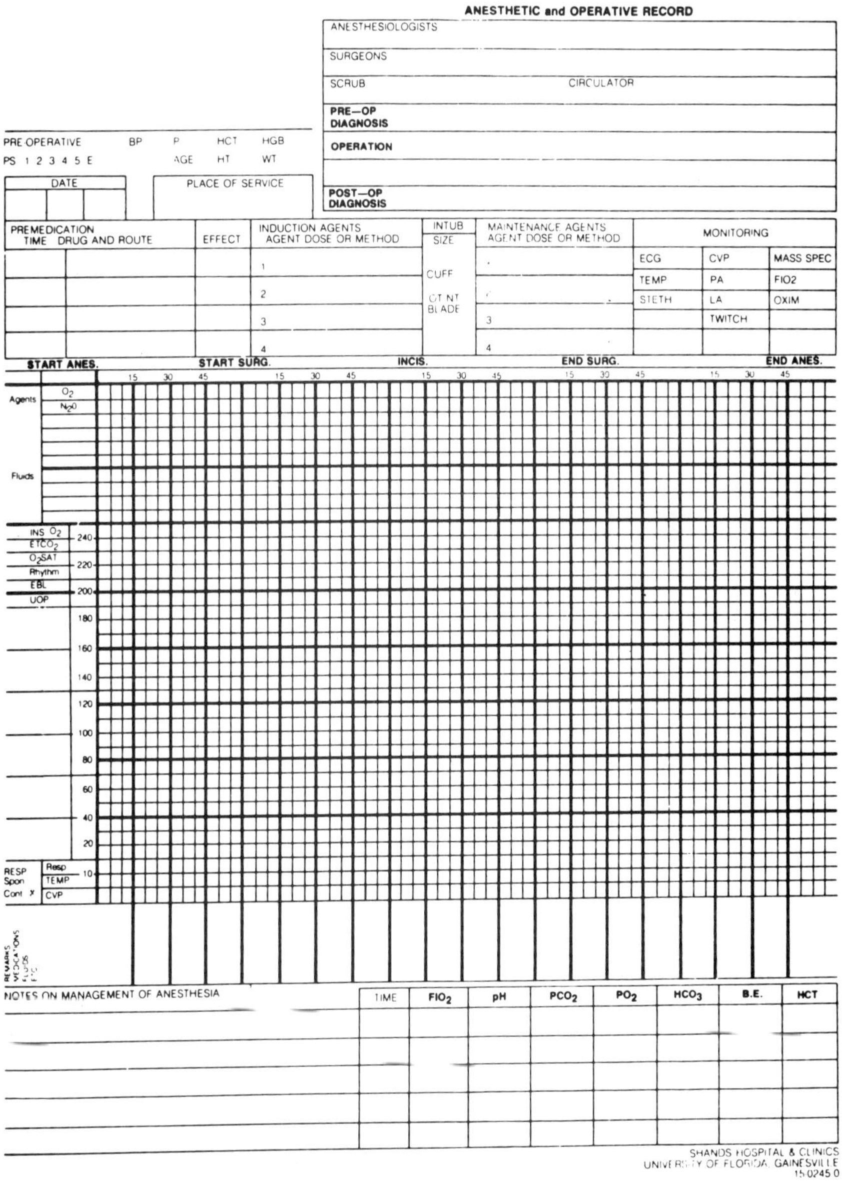

ANESTHETIC and OPERATIVE RECORD

ANESTHESIOLOGISTS

SURGEONS

SCRUB CIRCULATOR

PRE—OP DIAGNOSIS

OPERATION

POST—OP DIAGNOSIS

PRE OPERATIVE BP P HCT HGB

PS 1 2 3 4 5 E AGE HT WT

DATE	PLACE OF SERVICE

PREMEDICATION TIME	DRUG AND ROUTE	EFFECT	INDUCTION AGENTS AGENT DOSE OR METHOD	INTUB SIZE	MAINTENANCE AGENTS AGENT DOSE OR METHOD	MONITORING		
			1	CUFF		ECG	CVP	MASS SPEC
			2	OT NT BLADE		TEMP	PA	FIO2
			3		3	STETH	LA	OXIM
			4		4		TWITCH	

START ANES. START SURG. INCIS. END SURG. END ANES.

15 30 45 15 30 45 15 30 45 15 30 45 15 30 45

Agents: O_2, N_2O

Fluids

INS O_2
$ETCO_2$
O_2SAT
Rhythm
EBL
UOP

240
220
200
180
160
140
120
100
80
60
40
20
10

RESP Spon Cont X — Resp, TEMP, CVP

REMARKS MEDICATIONS FLUIDS ETC

NOTES ON MANAGEMENT OF ANESTHESIA

TIME	FIO_2	pH	PCO_2	PO_2	HCO_3	B.E.	HCT

SHANDS HOSPITAL & CLINICS
UNIVERSITY OF FLORIDA, GAINESVILLE
15 0245 0

Figure 15-3. Anesthesia record used at Shands Hospital at the University of Florida.

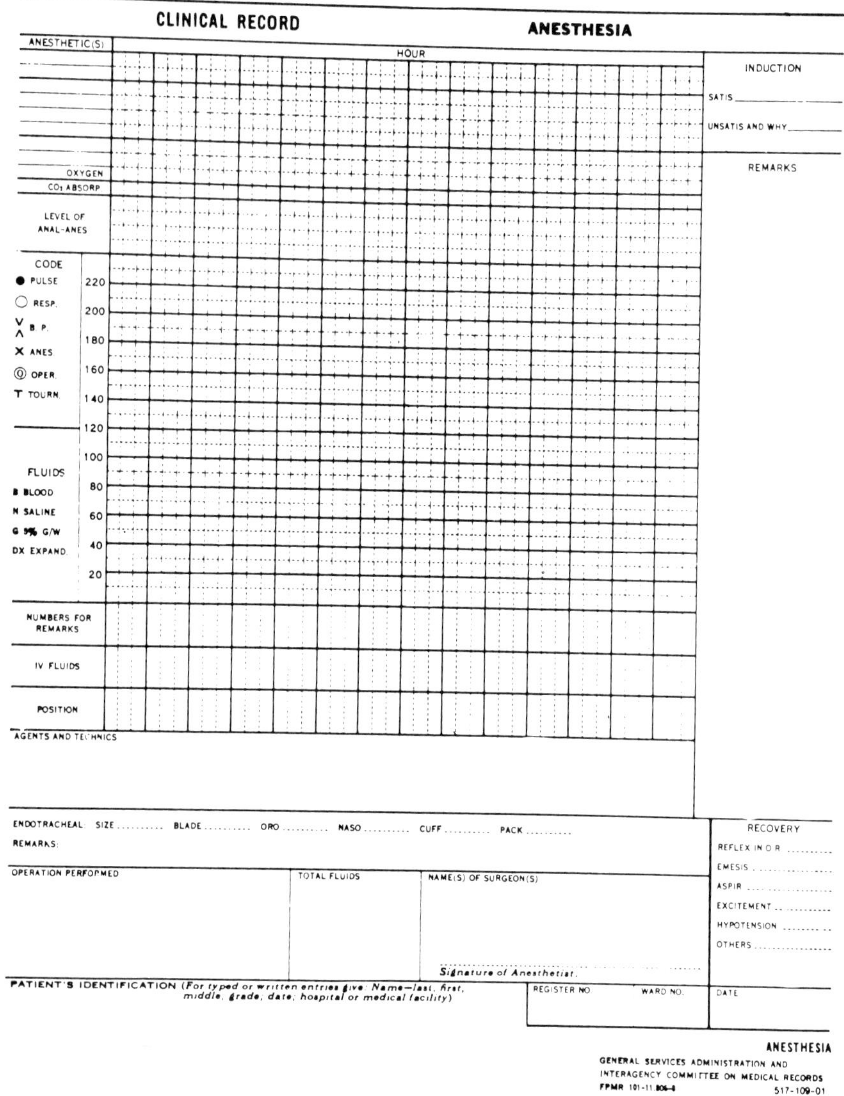

CLINICAL RECORD — ANESTHESIA

ANESTHETIC(S)

HOUR

OXYGEN

CO_2 ABSORP

LEVEL OF ANAL-ANES

CODE

● PULSE

○ RESP.

V Λ B. P.

X ANES.

◎ OPER.

T TOURN.

220, 200, 180, 160, 140, 120, 100, 80, 60, 40, 20

FLUIDS

B BLOOD

N SALINE

G 5% G/W

DX EXPAND.

NUMBERS FOR REMARKS

IV FLUIDS

POSITION

AGENTS AND TECHNICS

INDUCTION

SATIS.

UNSATIS AND WHY

REMARKS

ENDOTRACHEAL: SIZE .... BLADE .... ORO .... NASO .... CUFF .... PACK ....

REMARKS:

OPERATION PERFORMED

TOTAL FLUIDS

NAME(S) OF SURGEON(S)

Signature of Anesthetist.

RECOVERY

REFLEX IN O R ....

EMESIS ....

ASPIR ....

EXCITEMENT ....

HYPOTENSION ....

OTHERS ....

PATIENT'S IDENTIFICATION (*For typed or written entries give: Name—last, first, middle; grade, date; hospital or medical facility*)

REGISTER NO.

WARD NO.

DATE

ANESTHESIA

GENERAL SERVICES ADMINISTRATION AND INTERAGENCY COMMITTEE ON MEDICAL RECORDS

FPMR 101-11.806-8

517-109-01

OCTOBER 1975

Figure 15-4. Anesthesia record used in the Veterans Administration hospitals.

the graphic part of the anesthesia record and allows the anesthesiologist to enter by hand data relating to events such as drugs that have been administered or position changes. A system built by Ohmeda plots vital signs automatically and also provides for printing drug data, position changes, and other events with the help of a touch screen. These two automated anesthesia records signal a new development in anesthesia.

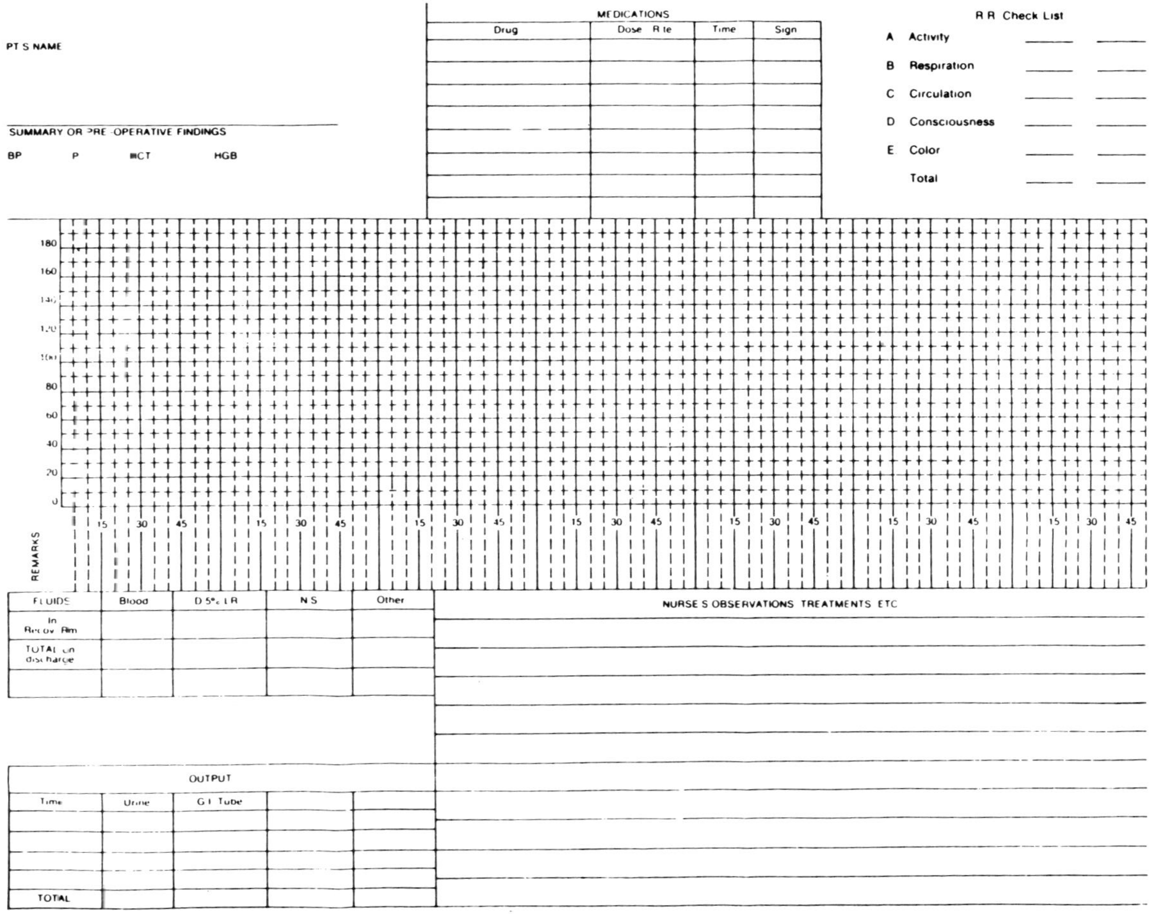

PT S NAME

SUMMARY OR PRE-OPERATIVE FINDINGS

BP P HCT HGB

MEDICATIONS

Drug	Dose Rte	Time	Sign

R R Check List

A	Activity		
B	Respiration		
C	Circulation		
D	Consciousness		
E	Color		
	Total		

180
160
140
120
100
80
60
40
20
0

15 30 45 15 30 45 15 30 45 15 30 45 15 30 45 15 30 45 15 30 45

REMARKS

FLUIDS	Blood	D 5% LR	N S	Other
In Recov Rm				
TOTAL on discharge				

OUTPUT

Time	Urine	G I Tube		
TOTAL				

NURSE S OBSERVATIONS TREATMENTS ETC

Figure 15-5. Recovery room record used at Shands Hospital at the University of Florida.

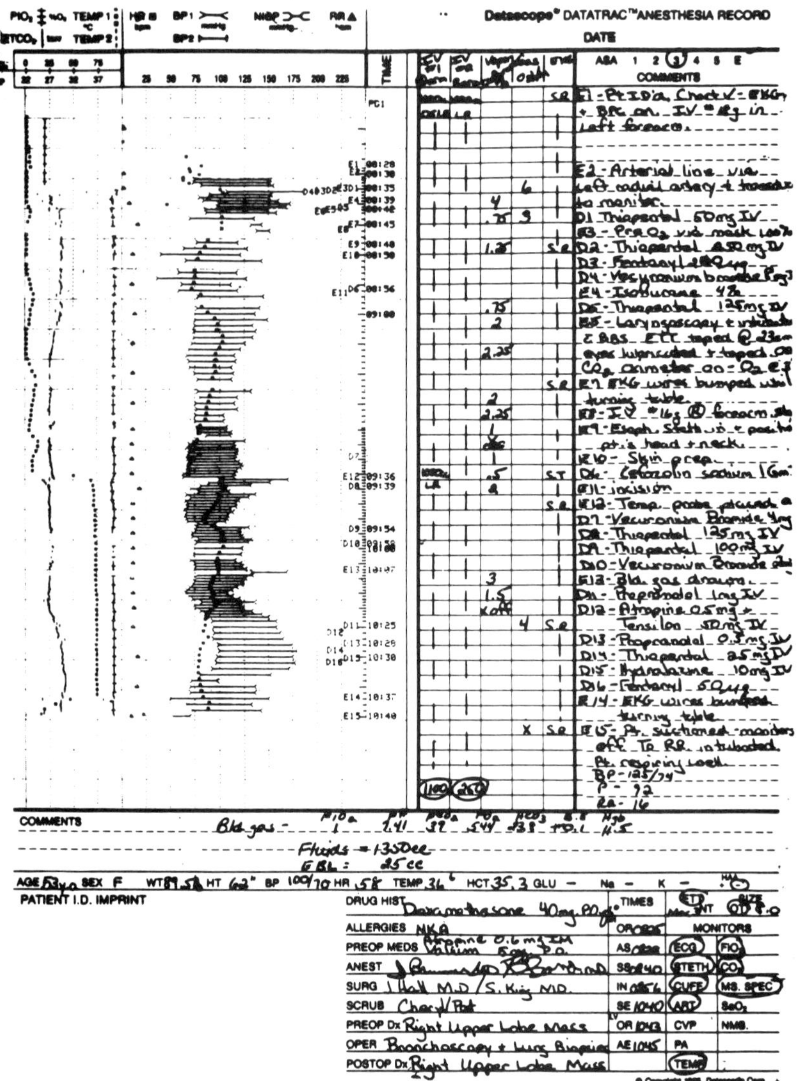

Datascope® DATATRAC™ ANESTHESIA RECORD

DATE

ASA 1 2 (3) 4 5 E

COMMENTS

E1 - Pt ID'd, Check ✓ - EKG + BP on. IV in left forearm.

E2 - Arterial line via left radial artery to monitor.

D1 Thiopental 50mg IV

E3 - Pre O₂ via mask 100%

D2 - Thiopental 250 mg IV

E4 - Isoflurane

D5 - Thiopental 125mg IV

E5 - Laryngoscopy

E7 EKG wires bumped while turning table.

E9 - Esoph. Steth

pt.'s head + neck.

E10 - Skin prep.

D6 - Cefazolin sodium 1 Gm

E11 - incision

E12 - Temp. probe placed

D7 - Vecuronium Bromide

D8 - Thiopental 125mg IV

D9 - Thiopental 100mg IV

D10 - Vecuronium Bromide

E13 - Bld. gas drawn.

D12 - Atropine 0.5mg + Tensilon IV

D14 - Thiopental IV

D15 - Hydralazine 10mg IV

D16 - Fentanyl

E14 - EKG wires bumped turning table

E15 - Pt. suctioned - monitors off. To RR intubated. Pt. respiring well.

BP - 125/74

P - 92

RR - 16

COMMENTS Bld gas - Fluids = 1350cc EBL: 25 cc

AGE 53 y.o. SEX F WT HT BP 100/70 HR 58 TEMP HCT 35.3 GLU – Na – K –

PATIENT I.D. IMPRINT

DRUG HIST Dexamethasone 40mg

ALLERGIES NKA

PREOP MEDS Atropine 0.6 mg IM, Valium P.O.

ANEST

SURG

SCRUB

PREOP Dx Right Upper Lobe Mass

OPER Bronchoscopy + Lung Biopsies

POSTOP Dx Right Upper Lobe Mass

TIMES: OR, AS, SS, IN, SE 1040, OR 1043, AE 1045

ETT, SIZE

MONITORS: ECG, FIO₂, STETH, CO₂, CUFF, MS. SPEC, ART, SaO₂, CVP, NMB, PA, TEMP

© Copyright 1985, Datascope Corp.

Figure 15-6. Semiautomatic anesthesia record. This semiautomatic record was generated by a Datatrac manufactured by Datascope (Paramus, NJ). The left side of the record with physiologic variables was generated automatically by the device; the right side was filled out by an anesthesiologist (see Fig. 15-7).

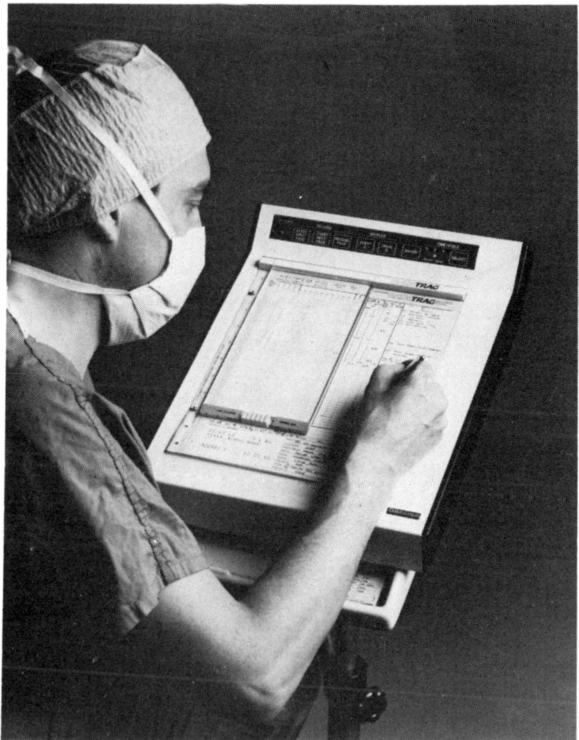

Figure 15-7. The Datatrac. The semiautomatic anesthesia recording device (Datascope, Paramus, NJ) provides for the printing of physiologic data including two pressures, heart rate, inspired O_2, end-tidal CO_2, and two temperatures. The printing head runs under the record and presses against the record from below, so that the record is never obscured. The right side is reserved for entries by hand, which are automatically timed and annotated with a D or E by pressing either the drug (D) or event (E) button.

Examples of automated records and the devices used to generate them are presented in Figures 15-6 to 15-9.

Equipment Checklist

Before beginning anesthesia the equipment must be checked for completeness and function with the help of a checklist. A sample is shown in Table 15-1. It is good practice even for experienced clinicians to use the checklist and not to rely on memory. The anesthesia record should show that a checkout procedure was completed and that all items on the checklist were found to be present and in working condition.

(Text continued on p. 385)

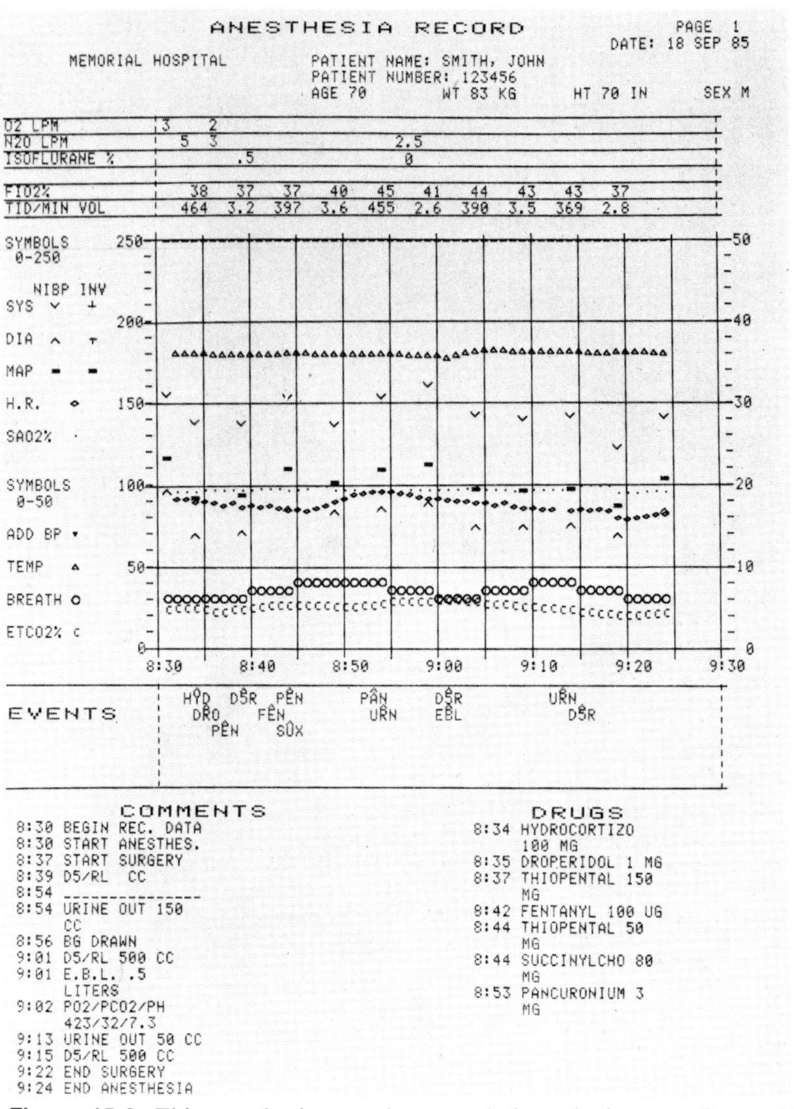

ANESTHESIA RECORD

PAGE 1
DATE: 18 SEP 85

MEMORIAL HOSPITAL

PATIENT NAME: SMITH, JOHN
PATIENT NUMBER: 123456
AGE 70 WT 83 KG HT 70 IN SEX M

O2 LPM	3	2								
N2O LPM	5	3				2.5				
ISOFLURANE %		.5				0				
FIO2%	38	37	37	40	45	41	44	43	43	37
TID/MIN VOL	464	3.2	397	3.6	455	2.6	390	3.5	369	2.8

COMMENTS

8:30 BEGIN REC. DATA
8:30 START ANESTHES.
8:37 START SURGERY
8:39 D5/RL CC
8:54 ----------------
8:54 URINE OUT 150 CC
8:56 BG DRAWN
9:01 D5/RL 500 CC
9:01 E.B.L. .5 LITERS
9:02 PO2/PCO2/PH 423/32/7.3
9:13 URINE OUT 50 CC
9:15 D5/RL 500 CC
9:22 END SURGERY
9:24 END ANESTHESIA

DRUGS

8:34 HYDROCORTIZO 100 MG
8:35 DROPERIDOL 1 MG
8:37 THIOPENTAL 150 MG
8:42 FENTANYL 100 UG
8:44 THIOPENTAL 50 MG
8:44 SUCCINYLCHO 80 MG
8:53 PANCURONIUM 3 MG

Figure 15-8. This anesthesia record was made by a device manufactured by Ohmeda. The physiologic variables are recorded automatically; the events are entered with the help of a touch screen (see Fig. 15-9). (Courtesy of Ohmeda, Madison, WI)

Table 15-1. EQUIPMENT CHECKLIST

Monitors	
†ECG monitor:	power on
†cable	ck
†leads	ck
†electrodes	ck
†B/P monitor:	power on
†cuff	ck size
†Precordial stethoscope	ck
§Esophageal stethoscope	ck
†Temperature probe	ck room temperature
†Pulse oximeter	power on
†Probe	ck
†Mass spectrometer or O_2/CO_2 meter	power on
Anesthesia Machine	power on
Gas supply:	
*O_2 wall	secure
machine	secure
§N_2O wall	secure
machine	secure
Auxiliary tanks:	
*O_2	ck 2200 psi
§N_2O	ck 745 psi
Flow meters:	
*O_2	ck moves freely
†N_2O	ck moves freely
*O_2 flush	ck on/off function
Breathing Circuit	
Common gas outlet hose	
*To circle system	ck attached/secure
†Soda lime	ck color
*Breathing hoses	ck attached; ck leaks
*Bag	ck attached; ck leaks
*Valve discs	ck present; ck moves
†Absorbant bypass	ck off
*Mask	ck attached; ck size
†Humidifier	ck
Ventilator	
§Power	ck source on/off
§Settings	ck set; ck function
†Hose to circuit	ck attached/secure
Vaporizers:	
†Fluid levels	ck
*Filling valves	ck closed
*Suction	ck on
*tip/catheter	ck ready
†Scavenging system	ck on

(Continued)

Table 15-1. (*continued*)

Supplies and Medications	
†Induction agent	ck labeled
†Muscle relaxant(s)	ck labeled
†Vasopressor	ck labeled
†Atropine	ck labeled
†Oral airway	ck size
†Tongue blade	ck
*Endotracheal tube	ck cuff; ck size
*Laryngoscope/blade	ck size; ck light
†Stylet	ck ready
§Tape	ck ready
†Fluids	ck

* Most important.
† Second priority—no instant death if not OK.
§ Third priority—delay not dangerous
(Paulus DA, Basta JW, Klie H, et al: Preanesthetic checklist. Anesth Analg 64:264, 1985)

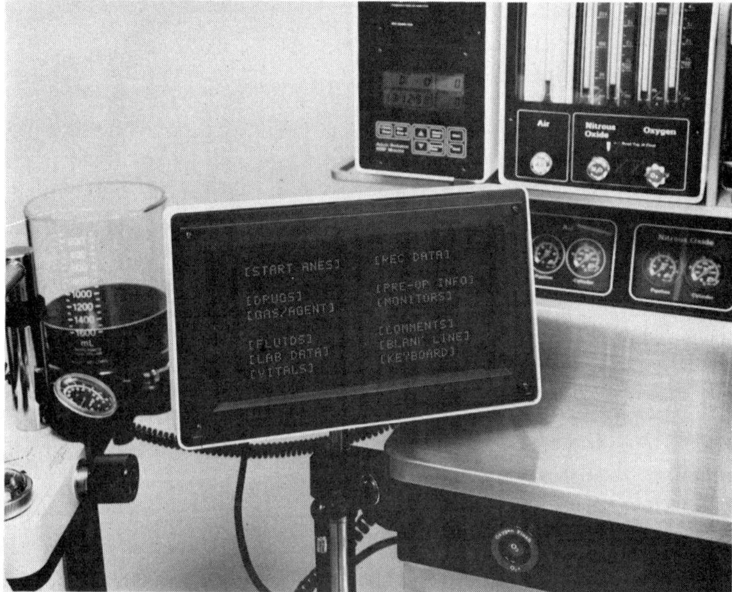

Figure 15-9. A data entry touch screen. The Ohmeda system has a record printing system incorporated into the table of the anesthesia machine. Hand entries are not required if the clinician avails himself of the touch screen that displays data and offers menus from which selection of entries can be made and commands for the operation of the device are given. (Courtesy of Ohmeda, Madison, WI)

Records in the Postanesthesia Recovery Room and Intensive Care Units

In the not too distant past, postanesthesia recovery rooms and intensive care units did not exist. They were established because all too often respiratory and cardiovascular complications overtook a patient soon after he had been returned to his room on the general ward. It became apparent that postoperative patients required more attention than busy ward nurses could give, yet less care than was available in the operating room. This perspective on the recovery room explains why the records there so clearly show their kinship to the anesthesia record (Fig. 15-5); indeed, the recovery room record is often printed on the back of the anesthesia record.

The intensive care unit is an extension of the recovery room and many of the variables monitored are the same as in operating and recovery rooms. However, the long stay of the patient in the intensive care unit brings with it the need to maintain extended records of fluid balance and respiratory management. Finally, attention to metabolic problems distinguishes the intensive care unit records from those of operating and recovery rooms.

REFERENCES

1. Beecher HK: The first anesthesia records. Surg Gynecol Obstet 71:689–693, 1940
2. Patient safety and risk management (film series). Park Ridge, IL, American Society of Anesthesiologists, and Washington, DC, US Food and Drug Administration, 1985
3. New classification of physical status. Anesthesiology 24:111, 1963
4. Owens WD, Felts JA, Spitznagel EL Jr: ASA physical classifications: A study of consistency of ratings. Anesthesiology 49:239, 1978
5. Aldrete JA, Kroulik D: A post-anesthetic score. Anesth Analg 49:294, 1970
6. Collins V: Principles of Anesthesiology, 2nd ed, p 191. Philadelphia, Lea & Febiger, 1976
7. Accreditation Manual for Hospitals (AMH/87), pp 1–8. Chicago, Joint Commission on Accreditation of Hospitals, 1986
8. Zollinger RM Jr, Kreul JF, Schneider AJ: Man-made versus computer-generated anesthesia records. J Surg Res 22:419, 1977
9. Schneider AJ: The validity of data from anesthesia records. In Grundy BL, Gravenstein JS (eds): The Quality of Care in Anesthesia, pp 100–113. Springfield, IL, Charles C Thomas, 1982
10. Paulus DA, van der Aa J, McLaughlin G, et al: A more accurate anesthesia record: The electronic clipboard (abstr). Anesthesiology 61:A178, 1984
11. Ream AK: In Gravenstein JS, Newbower RS, Ream AK, et al (eds): An Automated Anesthesia Record and Alarms. Boston, Butterworths, 1986

CHAPTER 16

Alarms and Computers

In the last decades, two newcomers have made important inroads in operating rooms and intensive care units: alarms and computers. The alarms came unheralded, introduced by the companies whose engineers thought that clinicians would appreciate an automatic alarm that could be set as desired. Soon many physiologic monitors had their alarms, and, almost as soon, they were silenced because the alarms were not as helpful as had been expected. Computers made their appearance initially in an unobtrusive way, namely hidden as microprocessors in many electronic devices. Their role in these monitors is secure and will surely expand in the next decade. In this short chapter, we will outline what alarms do, and what they ought to do. We will also discuss computers, since alarms need them in order to function successfully.

ALARMS

No clinician currently working with monitoring equipment has been spared feelings of frustration and annoyance with "modern" alarms. We have recently counted over 20 alarms that might have sounded in a single operating room. It often takes more than a few seconds of searching to discover the source of a single alarming buzz or beep, and much longer when two or more sound simultaneously. In intensive care units, the problem is multiplied because a warning buzz may come from any number of beds due to either monitored physiologic variables or mechanical devices.

Single Variable Alarms

In current operating rooms and intensive care units, several physiologic monitors and mechanical devices come with the option of having an alarm sound when a specific variable crosses a threshold. Table 16-1 presents a typical list of variables that can trigger an alarm.

Although it is easy to define single variables that would indicate a cardiac arrest, for instance, a flat ECG or ventricular fibrillation or no detectable blood pressure, it is quite difficult to define the border at which a single variable slips from normal to abnormal. Where, for instance, should we draw the limits between normotension and hypotension? This problem does not beset alarms monitoring certain machine functions where we are dealing with all-or-none phenomena, such as ventilator disconnect or ECG lead fault. Other variables on equipment, however, also have to be set to distinguish between normal and abnormal, such as a high pressure alarm of a ventilator or high temperature in a humidifier.

Alarms Based on Multiple Variables

Clinical decisions rarely depend on a single variable. Yet, current alarm technology has not yet constructed systems that examine several variables before sounding an alarm. Multiple variables could offer redundancy and allow the identification of states.

Redundancy

Today several monitors report heart rate from different sources, for instance, as obtained from ECGs, blood pressure monitors (both invasive and noninvasive), and pulse oximeters. Before triggering an alarm because the ECG heart rate exceeded preset limits, it would be helpful to check whether the redundant signals from the other units still reported acceptable heart rates. If this were the case, an alarm triggered by electrical interference with the ECG signal could be ignored, provided heart rates monitored by oximeter and blood pressure apparatus were still normal. So far, such already available redundancy is not exploited to reduce the incidence of false positive alarms. Other redundancies could also be incorporated into the system. For example, clinicians often operate two

Table 16-1. DEVICES THAT SOUND ALARMS

Monitor	Alarm Variable
ECG	Lead fault Heart rate low Heart rate high
Blood pressure device	Systolic or diastolic pressure low Systolic or diastolic pressure high Heart rate low Heart rate high
Oxygen analyzer	Oxygen in circuit low Oxygen in circuit high
Pulse oximeter	O_2 saturation low O_2 saturation high Heart rate low Heart rate high No pulse detected
Capnograph	Respiratory rate low Respiratory rate high No breath detected Bad waveform Inspired CO_2 high Expired CO_2 low Expired CO_2 high
Humidifier	Temperature high Temperature low
Mass spectrometer (in addition to repeating O_2 and CO_2 warnings, monitors anesthetic agent)	High
Electrocautery unit	Ground fault
Heating mattress	Temperature high Water level low Ground fault Incomplete circuit
Infusion apparatus	Air in tubing Obstruction Out of fluid Completed infusion

(In addition to these devices, respirometers, ventilators, and anesthesia machines, depending on make and model, have multiple alarms for gas pressures and volumes, etc.)

blood pressure measuring devices; many ventilator–anesthesia systems have two pressure gauges, others have two sources to monitor oxygen in the inspired gas.

The State

In the physiologic sense, a state is defined by a number of variables, the aggregate of which expresses a condition that is meaningful to the clinician. In clinical practice, a low arterial blood pressure with a low heart rate carries quite a different message (vagal stimulation? hypoxemia? sepsis?) than a low arterial pressure with a high heart rate (cardiac failure? hypovolemia?). As soon as a relevant third variable is added to the second one, additional refinement in differential diagnosis becomes possible. Thus, pulse oximetry could help to distinguish the state of hypoxemia from that of vagal stimulation.

In practice, this will probably be done with a hedge, that is, the computer—and it will take a computer—to print out a list of suggestions for consideration by the clinician. For the example of low arterial pressure and heart rate, the message might read: "check oxygenation; rule out hypoxemic bradycardia; vagal bradycardia." We believe that the future will bring such systems. But we have yet to define the different states that could be recognized by a computer-driven system and the thresholds for the different variables that would define any given state.

Another option is to look for the rate and extent of changes in a number of variables instead of looking for the crossing of thresholds. Thus, the clinician could be notified by computer when specific variables, such as blood pressure and heart rate changed and whether they changed rapidly or slowly, greatly or minimally, and whether the signal was steady or variable.[1] From such information one could also glean important information. For instance, a very rapid drop in systolic, mean, and diastolic pressure without a simultaneous change in heart rate or oximeter reading may mean nothing more than that the arterial catheter was turned off for the sampling of arterial blood. No alarm should sound. Experienced clinicians will be able to suggest many scenarios where rapid or slow, drastic or mild changes in this or that combination of variables connote alarming states or harmless occurrences.

The Priority

As yet we have few graded alarms of singly monitored variables. Examples are the Nellcor* and Ohmeda† pulse oximeters, which beep with

* Nellcor, Hayward, California
† Ohmeda, Boulder, Colorado

Table 16-2. THE DRÄGER SYSTEM HIERARCHY*

Class	Message	Priority	Condition	Audio	Visual
Warning	Apnea-vol	High	No volume detected in ventilator for 30 sec	Continuous	Flashing red
Caution	Apnea-vol	Medium	No volume detected in ventilator for 15 sec	Intermittent	Red
Advisory	O_2 sensor disconnected	Low	O_2 sensor unplugged	Single tone	Yellow
Advisory	Low tidal volume	Low	Tidal volume less than 70 ml	None	Yellow

* Extracted from a larger list

every pulse. This beep changes pitch as the oxygen saturation drops (or rises). Thus, an auditory as well as alphanumeric message serves to alert the clinician. But, to our knowledge, no monitor allows us to set two or three distinct thresholds corresponding to minimal, moderate, and extreme urgency.

Standard-setting agencies have also recognized these problems and at present the American Society for Testing and Materials (ASTM) defines three conditions that can trigger a warning signal: emergency, caution, and alert; there is also a general information category.[2] Few monitors in the operating room distinguish between the severities of the conditions. Since most alarms allow the setting of only a single threshold, our options are limited. Should there be violations of two or more thresholds simultaneously, would one not be likely to have priority over the other? Engineers designing monitoring equipment are beginning to respond to our needs for intelligent alarms. Particular praise should be given to North American Dräger,* the manufacturer not of a monitor *per se*, but of an anesthesia machine. Here, as far as we know for the first time, a hierarchy of warnings has been incorporated in the alarm system, the so-called Centralert. Its advantage is that it displays messages related to undesirable conditions of several indices. Table 16-2 shows examples of the hierarchy used by the Dräger system.[3]

With systems that integrate information from multiple variables, should some states not be given priority over others? An alarm sounded for a hypoxemic bradycardia with hypotension would call for a response

* North American Dräger, Allentown, Pennsylvania

with greater urgency than an alarm for vagal bradycardia secondary to the surgeon's tug on the mesentery. Before we can hope to get that type of sophistication in our alarms, the applications of models and expert systems (see below) will have to mature.

Sensitivity of Alarms

Only when set to be triggered by extreme values (*e.g.*, an exceedingly low blood pressure or heart rate) is a single variable alarm *consistently* helpful. At such a setting the alarm would have few if any false negatives; it would be said to exhibit high sensitivity. Fortunately, extreme values occur only rarely, but when they do trigger an alarm, the message is quite important. It would, therefore, make much sense to set alarms to extreme values rather than suffer the annoyance of frequent alerts that lead the users to disable the alarm and thus, lose any benefit from it. Monitoring redundant variables would reduce the incidence of false positives further, regardless of where the limits were set.

Introducing alarm technology that recognizes states would offer the advantage that alarm limits on single variables could be set at extreme values. When states are identified, these extreme values would not have to be reached. For example, when blood pressure is monitored, it might be useful to set an extreme alarm for a systolic pressure of 50 torr. That alarm would sound only with massive, sudden bleeding or a cardiac arrest, that is, only very rarely. But a pressure drop from 120 torr to 90 torr systolic, linked to an increase in heart rate from 80 beats to 100 beats per minute and coinciding with a decrease in central venous pressure from 7 cm to 3 cm H_2O, would generate a message labeled "check for hypovolemia" even though no single variable had reached extreme values or, indeed, values abnormal enough to cause concern when viewed individually rather than in the context of changes in other variables.*

COMPUTERS

Three abilities distinguish a computer:

1. It can add, compare, and select digital numbers very rapidly.
2. It can remember many numbers.
3. It can recall very rapidly what it has remembered.

These three abilities have been exploited in having computers carry out the most laborious calculations in fractions of a second. Such calculations often mean solving one set of problems, then using some of the results

* Values given here are examples and have not been established by scientific method.

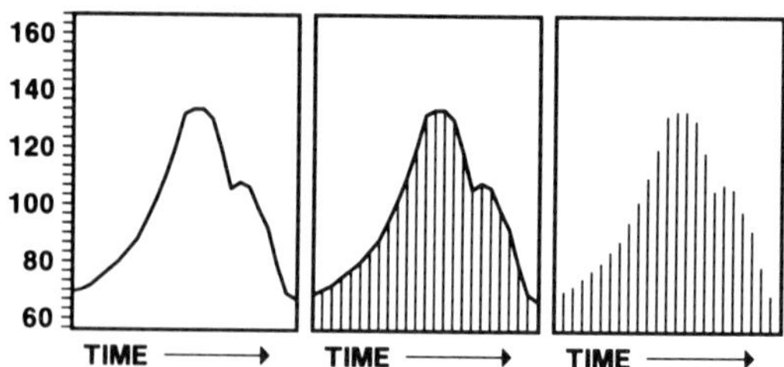

Figure 16-1. Analog to digital (A to D) conversion. Modern computers convert physiologic data such as blood pressure from their analog (curves describing the pressure changes during one cardiac cycle) into digital (numbers defining many points on the curve) formats. A to D conversion facilitates mathematical manipulation of data.

of the first set in the solution of a second, and so on for hundreds or thousands upon thousands of steps. This requires rapid reckoning, the ability to remember the results, and the capacity to recall them at a moment's notice for use in another step of computation, all of which is helpful not only when one has to calculate and recalculate the trajectory of a satellite or of Halley's comet, but also in a hospital.

Analog to Digital Conversion

In the operating room and intensive care unit, such prowess can also be exploited. For instance, the outline of a single blood pressure curve obtained invasively can be viewed as a series of measurements taken in rapid succession and then plotted with pressure on the *y* and time on the *x* axes (Fig. 16-1). Turning such a curve (an "analog curve") into a set of numbers is to digitize it. An instrument that converts analog signals into digital data is called an analog to digital or A/D converter.

Knowing the digital values for enough points of the pressure curve then permits the calculation of a mean pressure (the sum of them all averaged over time). Or one can have the computer compare all the values and let it name the lowest (diastolic), and the highest (systolic), or have it calculate the average systolic over 4 seconds, or 1 minute, or whatever. And this can be done for any measure that can be converted into numbers. Or, one can let it measure the rate of rise by letting it keep track of every value as long as they get bigger and bigger and at the same time count the time that has passed. For other curves the plateau can be measured and disturbances in the curve can be detected by letting the computer compare one value after the other.

Programming

For all of this one needs to give the computer a specific and detailed set of instructions, called programs. These can be laborious to write and newcomers who are awed by the speed of a computer are always suspicious when the programmers declare that it will take months to complete a program. Suspicion often turns to despair if after months the program does not perform as desired because "bugs" have nested in the program. To find and eliminate them takes more months. Unfortunately these bugs cannot be killed with an insecticide spray! Such sprays are not to be used on programmers! Bugs are usually small mistakes, sometimes amounting to nothing more than a "plus" instead of a "minus" in a command, which, however, sent the entire calculation in the wrong direction or to a wrong result.

The programs are referred to as *software*, in contrast to the wires and chips and electronic components of computers that are called *hardware*. By now we have software specialists and hardware experts, and then the rest of us who depend on their skills and patience.

The computer lives on numbers as we live on oxygen. Everything has to be reduced to numbers. Even wordprocessors, which masquerade as clever typewriters, are number machines, where every letter is converted into a number. That looks like an awkward system, but for computers with their prodigious speed and memory it is simple.

If computers do all of that, small wonder that the manufacturers of electronic monitoring equipment have incorporated little, and sometimes not so little, computers or computer components into their devices to calculate, average, remember, compare, announce, or display the results. Of course, instead of lighting up a display or causing words to be typed, the computer could throw a switch, start a pump, and calculate how much of a drug should be given. This, indeed, is likely to be something computers will be able to do better than people.

Models

When, for instance, we wish to lower the arterial pressure from a mean of 100 torr to a mean of 60 torr, the clinician titrates a vasodilator such as sodium nitroprusside. He would let it run in fast at first to budge the pressure and then would slow it down in order to avoid an overshoot. He would watch the pressure and dial in more or less drug to obtain the desired pressure. By necessity he will have to pay close attention to the blood pressure so that he can respond with a quick adjustment of the rate of infusion. But even close attention will not be enough to generate a smooth decline of the pressure without undershoot, to maintain a stable pressure during hypotension, and to return the pressure to a normal level without overshooting. Computers can do better. Not only can they pay unflagging attention, they also can calculate requirements and make adjustments in their calculations as they find that their initial conclusion led to all too rapid a decline or increase of pressure.[4]

Such calculation of how much to infuse initially and at what rate of infusion to stabilize the administration of the drug requires mathematical models of physiologic systems. These models have to be developed by scientists, but can be used "on the fly" only by computers fast enough to keep up with the required calculations even as the system changes in response to the treatment. A model designed, for instance, for the administration of sodium nitroprusside must be able to anticipate how the body of a specific patient (weight, blood volume, cardiac output, etc.) will distribute the drug, how quickly it will respond to the infusion, how much it will lower the pressure, and how long it will take to dissipate the effect. It must then be able to revise the calculations (the model "learns") as the response to the treatment can be assessed.[5]

Other models do not provide for adaptation, for instance, a model of the appearance of CO_2 in the expired gas that includes information about the CO_2 production, the volumes in which the CO_2 will distribute itself (lung, airways, ventilator system), the fresh gas flowing into the system, the pressure required to spill excess gas, the location of the overflow valve, the tidal volume and respiratory rate, the compliance of the system, and the resistance to gas flow in different components.[6] Any change in these variables will disturb the congruence of the mathematical model with the data gleaned from the patient and will call for a diagnosis of which variable might have changed to have caused the deviations from expected values.

The Expert System

Another approach that is being taken by computer buffs is the expert system. Here the designers are not attempting to define the model in physiologic detail but are content with observing experts at work. They then say, "Ah, every time the blood pressure drops by 30% and heart rate increases by 15% and CVP goes down by 50%, the expert lightens anesthesia and administers fluids."* Thus, the computer could be programmed to give a message on the monitoring screen saying "Check for indications to lighten anesthesia and give fluids" whenever it recognized such a set of circumstances, or in other words the state of hypovolemia as defined by the experts.

* Values given here are examples and have not been established by scientific method.

The Patient Bookkeeper

Computers make many appearances in devices where things need to be organized and plotted. Good examples of that are the automated records discussed in Chapter 15.

The least glamorous, but presently widest use of free-standing computers in hospitals (*i.e.,* not part of record keepers or CT scans or the like) is in the management of data: collecting them, storing them, ordering them this and that way, remembering them, and replaying them whenever commanded to do so. If there could ever be a computer revolution, it would come when the machines realized that we shamelessly exploit them to do menial things that require endless patience, a prodigious memory, and inurement to the most tedious repetitions.

REFERENCES

1. Beneken JEW, Gravenstein JS: Sophisticated alarms in patient monitoring. A methodology based upon systems engineering concepts. In Gravenstein JS, Newbower RS, Ream AK, et al (eds): The Automated Anesthesia Record and Alarm Systems. Boston, Butterworth. (in press)
2. Spraker T: Biomedical standards. In Gravenstein JS, Newbower RS, Ream AK, et al (eds): The Automated Anesthesia Record and Alarm Systems. Boston, Butterworth. (in press)
3. Schreiber P: Safety Guidelines for Anesthesia Systems, p. 87. Allentown, PA, North American Dräger, 1984
4. Sheppard LC: Computer control of the infusion of vasoactive drugs. Ann Biomed Eng 8:431–444, 1980
5. Pace NL, Westenshow DR: Computer regulated sodium nitroprusside infusion for blood pressure control. In Prakash O (ed): Computing in Anesthesia and Intensive Care, pp 292–301. Martinus Nyhoff, Boston, 1983
6. Beneken JEW, Gravenstein N, Gravenstein JS, et al: Capnography and the Bain circuit. I: A computer model. J Clin Monit 1:103–113, 1985

CHAPTER 17

Trace Gases in the Operating Room

Monitoring the level of anesthetic gases in the operating room is important for the protection of all personnel in the room. After long study, the American Society of Anesthesiologists published the most authoritative review of this subject. With their permission, a reprint of *Waste Anesthetic Gases in Operating Room Air: A Suggested Program to Reduce Personnel Exposure** follows:

Over the past 12 years, anesthesiologists have become aware that health hazards may exist consequent to working in the operating room environment. While the number of studies increases, the data remain

* This material was written by The American Society of Anesthesiologists, Ad Hoc Committee on Effects of Trace Anesthetic Agents on Health of Operating Room Personnel: Richard Mazze, MD, Chairman; Helmut Cascorbi, MD, PhD; Tom Jones, DDS; Jordan Katz, MD, and John Lecky, MD; Edited by John H Lecky, MD.

equivocal and a firm cause–effect relationship between chronic exposure to trace levels of anesthetic gases and disease entities in operating room personnel does not exist.

It is not the intent of this reprint to resolve the question regarding the scientific merit of the epidemiologic and laboratory studies. This booklet has been prepared in order to offer you a simple "how to do it" approach to reduce your and your co-worker's exposure to waste anesthetic gases. From the first suspicion that there might be an occupational hazard in the operating room, The American Society of Anesthesiologists has taken an active role in attempting to delineate the problem by initiating appropriate epidemiologic and laboratory studies and by supporting the development of information on how to reduce personnel exposure. This reprint represents one more ASA effort along these lines. It has been developed by a committee of your colleagues who have extensive experience in the design and use of scavenging systems and in the development of maintenance and monitoring procedures in the operating room.

While the authors feel that the data suggesting an operating room health hazard warrant the development and support of measures to reduce personnel exposure, we also feel that the issue must be kept in perspective: *The administration of anesthesia and the safety of the patient are our primary goals—pollution control must be of secondary concern.* Thus, we do not advocate marked alteration in anesthesia technique or the installation of complex scavenging systems which potentially compromise the administration of anesthesia or the safety of the patient. We do suggest a number of practical measures which can be taken to reduce exposure.

Lastly, some of you, after finishing this chapter may still have questions. A comprehensive reference list may be obtained from the ASA.* We hope that this reprint will allow you, with a minimum of effort, to institute and maintain an effective trace gas control program.

SCAVENGING OF EXCESS CIRCUIT GASES

The installation of an effective scavenging system is essential in reducing trace gas levels in the operating room. Scavenging alone can reduce pollution levels tenfold. There are three major components in an excess gas scavenging system: gas capturing assembly, disposal assembly, and interface.

* Write: American Society of Anesthesiologists, Anesthetic Contamination in the Operating Room Reference List, 515 Busse Highway, Park Ridge, Illinois 60068

Gas-Capturing Apparatus

The gas-capturing apparatus collects waste gases from the breathing circuit, ventilator, or extracorporeal pump oxygenator, enabling them to be conducted away from the breathing circuit for disposal. Such devices must not significantly alter circuit dynamics or delivered gas concentration.

Mechanical ventilators used during the administration of anesthesia must also be equipped with a means to capture and conduct effluent gases into the scavenging system for disposal. In some instances, however, the ventilator exhaust includes both the excess circuit gases and the driving gas. This may require a disposal system of high capacity. The ventilator manufacturer should clearly specify the scavenging system requirements necessary for effective scavenging with his particular ventilator, and whether it is compatible with the disposal system(s) available in the hospital.

The manufacturer of extracorporeal pump oxygenators should provide safe and effective means of evacuating the pump gas flow, if anesthesia is administered during cardiopulmonary bypass. In many cases, however, gas-capturing systems for oxygenators are still in the developmental stage. Because significant positive or negative pressure alteration at the gas outflow port can markedly alter oxygenator function, it is imperative to provide an effective scavenging interface system (see below) to ensure that excessive pressure swings do not occur at the oxygenator exhaust port.

Disposal System

Excess circuit gases may be disposed of by several routes: (1) nonrecirculating air conditioning system, (2) central vacuum system, (3) an independent system, (4) passive through-wall system, and (5) adsorber.

1. In operating rooms with effective nonrecirculating ventilation systems (100% fresh makeup air), the captured anesthetic gases may be conducted to an exhaust grill fixture. Flow around the fixture into the ventilation system effectively removes the anesthetic waste. Ideally, the disposal line to the exhaust grill should run overhead, so that the risk of occlusion is minimal. Should such a route be impractical, then the wall of the tubing should be reinforced, to avoid the possibility of occlusion by equipment wheels or someone standing on the tubing.

   Additionally, an interface should be included in the system, between the gas-capturing apparatus and the disposal line to ensure positive pressure relief in the event of accidental occlusion (see below).
2. Scavenging by means of a recirculating ventilation system results

in contamination of all the rooms on the common manifold. In this case, the central vacuum can be used as an alternate disposal route. (***Caution:*** Regulations of the National Fire Protection Association prohibit disposal of flammable agents into a central vacuum system.)

3. If neither the central vacuum nor the air conditioning system can be used, then an independent disposal system must be provided; such as a dedicated suction or blower system. Such independent anesthetic gas evacuation systems ought to be considered during renovation or in the design of new operating rooms. The system should be readily accessible to the anesthesia machine, and high volume (30–40 liters/min) flow (although not necessarily high vacuum) should be provided. As with all disposal routes, waste gases should be vented at a point where no possibility of personnel exposure exists.
4. Passive systems venting excess gas through a wall fitting to the outside are also acceptable, although these systems, too, must have positive pressure relief capability between the gas-capturing apparatus and the disposal line in the event of occlusion.

   If the central vacuum or an independent exhaust system is to be used, the hospital engineering department should be consulted regarding volume capacity and equipment resistance to corrosive chemicals. They should also be consulted to verify that the ventilation system is nonrecirculating, if that exhaust route is to be employed.
5. Activated charcoal adsorbers can remove halogenated agents from an excess anesthetic gas stream. These devices are relatively expensive, have a short life span (hours to days) and are ineffective in adsorbing N_2O. Their use, then, is limited to short-term elimination of halogenated agents.

Interface

Scavenging equipment adds complexity, and thus hazards, to the administration of anesthesia. In essence, a scavenging system extends the anesthetic circuit all the way to the final disposal point, so that any pressure alterations brought about by unopposed vacuum in or blockage of the scavenging system can be transferred to the anesthetic circuit, potentially harming the patient. With regard to safety, then, the most important component of an excess gas scavenging system is the interface, which relieves positive pressure in the event of scavenging system occlusion and prevents vacuum pressures from reaching the patient circuit when a blower or central suction system is used.

Manufacturers of scavenging systems which rely on a certain volume flow should clearly specify flow rate requirement and should suggest or provide some means of measuring it. A reservoir should be provided so that if circuit exhaust flows transiently exceed the ability of the disposal system to clear it, spillage will not occur. The major considerations in the design and selection of an interface, then, are adequate provision for protecting the patient from pressure fluxes by providing positive pressure relief and, if necessary, negative pressure relief and reservoir capacity to avoid spill of anesthetic agents when vacuum capacity is transiently exceeded.

ANTI-LEAK EQUIPMENT MAINTENANCE PROCEDURES

Anesthesia machines and their scavenging systems should routinely undergo servicing at regular intervals by a manufacturer's representative or equivalent. At those times, both the high and low pressure portions of the anesthesia machine should be examined and leakage corrected. Experience has been, however, that these routine service visits do not always identify or correct all of the high or low pressure leak points. In fact, significant leakage may remain after routine servicing. Additionally, leakage can develop suddenly; especially in the low pressure system. In-house monitoring by department personnel is necessary to ensure that leakage is minimized. It is unrealistic, in terms of time and cost, to expect manufacturers to maintain anesthesia equipment in a leakage-free state in the field.

Low Pressure System

The low pressure portion of the anesthesia machine extends from the flow meters to the patient and leakage from this portion of the anesthesia apparatus can be of sufficient magnitude to virtually negate scavenging. N_2O levels can reach the 200 parts per million to 300 parts per million (ppm) range, due to low pressure leakage alone! Thus, we recommend that leakage testing be incorporated into the routine check-out procedure before the start of every anesthetic. Frequent sites of low pressure leakage are presented in Figure 17-1.

To Test Low Pressure System Leakage

Close the relief valve ("pop-off valve") and occlude the Y-piece with your hand. Using a flow O_2 rotameter, note the O_2 inflow required to achieve and maintain a steady circuit pressure of 30 cm H_2O for 30 seconds with the reservoir bag in place. This flow rate represents the leakage rate. Circuit pressures during controlled ventilation average about 10 cm

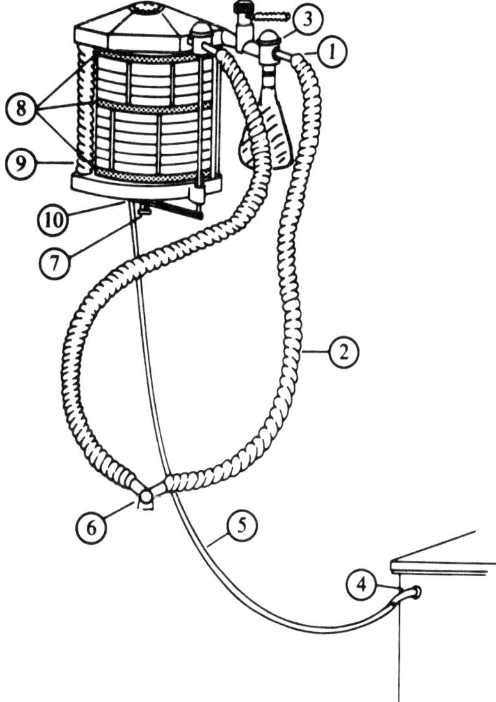

Figure 17-1. Major low pressure leak sites: (*1*) improper circle tubing connection; (*2*) perforated or cracked circle tubing; (*3*) leaking dome seals; (*4*) eccentric gas delivery hose–machine connection joint; (*5*) defective delivery hose; (*6*) leaking Y-connector; (*7*) improperly closed absorber; (*8*) improper cannister seal (gasket torn or kinked, soda lime granules spilled on gasket); (*9*) perforated or cracked bypass tubing; (*10*) leaking drain cock.

H_2O. Low pressure system leakage is roughly linear with pressure; thus, a 150 ml/min leak at 30 cm H_2O will produce approximately a 50 ml/min leak during controlled ventilation. The overall contribution to N_2O levels in the average operating room with a leak of this size should be less than 5 ppm. If the leak exceeds 150 ml/min, steps should be taken to detect and correct the leakage points. Leakage can be detected by trial and error or with the application of a soap solution (20% liquid soap, 80% H_2O) or an infrared (IR) N_2O analyzer. Defective delivery lines or circle and bypass tubing should be discarded. Other common causes of leakage include torn, cracked, or kinked cannister seals, and inadequate cannister tightening. Soda lime granules spilled on the gaskets can also prevent a tight seal.

High Pressure System

The high pressure N_2O system includes the central N_2O lines (at approximately 50 psi) and the anesthesia machine from the N_2O tanks (750 psi) to the flow meters. Leakage from these components causes elevated N_2O levels in the operating room even when no anesthesia is being given. With a recirculating ventilation system such leakage causes cross contamination between operating rooms (see The Ventilation System, below). These sources can produce concentrations in the hundreds of parts of NO_2 per million. With good maintenance procedures, however, high pressure leakage can be virtually eliminated.

Central N_2O Line Connectors

High pressure N_2O lines are made of flexible pressure tubing and are often provided with "quick connect" joints. Leakage usually occurs at the connectors; however, it can also occur at the fixed wall connection, inside a stand pipe or through defective tubing. Immersion in water, application of soap solution or use of an IR analyzer will usually identify these leaks. Once corrected, leakage can recur so that routine examination of high pressure lines and connectors should be performed quarterly.

Anesthesia Machine High Pressure Leakage

The N_2O tank yoke is an important source of leakage from the high pressure portion of the anesthesia machine. Tightening the clamp often seals an existing leak. Deformed, doubled, or absent washers are common leak sources and must be replaced. Soap solution applied to the yoke readily demonstrates a poor seal. The internal tubing, connections and valves, etc., are also potential, although rare, leakage sites.

TO TEST FOR HIGH PRESSURE GAS MACHINE LEAKAGE

Disconnect the anesthesia machine from the external N_2O source, close the rotameter valve, and open a tank of N_2O to pressurize the machine. Close the tank valve and record the N_2O tank pressure. One hour later, record the tank pressure again. If little or no pressure drop has occurred, the machine is tight. If it falls to zero, leakage is significant. With the exception of N_2O yoke leakage, most problems discovered in this system probably require a manufacturer's service representative for proper correction.

If leakage from the N_2O connectors is eliminated and the high pressure side of the anesthesia machine is tight, baseline N_2O levels should be less than 5 ppm in the area of the anesthesiologist. If N_2O connectors leak visibly when immersed in water and the high pressure side of the

A

Technician ______________

Date	Room No.	Machine No.	N_2O Connectors Mid	N_2O Connectors End	Machine Pressure Initial	Machine Pressure After 1 Hr.	Comments

B

Technician ______________

Date	Room No.	Machine No.	Initial Leak Rate	Corrected Rate	Leak Sites

Figure 17-2. (*A*) Sample high pressure test record and (*B*) sample low pressure test record (report leak rate in milliliters of O_2 per minute at a circuit pressure of 30 cm H_2O).

anesthesia machine fails to maintain its pressure over 2 hours, then significant baseline levels of N_2O can be anticipated. Infrared analyzers are also useful for the detection of baseline N_2O levels and in the identification of leakage sites (see Monitoring of Trace Anesthetic Gas Levels, below). Leak tests are best performed in the morning before the operating rooms are used and results of the tests should be recorded and maintained (Fig. 17-2*A*,*B*)

The above program is the mainstay of high and low pressure system leakage control. The individual supervising the maintenance program should always be notified immediately if any leaks are discovered that cannot be corrected during routine inspection.

REDUCTION OF TRACE ANESTHETIC LEVELS BY ALTERATION OF WORK PRACTICES

In addition to scavenging system malfunction and equipment leakage, the manner in which anesthetics are administered can contribute significantly to trace gas levels in the operating room. This section points out some of the work practices which lead to high levels of waste gases and suggests

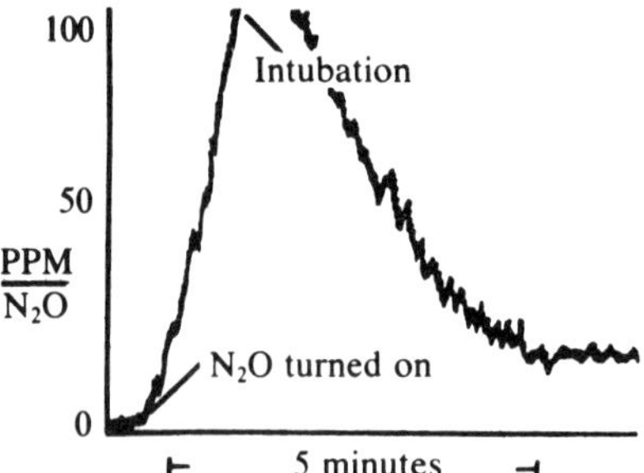

Figure 17-3. Unopposed gas spill during induction. Sequence: N_2O flow at 7 liters/min, thiopental administered, mask placed on patient, intubation.

minor changes in work practices which can reduce operating room contamination without compromising patient safety.

Trace gas contamination resulting from work practices tends to be transient, but can reach quite high levels and in the case of a loosely fitted face mask such levels can persist throughout a case. With careful work practices and proper scavenging, very low intraoperative levels have been reported.

It is quite possible to alter work practices to avoid gas spill, yet not compromise the safe administration of anesthesia. The following is a list of suggestions that can substantially reduce anesthetic spillage. Where applicable, tracings obtained in the breathing zone of the anesthesiologist using an IR N_2O analyzer are included, to illustrate the effect of some of these work practices on N_2O levels.

Suggestion 1

Unless warranted by the clinical situation, avoid turning on the N_2O or volatile agent until the mask is properly fitted, or the trachea is intubated and the endotracheal tube is connected to the circuit. By doing this, excess gas enters the scavenging system and room contamination is minimized (Figs. 17-3, 17-4).

Suggestion 2

Where reasonable, discontinue anesthetic gas flows and empty the reservoir bag into the scavenging system prior to suctioning or intubation to prevent gas spillage (Fig. 17-5).

Suggestion 3

At the end of a case, before extubation or removal of the mask, administer 100% O_2 for as long as possible, so that the washed out anesthetic gas

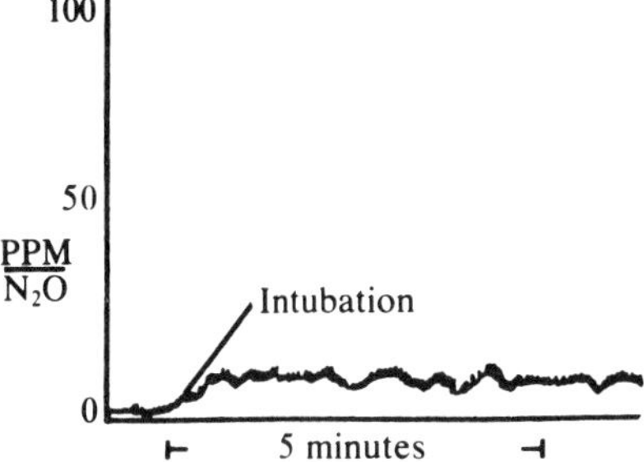

Figure 17-4. N_2O levels during induction. Sequence: trachea intubated, circuit connected. N_2O administration begun.

can be removed by the scavenging system. As well as benefitting the patient, this keeps contamination to a minimum (Fig. 17-6).

Suggestion 4

Exercise care in filling vaporizers. Spillage of even small amounts of volatile agents results in markedly elevated levels (1 ml of a volatile anesthetic vaporizes to approx. 200 ml of gas). The olfactory threshold for most volatile agents is 50 ppm; if you can smell it, you are being exposed to very high levels.

Suggestion 5

Mask fit is critical. It is possible to run quite low trace gas levels during a case, using a mask and assisted or controlled ventilation. Loose mask fit, however, can result in high levels of waste anesthetic gases (Fig.

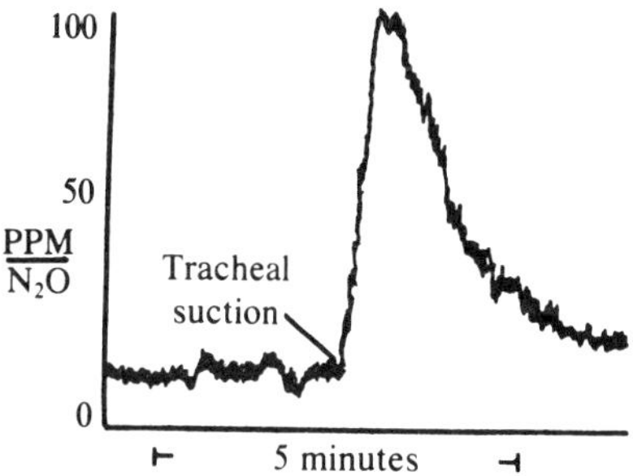

Figure 17-5. Effect on N_2O levels of continued gas flow during suctioning.

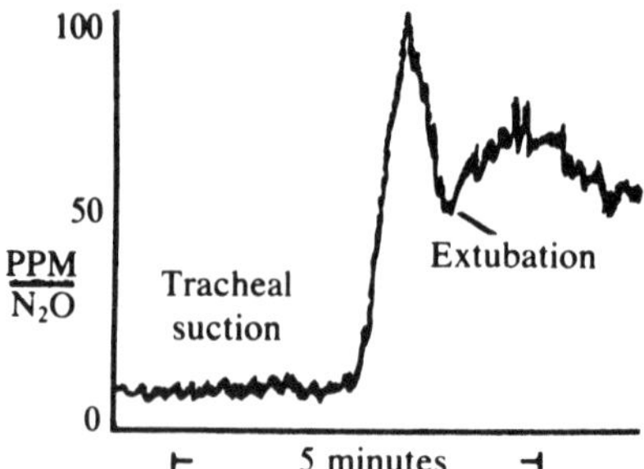

Figure 17-6. N_2O levels resulting from suctioning and extubation without prior O_2 breathing.

17-7). Often, very small changes in mask angle can mean the difference between a poor and a tight fit.

Adherence to the above suggestions can significantly reduce operating room contamination. They are intended as suggestions only and obviously become of secondary importance when patient safety is in question. You should be able to follow these suggestions most of the time, however, without interfering with the safe administration of anesthesia.

THE VENTILATION SYSTEM

Two basic types of ventilation systems are used in hospitals. With a non-recirculating type, all of the air which enters the operating room is brought into the building, passed through filters, into the operating room and is then exhausted to the outside. Such a system is suitable for anesthetic gas disposal (see Scavenging of Excess Circuit Gases, above). However, it has the disadvantage that all of the air must be heated or cooled (which can be very costly). A recirculating system is employed by many hospitals

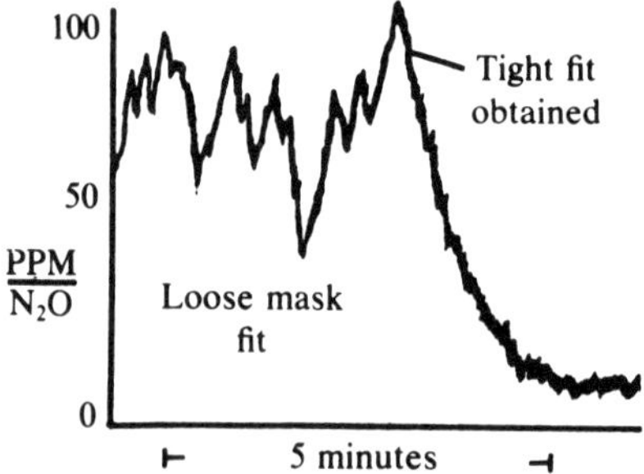

Figure 17-7. Effect of mask fit on N_2O levels.

and the amount of added fresh air will vary as a function of the outside temperature. Air exhausted from a room is filtered for particulate matter and bacteria, not anesthetic gases, and is then recirculated through several rooms by means of a common mixing (plenum) chamber. In this process, some fresh air is added and an equal amount of recirculating air is exhausted. With such a system, when anesthetic gas contamination occurs in one room, all of the rooms on the common system will become cross contaminated. Thus, reduction of trace gas levels in each room becomes all the more important with a recirculating system to avoid cross contamination of other operating rooms.

Once spilled into the room, anesthetic gases are removed slowly by the air conditioning system. Under no circumstances can the ventilation system be expected to adequately purge a room in the absence of effective scavenging.

The efficiency of ventilation in each operating room should be checked periodically to ensure that filters have not become clogged and that flows are appropriately balanced.

MONITORING OF TRACE ANESTHETIC GAS LEVELS

Trace gas levels can be determined by several methods, each with its own advantages and disadvantages. In this section, we will discuss several monitoring techniques and their applications. We will also present the major considerations in selecting a trace gas monitoring system and in deciding whether to perform on-site analysis or to use the services of a central testing facility.

Trace gas contamination in the operating room is the net result of four main factors:

1. High pressure system leakage
2. Low pressure system leakage
3. Technique-induced spillage
4. Scavenging system malfunction

The final assessment of a control program's effectiveness is the determination of intraoperative trace gas levels. These measurements achieve two objectives: (1) they reflect how well the four factors mentioned above are controlled, and (2) they document the concentrations found.

How Are Trace Gas Levels Described?

Low concentrations of gas are expressed on a volume/volume basis as parts per million. Thus, 100% of a gas equals 1,000,000 ppm and 1% of a gas equals 10,000 ppm.

Table 17-1. CONCENTRATIONS (ppm) OF N_2O IN BREATHING ZONE STUDIES*

Technique	Measurement	Anesthetist Zone	Circulating Nurse Zone	Scrub Nurse Zone
Mask + endotracheal	Mean ppm ± SE	50 ± 6.5	29 ± 3.6	30 ± 3.8
	ppm range	1 to 400	1 to 230	1 to 310
	n	190	190	190
	% ppm < 25	69	74	73
	% ppm > 100	26	19	9
Mask	Mean ppm ± SE	180 ± 25	100 ± 14	100 ± 14
	ppm range	23 to 430	9 to 230	9 to 250
	n	26	25	26
	% ppm < 25	4	8	8
	% ppm > 100	62	44	42
Endotracheal	Mean ppm ± SE	16 ± 5	9 ± 2	8 ± 1
	ppm range	12 to 370	0.5 to 80	0.5 to 69
	n	72	71	70
	% ppm < 25	93	95	97
	% ppm > 100	1	0	0

* Conducted in 11 air-conditioned operating rooms with anesthesia in progress—an effective anti-leakage equipment maintenance program was in effect. (Whitcher C: Occupational exposure, education and sampling methods. Anesthesiology 51 (suppl):S336, 1979)

What Levels Are Seen in the Operating Room?

In operating rooms in which no attempt has been made to reduce leakage or to scavenge waste gases, trace gas levels can approximate 500 ppm for N_2O and 10 ppm for halothane (or other halogenated agents). Effective scavenging can reduce these levels more than tenfold.

What Are Acceptable Levels?

At present, the National Institute for Occupational Safety and Health (NIOSH) Criteria Document proposes standards of less than 25 ppm N_2O and 0.5 ppm for halogenated agents or 2 ppm for halogenated agents when they are used alone. It is not known whether these are "safe" levels; they are based upon early studies suggesting that they are "readily achievable." More recent studies, however, lead us to question whether they are consistently achievable in the average hospital setting. In fact, N_2O levels averaging as high as 180 ppm have been reported, depending on work practices (Table 17-1). It is desirable to achieve the lowest possible levels (see above), accepting the fact that reasonable anesthesia practice (pediatric induction "steal," mask anesthesia, etc.) may result in levels above those that can be achieved in the ideal situation.

What Monitoring Options Exist?

There are three general approaches to gas sampling:

The Instantaneous or "Grab" Sample

The "grab" sample is best employed for analysis of steady state contamination, for example, high pressure leakage from N_2O hoses which produces baseline N_2O levels. Using a sampling syringe or other leak-free container, air samples can be obtained for subsequent analysis, either chromatographic or infrared. The container must not absorb the anesthetic and must not leak. Glass syringes are suitable, but only if the analysis is performed soon after sampling because they may leak. If samples are to be sent to a central testing facility, a leak-proof, inert container is mandatory.

Grab samples may also be used to measure intraoperative trace gas levels. In most instances, pollution levels tend to rise during the first half-hour of a case, then equilibrate about a level that represents the net effect of system leakage, air conditioning flow, anesthetic technique, and scavenging efficiency. Under these conditions, a grab sample, 30 minutes after induction of anesthesia, can afford a spot check on intraoperative levels, closely reflecting time-weighted average determinations a majority of the time. More elaborate and precise analysis methods are available and may be desirable and cost-effective.

Continuous Monitoring

Infrared monitors capable of continuous sampling, while expensive in terms of initial cost and maintenance, are useful for the rapid detection of leaks and for determining the effects of anesthetic technique on pollution levels. For the hospital with a large number of operating rooms (more than seven or eight) or a teaching program, the convenience and the immediate feedback provided by a continuous monitor may outweigh its expense. In the small hospital, the dental operatory, or the veterinary office, the time, expense, and staff required to maintain analyzing equipment may make possession of a continuous monitor uneconomical. In such circumstances, several institutions or individuals might consider sharing an instrument or a manufacturer's service representative might utilize one during his routine quarterly maintenance calls.

The Time-Weighted Average Sample

Time-weighted average (TWA) sampling is frequently employed for checking air contamination. A TWA sample is obtained by pumping ambient air continuously into an inert bag at constant low flow rates; the bag concentration then represents average exposure. The integrated output of an infrared analyzer will also provide a TWA.

How Often Should An Operating Room Be Tested?

After initiating the steps outlined previously, we recommend the following: (1) Baseline N_2O levels should be measured quarterly in each operating room after it has been out of service for at least 2 hours using either a grab sample method or an IR analyzer. (2) On the same day as #1, obtain a grab sample from the breathing zone of the anesthesiologist 30 minutes into a case. The sample should be analyzed based on the considerations previously outlined. For greater precision, several grab samples could be obtained during a case, TWA or continuous monitoring might be employed, or rooms could be sampled more frequently than on a quarterly basis. Such measurements should also be obtained in each operating room whenever major renovation or equipment alteration has occurred.

What If Trace Gas Levels Are High?

If baseline levels are above 5 ppm, then the anti-leak equipment maintenance procedures should be followed to correct leakage (see above).

If intraoperative levels are above 180 ppm with mask techniques (they should be lower with endotracheal techniques; Table 17-1), then the material in this chapter should be reviewed. You may determine that your trace gas levels are appropriate for your practice and, thus, are irreducible. On the other hand, elimination of leakage and simple changes in work practices may result in significant reduction in contaminant levels.

It should be noted that the levels selected are arbitrary. They are not known to be safe or, for that matter, toxic. They should, however, be obtainable in operating rooms where good scavenging and equipment maintenance procedures are followed. A sample data sheet for recording levels is presented in Figure 17-8.

ANESTHESIA DEPARTMENT INVOLVEMENT

It is important to remind Department of Anesthesia personnel that their efforts are the key to reducing not only their own exposure but that of their co-workers. The need for periodic reminders will vary from insti-

Date_______ O.R. No.______ Machine No.______ Technician______________

Ventilator_______ Low Pressure Leak Rate______ Scavenger Checked ______

"GRAB" SAMPLE

Time	PPM N_2O	PPM___	PPM___

TWA SAMPLE

Site	Time Span	PPM N_2O	PPM___	PPM___

Figure 17-8. Intraoperative trace gas monitoring report.

tution to institution. Large teaching hospitals where residents in training rotate through several hospitals will obviously require frequent reminders; none may be necessary in a smaller hospital with a more cohesive anesthesia group. Thus, both the tone and frequency with which anesthesia personnel are reminded of their role in reducing trace levels of anesthetic agents is a matter of judgment. A letter which can be used, if appropriate, for your institution follows: The use of such a letter not only enlists the aid of your personnel in this issue but also serves as an indication of your department's concern and of its attempts to control contaminant levels, further underscoring your role as a responsible employer.

To: Department of Anesthesia Staff
Re: Anesthetic Pollution Control

It is our intention with this letter to remind you of the health hazards that may result from chronic exposure to trace levels of anesthetic gases in the operating room and what you can do to reduce your and your co-workers exposure. However, before we continue, it is important to point out that our primary goal is the safe administration of anesthesia. Patient safety should never be compromised in the interest of pollution control.

There are three major sources of operating room contamination: (1) excess circuit gases—which should be captured by the scavenger, (2) equipment leakage, and (3) work practices. The following practices will help to reduce contamination by waste anesthetic gases.

1. Before starting an anesthetic, check to see that the scavenger is connected to an operating suction or other disposal route. Although there have been reports in the literature about hazards to the patient of

scavenging, well designed, operated, and maintained scavenging equipment poses little threat to the safe administration of anesthesia.

2. If a ventilator is to be used, ensure that it is appropriately connected to the scavenging system.
3. Check your anesthetic equipment for low pressure leakage prior to starting a case.
4. Try to avoid unnecessary spill of anesthetic gases into the room. Examine your practice of turning on the anesthetic gas flows. It is often unnecessary to turn on the gases before giving intravenous induction drugs and volatile agents to the patient. Such practice spills tremendous amounts of nitrous oxide into the room. Where the patient's condition or your plan warrants, try to have the mask on the patient's face before the anesthetic is begun. Where possible, connect the circle to the endotracheal tube before the anesthetic flows are begun so that excess gases are dumped into the scavenging system rather than into the room.
5. Where possible, discontinue anesthetic gas flows and empty the reservoir bag prior to suctioning or intubation.
6. At the end of a case, before extubation or removal of the mask, administer O_2 as long as possible so that the scavenging system can eliminate the washed out anesthetic gases. As well as benefiting the patient, this minimizes contamination.

Your efforts will contribute greatly to reduced exposure for all of us in the operating room. Thank you for your help.

NOTIFICATION OF EXPOSED PERSONNEL

Operating room pollution by anesthetic gases and the possibility that this pollution may cause a variety of disease entities in operating room workers often engenders emotional responses, far in excess of what is warranted. Our Committee has taken the position that even though data regarding the health hazards of waste anesthetic gases are equivocal, levels should be reduced and that we should inform our co-workers of the possible hazards of working in operating rooms.

A letter is presented below which might serve as a model for your hospital to use in dealing with potentially exposed members of the surgical, housekeeping, nursing, and anesthesia departments. This communication should be sent out annually and given to all new employees. In addition, in-service programs putting the equivocal nature of the health hazard data into perspective, pointing out what measures are being taken to reduce and monitor trace gas exposure, and indicating that personnel will be kept informed of major developments in the literature may be of value in your institution.

PERSONNEL NOTICE

Notice to Employees on the Possible Potential Health Hazards Associated with Occupational Exposure to Anesthetics

Our concern about your health and the quality of our environment requires that we periodically bring to your attention the suspected occupational health hazards associated with working in anesthetizing locations such as the operating room.

Epidemiologic surveys suggest that there may be increased incidences of some diseases, particularly those associated with the reproductive process, in operating room employees.

While chronic occupational exposure to trace concentrations of anesthetic gases is a suspected cause of these disease entities, the evidence is equivocal. Thus, conclusive proof of cause is presently not available. Indeed, other factors such as the stress of working in the operating room have also been proposed as causes of these health hazards.

Fortunately, anesthetic exposure can be reduced substantially. A comprehensive protection program is in effect in all of our surgical and obstetric operating rooms: equipment maintenance has reduced leakage to a minimum; excess anesthetic circuit gases are captured and vented at a point where no personnel exposure occurs; and the operating room air is monitored to document that the trace gas control program is effective and that low levels really are being maintained.

A question frequently raised is whether women who are pregnant or who are contemplating pregnancy should work in the operating room. A definite answer cannot be given, and the data are not strong enough to remove categorically all such women from the operating rooms. With the above factors in mind, we have attempted to make our operating suites as safe as possible by our concerted efforts to hold anesthetic exposure to a minimum. However, no "safe" exposure level below which we can be sure that adverse effects will not occur has yet been identified. You must decide whether to accept the potential risks of working in anesthetizing areas. Should you have any questions or concerns, we urge that you consult your obstetrician or a knowledgeable anesthesia department member.

Whether pregnant or not, if you prefer not to have any exposure to trace gases, then you may request to work elsewhere in the hospital. The staff in the Anesthesia, Surgical, Nursing and Housekeeping Departments will make every effort to accommodate the wishes of concerned persons.

To show that you have received and understand this notice, please sign below and return it to us.

Thank you for your cooperation.

I have read and understand this notice.

Name Date

The ASA Ad Hoc Committee on Effects of Trace Anesthetic Agents on Health of Operating Room Personnel hopes that you find this materal helpful in developing your hospital's program to reduce personnel exposure to waste anesthetic gases in the operating room. Our suggestions are based on our views of the presently available health hazard data and on our experience in the practical means of reducing personnel exposure. We have outlined a basic acceptable program which when implemented should significantly reduce exposure to waste anesthetic gases. Where personnel and financial resources permit, a more sophisticated and comprehensive program may be developed. Each of you must design your own program based upon your needs and the resources available to you.

We will keep you informed and, if necessary, will amend our recommendations as technology changes and as the merits of the health hazard data warrant.

CHAPTER 18

Safety and Maintenance of Electrical Equipment

In operating rooms and intensive care suites, electrical equipment has proliferated. Because the pieces of electrical apparatus used in these environments pose considerable hazards, yet are not well understood by clinicians, we shall discuss the safety and maintenance of electrical equipment.

PRINCIPLES OF ELECTRICITY

Electrical energy comes into the operating room as direct current (DC), for instance in batteries, or as alternating current (AC), from the outside power net. As shown in Figure 18-1, with direct current, electrons always flow in the same direction through a conductor. Although this flow may be intermittent, it is always in the same direction. An alternating current, as shown in Figure 18-2, oscillates around zero, that is, the electricity flows intermittently in one and then the other direction. When the flow

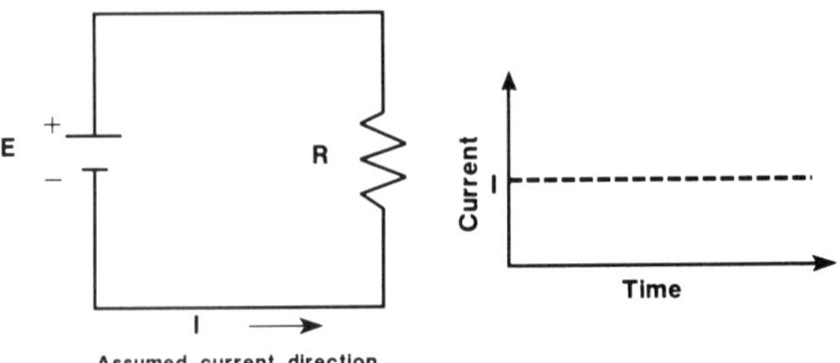

Figure 18-1. Simple circuit for direct current with electricity flowing in one direction. (I = current, R = resistance, E = voltage.)

is recorded, these oscillations resemble those of sine waves. The alternating current delivered to electrical outlets in our homes and hospitals in the United States changes direction 60 times per second, called 60 cycles per second or 60 Hz. In many other countries 50 Hz is the norm.

The wires in an electrical system are color coded (Fig. 18-3). The black wire is connected to the power source's generator and accepts the current there and carries it to the user. It is therefore called the "hot" wire. The white wire is called "neutral," but it is still potentially dangerous because in order for current to flow through the hot wire, a circuit has to be completed. The white wire completes the circuit and, thus, also carries electricity, which is eventually grounded. The third wire, green, is a safety wire and provides an extra ground through which any leakage of current can escape. In older structures, the electrical wiring includes no third (green) safety wire. All modern hospital systems must have this third ground wire.

The flow of electricity is measured in amperes. An ampere is the quantity of electricity that flows through a conductor in 1 second. In an analogy to the cardiovascular system, an ampere would be the cardiac output measured in liters of blood per minute. Just as blood flowing

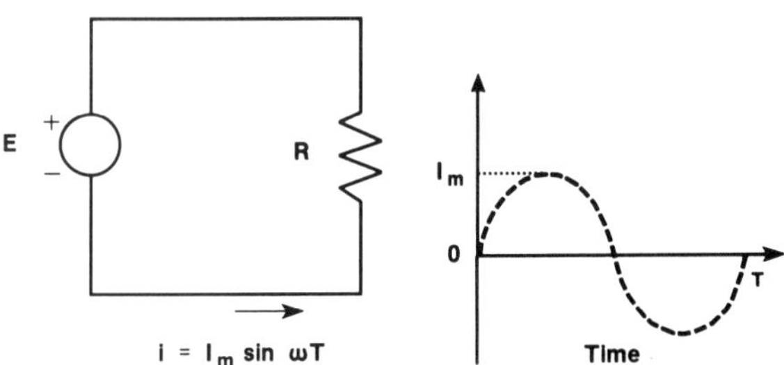

Figure 18-2. Simple circuit for alternating current with current direction and amount changing.

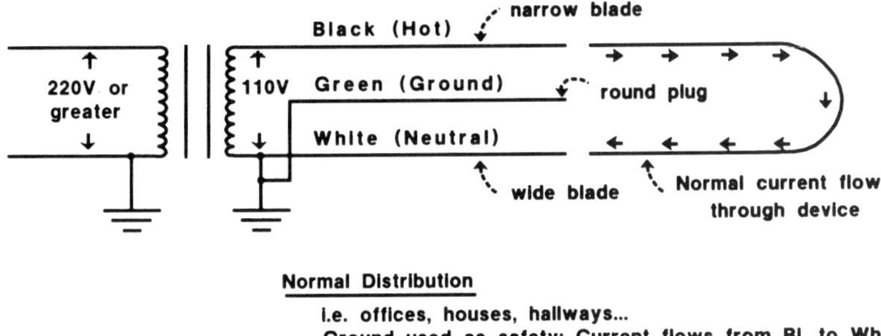

Figure 18-3. Normal distribution: *i.e.*, offices, houses, hallways. . . . Ground used as safety; current flows from black to white (Courtesy of C. Kemmerer)

through the arterioles meets with resistance, electricity flowing through a conductor also meets with resistance, which is measured in ohms. The pressure lost as electricity (*i.e.*, electrons) flows against resistance is expressed in volts. The hemodynamic analogy to voltage is the pressure dissipated, for example, between the aorta to the right atrium. Ohm's law: $E = IR$, defines the relationship that exists between voltage, current flow, and resistance. In this simple mathematical equation, by convention, E represents voltage drop (volts), I the current flow (amperes), and R the resistance (ohms).

Power defines the rate at which work is done. We determine power (watts) by multiplying voltage by amperes:

1 ampere × 1 volt = 1 watt of power

When we wish to assess the value of energy, we multiply power by the time over which it is applied, and obtain the watt-second or the watt-hour. An extension of this concept generates the joule, that is, the meter-kilogram-second of energy.

The last term we will need to know is current density. Current density represents the concentration of current traveling through a conductor.

ELECTRICAL SHOCK

Physiology

The human body consists largely of electrolyte solution enclosed in skin which, when dry, tends to resist current flow. The resistance (ohms) of the skin can be reduced by two orders of magnitude by simply breaking the skin and exposing electrolyte-containing plasma and tissue to a current. This lowered resistance allows much higher current (amperes) to flow and current density can increase significantly. Increased current density can cause injury, as we shall see.

Electric current threatens us in two ways. First, if dense enough, it can raise temperature enough to burn (therefore, low amperage, battery-powered devices are usually safe). The second threat of electricity is the excitation of nerve and muscle.

All of us, at one time or another, have felt a tingling sensation when we have come into contact with electricity without the protection of an insulated covering. In this instance, current flowed from one contact point, through a second contact point, and during the course, stimulated the sensory nerves. If motor nerves are also depolarized, involuntary muscle activity arises, and if the current is of a sufficient density, it will activate whole muscle groups, leading to tetanic contraction of respiratory muscles and respiratory arrest. If an electrical current enters and leaves the body through the same extremity, respiratory and heart muscles will be little affected. However, if during the course traveled from its entry point in one extremity to its exit from another extremity, sufficient current flows through the heart and the respiratory muscles, extrasystoles may be triggered, causing ventricular fibrillation and respiratory arrest.

The heart is most sensitive to electricity. Cellular response to alternating current depends upon the duration and frequency of exposure to the current. Commonly used voltages for electrocautery are delivered at frequencies in the megahertz range, with current duration too short to cause fibrillation. To cause a single twitch of heart muscle, the shock must be of sufficient duration (at least 0.0001 sec) and intensity (at least 2 μA) when applied directly to the myocardium, for instance, through a wire catheter lying in one of the cardiac chambers.[1] After a single contraction, the myocardium will then usually resume its rhythmic contractions. Low current densities will also cause extrasystoles until the energy source is removed, while a more prolonged exposure can result in cardiac fibrillation, which will continue even after the cessation of current flow. Tables 18-1 and 18-2 show the levels of current necessary to cause various phenomena and demonstrate the critical location and current density of alternating current on the patient.[2,3] Observe that current at very low levels, imperceptible to the patient or person in contact with him, can still cause ventricular fibrillation if it is applied directly to the heart. A saline-filled catheter or a transvenous pacemaker provides an excellent conduit for such current.

Physical Factors

Electrical energy is usually generated by remote stations and sent along transmission lines at very high voltages (100,000 V). Substations reduce the voltage for local delivery, until it arrives in our homes or hospital

Table 18-1. PHYSIOLOGICAL EFFECTS OF ELECTRICAL CURRENT ON HUMAN SKIN (1 SEC DURATION AT 60 Hz)

Current	Effect
500 μA	Threshold of perception
5 mA	Accepted safe level
10–20 mA	Maximum "let go"
75 mA	Ventricular fibrillation threshold
100 mA	Respiratory paralysis threshold

(Cromwell L, et al: Biomedical Instrumentation and Measurement, p. 434. Englewood Cliffs, NJ, Prentice-Hall, 1980.)

rooms at 220 or 110 V. For defective equipment to deliver a painful or even lethal shock a "first" and "second" contact must be made between the patient and the defective equipment: the first contact between a wire carrying current and the instrument case or a probe occurs when moisture or mechanical damage has bridged the insulation; the second contact when the patient touches the surface of the case or the probe and establishes a pathway for the current to flow through the body. Birds can sit and sing on suspended overland high voltage wires because they make only one of the two required contacts—fortunately!

Figure 18-4 depicts a "short" between the hot wire and the case of the instrument.[1] Now, let the patient be grounded, for instance, by touching metal on the operating table, and at the same time the instrument case or defective probe, and the ingredients for a disaster are present. Current will flow only at a rate inversely proportional to the resistances in the circuit. For example, if the patient is connected to the ground through a dry rubber mattress, much less current will flow into him than if he were lying on the wet steel of a table. The point is that preventive measures must be applied at two sites: the instrument itself (do not tolerate defective

Table 18-2. PHYSIOLOGICAL EFFECTS OF ELECTRICAL CURRENT ON HUMAN MYOCARDIUM (2 SEC DURATION AT 60 Hz)

Electrode Diameter (cm)	Mean Current (mA)	Range (mA)	Effect
2.5	3366	1500–6000	Fibrillation
0.25	583	180–1500	Fibrillation

(Bruner JMR: Hazards of electrical apparatus. Anesthesiology 28:402, 1967)

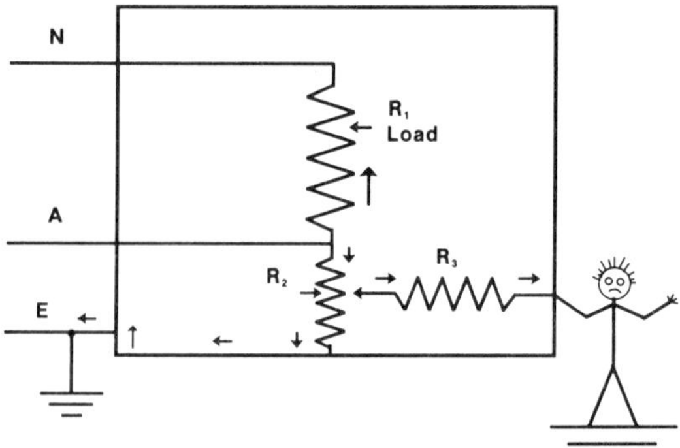

Figure 18-4. A fault exists between the hot or active wire and the case of the instrument. The case is now "live," so electricity can flow through a person in touch with the case and ground. How much current will flow depends partially on the values of R_1, R_2, R_3. (Used with permission of Kerr DR, Malhatra IV: Electrical design and safety in the operating room and intensive care unit. Int Anesth Clin 19[2]:27–48, 1981)

equipment), and the patient's contact with equipment (limit it to the essential).

PREVENTION OF ELECTRICAL ACCIDENTS

Several methods are used to reduce the likelihood of an electrical accident. However, all either try to isolate the instrument from the electrical hazard or ground it so that current, which always follows the path of least resistance, flows harmlessly into the ground.

Grounding

Figure 18-4 shows the advantage of keeping the resistance between the hot wire and ground minimal; as the hot wire touches the instrument case, current will preferentially flow to the ground (least resistance) and not through the patient (greater resistance). This requires that the green ground wire be attached directly to the case, which is done in many instruments. Another safety feature enters here. Excessive current interrupts a protective device called a circuit breaker or fuse, thereby cutting off current flow immediately to all points distal to the breaker. On the one hand, protection against electrocution would demand very sensitive circuit breakers to interrupt the current at relatively low levels of electrical disturbances; on the other hand, loss of power to all devices may jeopardize the patient whose life may depend on the functioning of the very electrical device that is being deprived of its power by a tripped circuit breaker. For example, we recently suffered a loss of power in the operating rooms of our modern hospital. For over 20 minutes we depended on batteries because, due to a fluke in the emergency system, electricity failed to be delivered. Fortunately, no tragedies resulted, but the need for functional emergency equipment was driven home forcefully.

Double Insulation

Insulation is accomplished by covering the conductive portion of the equipment with a nonconductive material such as plastic. When the casing is also nonconductive, the equipment is considered to be doubly insulated. Popular for hand-held tools, this method fails when, for example, conductive fluids are poured over the equipment, allowing contact between the conductive material and the surface of the outer case.

Low Voltage

Battery-operated appliances are electrically safer than equipment requiring 110 V because low voltage generates little current. Hand-held ophthalmoscopes and portable, battery-operated radiographic equipment and nerve stimulators serve as examples of low-voltage equipment.

Ground-Fault Interrupter

If the patient is totally isolated from contact with any electricity, then there is no chance of current running through him. Similarly, if no leakage of current is present, no current will flow to the ground and the current flowing in both the black (hot) and white (neutral) wires should be equal. Through a break in insulation, some current can leak from the hot wire to the green ground wire. This can be detected with the help of a differential transformer and electronic amplifier that constantly measure the difference between the hot and neutral wire currents. If the difference exceeds 5 mA, a circuit breaker is triggered to interrupt current flow, thus minimizing the possibility of shocking the patient.

Isolation of the Patient

Another means of protecting the patient from shock is to isolate the ECG and any other present circuits from the power line, the ground wire, and any other components of the instrument. Figure 18-5 shows how this can be accomplished by isolating the power supply of the ECG circuit via an isolation transformer that separates this circuit from the monitor's power supply. Instead of sending the ECG signal from patient to the display through conducting wires (which could also conduct higher currents in

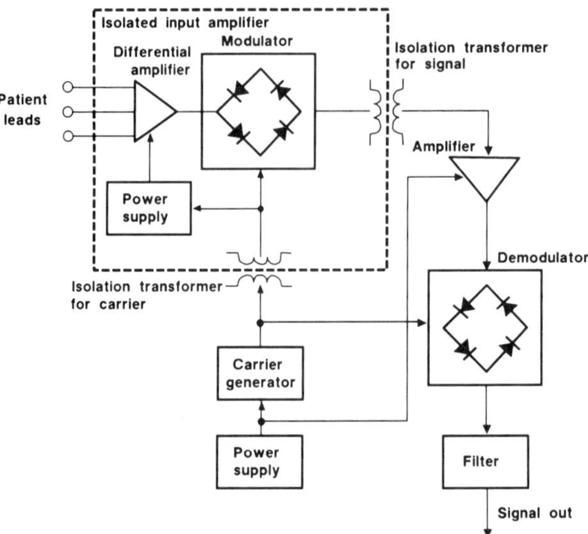

Figure 18-5. Isolated patient leads offer electrical safety by isolating with use of a carrier amplifier. (Used with permission of Cromwell L, Weibell, FJ, Pfeiffer EA [eds]: Biomedical Instrumentation and Measurements, 2nd ed, p 433. Englewood Cliffs, NJ, Prentice-Hall, 1980)

the opposite direction to the patient), the ECG signal is processed and transmitted through an isolation transformer. What is done for the ECG signal can be done for any other physiologic signal.

A second means of minimizing shock hazard is by isolating the power supply from the ground, again using an isolation transformer. As depicted in Figure 18-6, only the primary side of the transformer is grounded. If the case of the instrument supplied by the secondary winding is shorted to one of the wires, current will not flow because neither wire is connected to the ground. In the operating room, the adequacy of isolation is constantly monitored by an isolation monitor which alternately checks each wire for isolation from the ground. When isolation falls below a predetermined level, a green light turns red. Another method of separating the patient from potential leakage currents gaining access to him (e.g., through an ECG monitor) employs magnetic or optical coupling. In either case no direct mechanical connection exists between primary and secondary coils of the electrical device close to the patient. Instead, either light or magnetic energy is used to transmit information from one piece of monitoring equipment to another.

Telemetry, the measuring of a quantity and its transmission to another station (usually by radio), is another available method that enhances mobility and makes leakage currents from monitoring device to patient im-

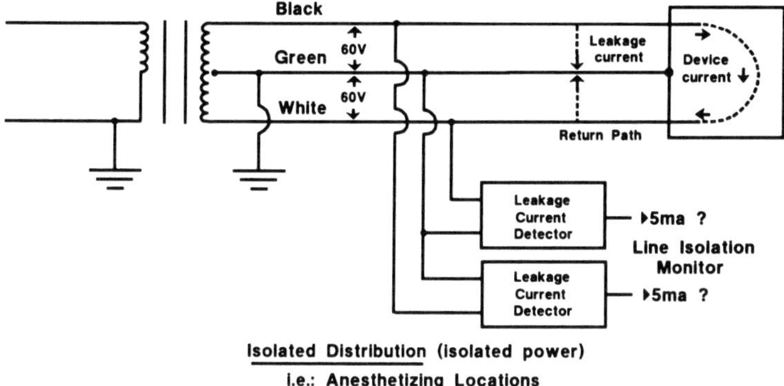

Figure 18-6. Isolated power supply. (Courtesy of C. Kemmerer)

possible. The patient is attached to a transmitter that is connected by telemetry to a receiver.

ELECTROSURGERY

In 1928, Cushing commented on the usefulness of electrosurgery, and since that time its use has expanded. Electrosurgery utilizes electrical frequencies of hundreds of thousands to millions of hertz. The intense concentration of electricity at this frequency creates temperatures in excess of 1000°C which literally explode the tissue cells and, depending on the waveform used, can cut or coagulate. The active cutting or coagulating electrode concentrates the current at a very small point operated by the surgeon. To close the circuit a second electrode is needed; this is kept large so as to disperse and render harmless the intense current. In order to safely perform electrocautery, several precautions must be taken:

Selection of Site for the Dispersive Electrode

Select a site away from long protuberances to ensure the effective adherence of the electrode. Avoid tissue folds, and position the electrode so that fluids will not be trapped. Pick a location close to the surgical site to shorten the path from cutting to dispersive electrode and avoid putting the heart between dispersive and cutting (coagulating) electrode.

Preparation of Site for Dispersive Electrode

The site should allow good skin contact with the dispersive electrode. Hair, cosmetics, dirt, and perspiration all affect the quality of contact. Apply conductive gels evenly. Since blood flow carries heat away from the skin, the dispersive electrode should be placed where blood flow is not restricted.

Alternate Return Paths

Since electrosurgical energy will follow the path of least impedance, it is important to reduce the likelihood that current will flow to sites other than the dispersive electrode. This is called the alternate path hazard. This hazard is reduced by (1) insulating the patient from metal devices, (2) using ECG cables specially designed to cope with electrosurgical energy, (3) placing the dispersive electrode close to the surgical site, and (4) keeping ECG electrodes as far from the active site as possible.

ENDOSCOPES

Endoscopic procedures with electrosurgery (such as the common transurethral resection of the prostate) should use low-voltage generators and conductive sleeves. Adequate irrigation with a nonconductive fluid is essential.

PACEMAKERS

Monitor the patient's ECG continuously. Also, be sure that the path from active electrode to dispersive electrode is short and that it does not pass through the vicinity of the heart. Be ready to convert a demand pacemaker to a nondemand mode (Chap. 3).

ELECTRICAL SAFETY CHECKS

All electrical equipment used in the vicinity of patients must be checked for electrical safety at least every 12 months, and before being put into service.[4] Hospital technicians should first check the physical integrity of the power cord. Then, electrical measurements are made that include the following:

1. The resistance between the device's chassis or other exposed conductive surfaces and the ground pin of the attachment plug should be less than 0.5 Ω.
2. Leakage current from the chassis to the ground for cord-connected devices should be no more than 100 μA.
3. The leakage current between patient leads connected together and the ground must not excced 100 μA.
4. When the external power is turned on and 60 Hz current at 110 V

is driven into the patient leads and the ground, skin current must not exceed 20 μA.

5. The leakage current between leads must not exceed 50 μA if the input is nonisolated, and 10 μA if it is isolated.

CHECK-IN AND MAINTENANCE OF EQUIPMENT

The maintenance of monitoring equipment in hospitals has become increasingly important and difficult as monitors have proliferated and grown in complexity. Not too long ago maintenance and electrical safety of electronic equipment were treated as two components of the same problem. Although concerns about electrical safety remain important, a greater hazard faces the patient from poorly maintained equipment that does not function as it was designed to; that is, the equipment does not work at all when needed or—what may be worse—gives misleading data. Poorly maintained equipment can be extraordinarily expensive to the institution and its physicians when scheduled cases have to be cancelled or procedures delayed. In many American hospitals, a 10-minute delay may cost hundreds of dolllars when personnel have to stay longer and an expensive facility sits idle.

The Check-In Procedure

When a piece of equipment is first purchased or has undergone major repairs, modifications, or overhaul, it must undergo an "acceptance test" to ensure that it performs safely and according to expectations. Performance should conform to the manufacturer's specifications. Sometimes specific performance criteria are detailed in a purchase order because added functions or features demand a particularly attentive acceptance test that is not accorded the standard edition of the item.

Acceptance tests must comply with local and state requirements, as well as requirements formulated by the Joint Commission on Accreditation of Hospitals (JCAH).[5] A properly completed and well-documented acceptance test protects not only the patient from harm, but can also shield the hospital, its personnel, and the physicians from certain claims of negligence. Conversely, omitting or not documenting an acceptance test, or putting into service a unit that has failed such a test, exposes the hospital and its physicians to considerable legal risks. As an additional precaution, one may wish to delay final payment of the vendor until the acceptance test has demonstrated that the instrument performs up to expectations.

Once the acceptance test is completed, the unit should not be placed into service until the personnel that will use the item have been trained in its operation. This obvious precaution is often ignored. We all tend to turn on a unit before reading the instructions, not only because we assume that we are intelligent enough to operate just about anything, but also because the manuals that come with the equipment are often poorly written, lengthy, and not geared to the clinician. This common weakness is magnified when the unit has been in operation for some time and a new employee takes the place of the former operator. Often the manual can no longer be found, and even if it is found, it may be not helpful without a company representative who can amplify and interpret the opaque instructions. Manufacturers could be more helpful in lavishing greater attention on the operator's manuals, perhaps reissuing them periodically. When possible, with units that have electronic screens, it would be helpful to offer key instructions on demand concerning alphanumeric displays. This could include reminders about inspections that fall due. As long as this is not available, the clinician, nursing service, or clinical engineering personnel should keep a calendar with reminders of when to inspect equipment in use and document in that calendar the dates and results of inspection.

Calibration

While calibration may be carried out as part of an acceptance test, it must be repeated much more often than regular inspections are. Just because an instrument is new, it is not wise to assume that the calibration is satisfactory. Calibrations should cover the full range of measurements of the instrument. For example, a blood pressure measuring device should be checked from 0 torr to 200 torr, because it is not uncommon for instruments to measure accurately only over a portion of the clinically significant range.

Preventive Maintenance

In addition to the routine, daily inspection of an instrument before it is put to use, preventive maintenance should be scheduled on a regular basis. Typically, this consists of a visual examination, thorough cleaning, lubrication where necessary, replacement of cracked housing or cover plates over dials, and replacement of worn wires or other parts that have a limited life. Screws are tightened, cathode-ray tubes aligned, worn out bulbs and batteries replaced.

Once machines have gathered stains from body fluids, dust, and residue from old tape, and their paint or lacquer shows the scars of rough handling, the care with which they are used diminishes markedly. One way to reduce the accumulation of adhesive tape residue is to provide a holding clamp or other attachment mechanisms. We follow the recommendations of the Emergency Care Research Institute (ECRI) for cleaning the exterior of devices, using only alcohol in well-ventilated places or water (Table 18-3).[6] For the exterior of the instrument, we recommend the use of soap or a mild detergent using a damp cloth. This will remove most of the offending stains. For cleaning the interior, we rely on the expertise of biomedical engineering technicians.

Frequency of Preventive Maintenance

Although it is difficult to define optimal intervals at which instruments should be inspected from both clinical and legal standpoints, it is wise to lean toward too many inspections rather than too few. We make use of factory-authorized technicians in maintaining our devices. This has several advantages: an expert carries out the maintenance, the proper spare parts are available, and the maintenance will be carried out without the need to consult a calendar and monitor compliance by local hospital personnel. Depending on the maintenance contract which the hospital or clinical service has made with the vendor or manufacturer's representative, maintenance carried out under contract may also offer some legal protection.

The 1987 JCAH Accreditation Manual recommends that a testing interval of 6 months should never be exceeded[5]—a goal that is reached by few hospitals for all monitoring items that warrant preventive maintenance. The National Fire Prevention Association (NFPA) states that an electrical safety check must also be performed for repairs that may have compromised electrical isolation or safety of the patient.[4] Furthermore, they suggest that the testing be done annually for general care area equipment, and semiannually for equipment used in critical care areas, such as operating rooms and intensive care units. ECRI suggests that your own experience and special circumstances are important factors in determining the intervals between inspections.[6] They suggest that if only 2% to 5% of inspections reveal significant deficiencies, the intervals are probably sufficient. It must be emphasized, however, that the manufacturer's design and materials, the frequency of clinical use, the potential hazard associated with the use of the equipment, and the appearance and condition of the equipment are all factors that may persuade the hospital to insist on a more frequent preventive maintenance routine. Tables 18-4 and 18-5 offer guidelines for assessing inspection and preventive maintenance intervals for equipment used in the care of patients.

A special position is occupied by devices that are not used regularly, but that must function properly when suddenly needed, such as resuscitation equipment, defibrillators, and pacemakers. Some components should be checked daily, for instance, the batteries in laryngoscopes, and others at least weekly or monthly. The main parts of a system should undergo quarterly preventive maintenance.

Table 18-3. EQUIPMENT CLEANING GUIDE

	Suggested Materials
Common Residues	
Adhesive tape	Alcohol, tape residue removal pad, naphtha, trichlorethylene, proprietary solvent*
Dried blood	General cleaner, alcohol, fine abrasive
Urine	General cleaner, baking soda
Exterior	
Housing	Vacuum cleaner, general cleaner, alcohol
CRT window, grid, filter	Vacuum cleaner, general cleaner, anti-static compound
Meter window, cover	Vacuum cleaner, general cleaner, anti-static compound
Magnetic tape heads	Alcohol, trichlorethylene, head cleaner
Interior	Vacuum cleaner, proprietary solvent*
Mechanical	
Drive system	Proprietary solvent,* lubricant
Rubber rollers	Alcohol
Hinges, latches	General cleaner, alcohol, lubricant
Wheels, casters	Vacuum cleaner, general cleaner, alcohol, lubricant
Conductive wheels, casters	Vacuum cleaner, general cleaner, alcohol, graphited oil
Electrical	
PC boards	Vacuum cleaner, general cleaner, alcohol, trichlorethylene, proprietary solvent,* eraser, deionized water
Connectors	Alcohol, trichlorethylene, contact cleaner, eraser
Switch and relay contacts	Proprietary solvent,* contact cleaner, burnishing tool, lubricant
Pitted heavy duty contacts	Proprietary solvent,* contact cleaner, fine abrasive, burnishing tool, lubricant
Potentiometers	Proprietary solvent,* contact cleaner, lubricant
Insulators	Vacuum cleaner, general cleaner, alcohol, trichlorethylene, surface sealant
Heat sinks	Vacuum cleaner, general cleaner, alcohol

* Check manufacturers' instructions for application details and specific suggestions. (Health Devices Inspection and Preventive Maintenance System, p 28. Plymouth Meeting, PA, Emergency Care Research Institute, 1984. Copyright © ECRI. Reproduced with permission.)

Table 18-4. GUIDELINES FOR ASSESSING INSPECTION AND PREVENTIVE MAINTENANCE INTERVALS

	Too High	Effective	Too Low
Calibration	Always correct at inspection	Slightly off; does not affect patient care	Often out of calibration/erroneous results/improper therapy
Performance of subsystems	Within accepted norms	Within accepted norms	Outside accepted norms/potential for catastrophe
Cleanliness	Requires no cleaning/lubrication	Requires some cleaning/lubrication/hardware needs some tightening	Often dirty, inadequate lubrication/loose or missing hardware
Downtime/operation	Downtime low/smooth operation	Infrequent complaints/downtime	Frequent complaints/downtime
Emergency repair	Infrequent need	Infrequent need	Frequent need/breakdown costs high
Equipment condition	Always safe and ready for use	Safe/maintenance time does not usually affect use	Possibility of injuries/delayed, improper diagnosis and therapy

(Webster J, Cook A: Clinical Engineering: Principles and Practices, © 1979, p. 282. Reprinted by permission of Prentice-Hall, Englewood Cliffs, N.J. Adapted in Health Devices Inspection and Preventive Maintenance System, p 12. Plymouth Meeting, PA, Emergency Care Research Institute, 1984. Copyright © ECRI. Reproduced by permission.)

Table 18-5. GUIDELINES FOR INSPECTION/PREVENTIVE MAINTENANCE INTERVALS

Device Type	Interval	General Criteria
Line-powered electronic devices	Annual	Major inspection consisting of visual inspection, electrical safety, performance/minimal preventive maintenance; minor inspection consisting of qualitative inspection/ electrical safety if necessary
Battery-powered devices	Annual	Major inspection consisting of visual inspection, electrical safety, performance/minimal preventive maintenance/test battery capacity or voltage; minor inspection consisting of qualitative inspection/ electrical safety if necessary/test battery capacity or voltage
Mechanical/electromechanical/ pneumatic/fluidic powered or controlled devices	Semiannually or quarterly	Inspection consisting of visual inspection/safety and performance test/cleaning and lubrication/other preventive maintenance; subdivision into major and minor procedures depends on class of service
Life-support/resuscitation devices	Quarterly or semiannually	More frequent inspection required/at least semiannually
Devices in special care areas	Quarterly or semiannually	More frequent inspection usually required
Clinical monitoring devices	Annually or semiannually	Most component failures random/inspection frequency has little or no effect on occurrence

(Health Devices Inspection and Preventive Maintenance System, p 13. Plymouth Meeting, PA, Emergency Care Research Institute, 1984. Copyright © ECRI. Reproduced by permission.)

Establishing a Maintenance Program

Most hospitals have a substantial amount of equipment whose maintenance is beyond the capability of the "in-house" electrical and mechanical technicians. For this reason, many hospitals set up their own biomedical engineering technician service, which may assume overall rcsponsibility or share this responsibility with qualified service representatives. An example of one such service for anesthesia equipment is that described by Duberman for a large metropolitan hospital.[7]

REFERENCES

1. Kerr DR, Malhotra IV: Electrical design and safety in the operating room and intensive care unit. Int Anesth Clin 19(2):27–48, 1981
2. Cromwell L, Weibell FJ, Pfeiffer EA: Biomedical Instrumentation and Measurements, p 434. Englewood Cliffs, NJ, Prentice-Hall, 1980
3. Bruner JMR: Hazards of electrical apparatus. Anesthesiology 28:402, 1967
4. Safe use of electricity in patient care areas. In Standards for Health Care Facilities 99, pp 63–77. Quincy, MA, National Fire Prevention Association, 1984
5. Accreditation Manual for Hospitals (AMH/87), pp 199–200. Chicago, Joint Commission on Accreditation of Hospitals, 1986
6. Health Devices Inspection and Preventive Maintenance Systems, pp 11–13, 26. Plymouth Meeting, PA, Emergency Case Research Institute, 1985
7. Duberman S: An integrated quality control program for anesthesia equipment. J Quality Assurance 9:328–336, 1983

Index

Numbers followed by *f* indicate a figure; *t* following a page number indicates tabular material.